Danilo Jankovic
Christopher Wells

Regional Nerve Blocks

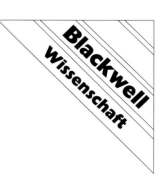

Danilo Jankovic
Christopher Wells

Regional Nerve Blocks
Textbook and Color Atlas

Second edition

Over 400 illustrations and 17 tables

Blackwell Science Berlin · Vienna 2001

Edinburgh · Boston · Copenhagen · London · Melbourne · Oxford · Tokyo

English edition 2001 by Blackwell
Wissenschafts-Verlag Berlin Vienna

First German-language edition (1997) and
Second German-language edition (1999)
© by Blackwell Wissenschafts-Verlag Berlin • Vienna

Editorial Offices:
Blackwell Wissenschafts-Verlag GmbH
Kurfürstendamm 57, 10707 Berlin, Germany
Firmiangasse 7, 1130 Vienna, Austria

Other Editorial Offices:
Blackwell Science Ltd
Osney Mead, Oxford OX2 0EL
25 John Street, London WC1N 2BL
23 Ainslie Place, Edinburgh EH3 6AJ
Commerce Place, 350 Main Street,
    Malden, MA 02148-5018, USA
54 University Street, Carlton,
    Victoria 3053, Australia
10, rue Casimir Delavigne, 75006 Paris, France

Blackwell Science KK
MG-Kodemmacho Building, 3F
7-10 Kodemmacho Nihonbashi
Chuo-ku,Tokyo 103-0001, Japan

Iowa State University Press
A Blackwell Science Company
2121 S. State Avenue
Ames, Iowa 50014-8300, USA

Authors' addresses:
Dr. med. Danilo Jankovic
Sana-Klinik
50354 Köln-Hürth (Cologne-Huerth)
Germany

Dr Christopher Wells
45a Rodney Street
Liverpool L1 9EW
United Kingdom

English translation by:
Michael Robertson, Augsburg, Germany

The right of the Authors to be identified as the Authors
of this work has been asserted in accordance with the
German Copyright Law of September 9, 1965, in its version
of June 24, 1985.

DISTRIBUTORS

Marston Book Services Ltd
PO Box 269
Abingdon
Oxon OX14 4YN
(*Orders:* Tel: 01235 465500
            Fax: 01235 465555)

USA
Blackwell Science, Inc.
Commerce Place
350 Main Street
Malden, MA 02148-5018
(*Orders:* Tel: 800 759-6102
                   781 388-8250
            Fax: 781 388-8255)

Canada
Login Brothers Book Company
324 Saulteaux Crescent
Winnipeg, Manitoba R3J 3T2
(*Orders:* Tel.: 204 837-2987
            Fax: 204 837-3116)

Australia
Blackwell Science Pty Ltd
54 University Street
Carlton, Victoria 3053
(*Orders:* Tel: 3 9347-0300
            Fax: 3 9347-5001)

A catalogue record for this title is available from
the British Library

ISBN 0-632-05557-X

Library of Congress Cataloging-in-Publication Data

Set by Type-Design, Berlin, Germany
Printed and bound by Druckhaus Mitte, Berlin

For further information on Blackwell Science visit our web-
site: www.blackwell-science.com

Foreword

There has been a marked growth of interest in regional anesthesia in the last 30 years. Attention has been given to the practical applications required to carry out the appropriate techniques. This has led to a strong demand for specialist textbooks and atlases, capable of meeting the highest educational standards. Effective regional anesthesia requires not only good anatomical knowledge, but also optimal patient positioning, precise localization, and good technical precision on the part of the trained anesthetist in administering an accurate dose of local anesthetic. The doctor attending the patient must also be able to recognize potential side effects or complications, and to treat them immediately. When all of these requirements are met, regional nerve blocks can be used as a standard procedure during surgery. Unfortunately these techniques are still used infrequently, in spite of the well-known benefits.

In this book, Dr Danilo Jankovic and Dr Chris Wells have helped close a significant gap in the literature concerning regional anesthesia. The book contains precise anatomical drawings and illustrations, and also provides detailed instructions on how to apply local anesthesia. This allows the anesthetist concerned to proceed according to clear guidelines, and to improve the quality of treatment, all for the benefit of the patient.

The book is practically oriented, and could almost be taken to the operating room and used as a guide. It covers anatomy, indications, contraindications, dosages, explanations of individual drugs, as well as complications, caveats, and potential adverse side effects, and how to avoid them or treat them. In addition it provides information on technical aspects of materials.

The second edition has been substantially expanded, with the number of chapters increased from 12 to 41. Each procedure is explained step by step, and presented in a suitable educational form, using numerous illustrations and photographs – more than 400 in all.

For each procedure, a specific form (record and checklist) is provided for recording the individual treatment steps. These checklists make the techniques taken at any point in time easy to comprehend and reconstruct, so that potential complications can be analyzed and avoided. The authors present both familiar and new therapeutic techniques, for both the treatment of pain and regional nerve blocks during surgery. In addition, the most recent local anesthetics and additives are discussed, with particular reference to the relevant indications and dosages.

A detailed list of the materials used, with information on their manufacturers, makes it easier for the user to select the most appropriate needles for each particular block.

The technique of regional block provides a wide range of opportunities for improved patient care in the field of anesthesia. In this volume Dr Jankovic and Dr Wells have made a valuable contribution to the broader application of this form of treatment to our patients, and we must make the same full and vigilant efforts to care for our patients that we are accustomed to applying in general anesthesia.

André van Zundert, MD, PhD
President of ESRA

Eindhoven,
Autumn 2000

Preface to the second edition

At the start of the new millennium, modern medicine has become highly specialized. Complex therapeutic techniques require elaborate equipment and precise knowledge. The opportunities provided by such forms of treatment, and their limitations, become evident very quickly. Today, rational and successful treatment of pain has become the focus of a wide variety of specialist disciplines; and most importantly, it is very much in the patient's interest.

Regional nerve blocks can be used with a high degree of success, both for surgical procedures and in modern pain treatment. They can be used for diagnosis, prognosis and therapy. Unfortunately, familiarity with the techniques of regional blocks and their indications, together with awareness of the complications, is not sufficiently widespread. The techniques are consequently underused, and sometimes more elaborate and invasive forms of anesthesia expose the patient to unnecessary risks.

There has been an excellent response to the first edition of this book from the scientific press, and the many letters Dr Jankovic has received from readers show that there is strong interest in further training in the techniques of regional anesthesia. This has encouraged us to present a revised and translated version of this already tried and tested handbook – substantially expanding the range of topics covered – some three and a half years after publication of the first edition.

Once again, we have given special attention to educational aspects. The aim has been to ensure that each individual step of treatment is understandable. This is the only way to avoid mistakes and to recognize and remedy any complications quickly. The numerous illustrations serve to clarify the matters being dealt with and provide additional information. With a good knowledge of topographic anatomy, the reader will be enabled to work independently and safely with the patient.

Due to the many additions made in this edition, preparing and producing it involved very considerable efforts. I would therefore like to express my deep gratitude to all those who have made patient and constructive contributions to the success of this book. I would also like to thank the numerous colleagues and friends who provided advice, information and ideas. My heartfelt thanks go to Mr H. Kreuzner for the immense patience and expertise he showed in his work with me and for his outstanding photography. Last, but not least, I owe thanks to my family, who have once again stood by me with all their strength and care.

I shall of course continue to welcome further suggestions, tips and constructive criticism. This is the only way in which scientific innovations and years of experience can be constantly updated and transferred into practice as widely as possible.

Danilo Jankovic   *Cologne, Autumn 2000*

Preface to the first edition

This book presents a practical summary of the most important block techniques used in diagnostic and therapeutic and local anesthesia in the upper body. This work is based on my many years' experience in clinical practice.

The book is aimed at the many specialist disciplines whose work involves pain therapy. This includes anesthetists, orthopedic surgeons, general surgeons, neurosurgeons, ENT surgeons, radiologists and fascia maxillary surgeons. The techniques presented here in the illustrations and text are an essential component of the modern multidisciplinary approach to pain therapy. Each individual block is discussed step by step and the way in which it is carried out is rendered easier to grasp through the use of specially developed record forms and checklists. At the same time, the physician concerned is informed about the relevant regulations that need to be observed. The focus is on the description and discussion of potential complications – how to recognize them quickly, how to prevent them and how to treat them in a timely fashion. I recommend those unfamiliar with this branch of pain therapy start by familiarizing themselves thoroughly with the anatomy of the region and the pharmacological properties of the most frequently used local anesthetics.

The underlying concept for this book was the idea of presenting, in a clear and practical fashion, ways of carrying out a block with optimal efficacy while at the same time ensuring the patient's complete safety.

Special thanks go to my teacher, Prof. Hans Ulrich Gerbershagen. I would also like to thank the numerous colleagues and friends who have provided advice, information and ideas – particularly Dr. Günter Datz for his tremendous assistance, as well as my colleagues in my immediate area of work, particularly Ms. Gabriele Haarmann and Mr. Peter Kaufmann. Thanks also go to my family for their understanding, patience and support.

Last, but not least, I should like to express my gratitude to the publishers, Blackwell Science, for their helpful collaboration and for the excellent design and presentation of the book.

I shall welcome and gratefully take account of any suggestions, tips and constructive criticism from readers of this book.

Danilo Jankovic   *Cologne, December 1996*

Contents

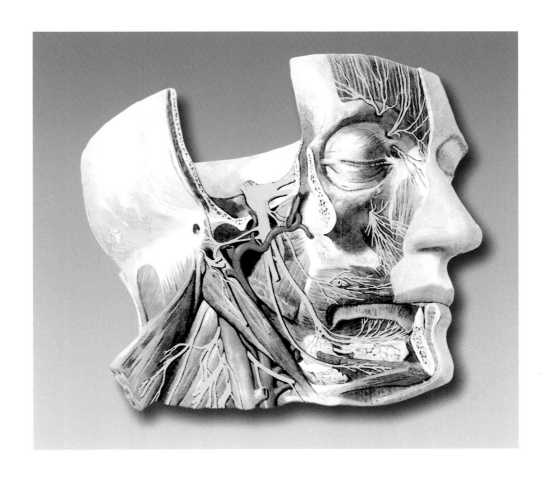

1 Regional nerve blocks in clinical practice

Introduction

Regional anesthesia involves the reversible interruption of nerve conduction using specific drugs (local anesthetics). This interruption of impulse conduction can be carried out in every region of the body in which the nerves are accessible to an external approach.
Indications include:
1. Clinical anesthesia.
Particularly in trauma, orthopedics, urology, gynecology, as well as for abdominal surgery with continuous epidural or spinal anesthesia.
2. Obstetrics.
3. Post-operative analgesia.
Regional anesthesia is probably the most appropriate technique to produce initial post-operative analgesia. A combination of local anesthetics with opioids or other substances can also be applied, with well-established long-term efficacy.
4. Pain therapy.
The diagnosis or prognosis as well as treatment.

In 1979 a commission set up by the International Association for the Study of Pain (IASP) defined pain as "an unpleasant sensory and emotional experience, linked to actual or potential tissue damage". Acute pain is caused by stimulation of pain receptors. This stimulation is transient, and sets in motion biologically useful protective mechanisms. The ideal way of relieving it is to treat the cause. However, obviously when the cause is necessary surgery, other techniques must be employed.
Chronic pain is regarded as a pathological state. It can arise as a result of constant stimulation of pain receptive afferents or can develop as neuropathic pain after injury or damage to the nervous system [4, 5, 8].
Chronic pain can often lead to alterations in the patients' living habits, their physical function, and their personality. Its management requires a coordinated interdisciplinary approach. This, in turn, presupposes a clear assessment and diagnosis, based on a full general pain history, physical examination and full assessment.
Many techniques exist to control pain. These include pharmacological therapy, physical and manipulative procedures, neurological and neurosurgical methods, physiotherapy and psychosocial management strategies. How-

ever, the use of nerve blocks, both temporary and permanent, is firmly established as part of pain therapy. In quantitative terms, regional blocks have only a small part to play in the management of chronic pain. However, qualitatively they can produce good results when used in the correct circumstances.

Nerve Blocks in Surgery and Pain Therapy

The application of regional anesthesia methods for temporary interruption of stimulus conduction in a nerve or plexus, as described in the following chapters, requires well established indications and the implementation of an agreed therapeutic approach. These blocks can be administered for surgery, diagnosis, prognosis and therapy [2].
Surgical blocks are administered with high-dose local anesthetics for targeted isolation of a specific body region in order to carry out an operation.
Diagnostic blocks using low-dose local anesthetics are appropriate for differential diagnosis of pain syndromes. They allow the affected conduction pathways to be recognized, and make it possible to identify the causes of the pain. Diagnostic blocks can also be used to clarify the question of whether the source of the pain is peripheral or central.
Prognostic blocks allow predictions to be made regarding the potential efficacy of semi-permanent nerve block, neurolysis, or surgical sympathectomy. They should also be used to prepare the patient for the effects of a permanent block.
Therapeutic blocks are applied in the treatment of various pain conditions. Typical examples of this are post-traumatic and postoperative pain, complex regional pain syndrome (CRPS) types I and II (reflex sympathetic dystrophy and causalgia), joint mobilization, post-herpetic neuralgia and malignant pain.

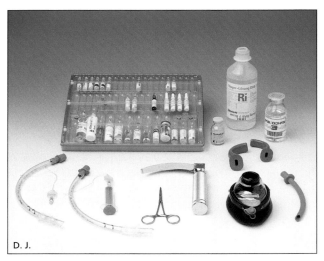

Fig. 1.1 Emergency equipment

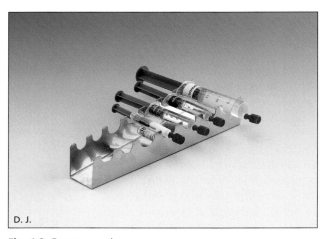

Fig. 1.2 Emergency drugs

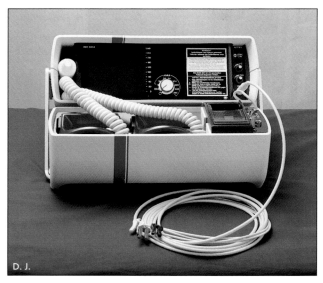

Fig. 1.3 Defibrillator

Technical requirements

The doctors carrying out these procedures in surgery and pain therapy will require appropriate technical equipment and experience in the use of all of the instruments concerned. This book describes appropriate patient positioning, the importance of aseptic conditions, and the type of equipment appropriate. This includes syringes, needle types and other supplies.

Obviously, full resuscitation equipment must be available, along with equipment and monitor therapy, to treat the various adverse events or complications that might occur.

Accessories for primary care

▨ *Emergency equipment* (Figs. 1.1 and 1.2)
- Intubation and ventilation facilities
- Oxygen source (breathing apparatus)
- Ventilation bag with 2 masks (large, medium)
- Guedel tubes nos. 3, 4, 5
- Wendel tubes nos. 26–32
- Endotracheal tubes nos. 28–36
- Tube clamp, blocker syringe (10 ml)
- Laryngoscope with batteries (replacement batteries and replacement bulbs), spatula
- Magill forceps, mouth wedge, 1 tube 2% lignocaine gel
- Suction device
- Infusion equipment
- 2 sets of infusion instruments
- 5 plastic indwelling catheters
- Syringes (2 ml, 5 ml, 10 ml), plaster, gauze bandages

▨ *Infusion solutions*
- 1 bottle each of Ringer's solution, plasma expander, 8.4 % sodium bicarbonate (100 ml)

▨ *Defibrillator* (Fig. 1.3)
▨ *Drugs for emergency treatment*

When blocks are being administered, a sedative (Valium®), a vasopressor (ephedrine) and a vagolytic (atropine) should be available for immediate injection. All other emergency medications should also be on hand:
- 5 ampoules of atropine
- 2 ampoules of Alupent®
- 2 ampoules of ephedrine (1 phenyl-2-methylamino-1-propanol)
- 3 ampoules 0.1 % Suprarenin® (epinephrine) (1 : 1000)
- 2 prepared syringes of Suprarenin® (1 : 10 000, 10 ml)
- 2 ampoules of dopamine
- 1 ampoule 10 % calcium gluconate
- 1 ampoule dimethindene maleate (Fenistil®)

- Prednisolone (Solu-Decortin®) (50 mg, 250 mg, 1000 mg)
- 5 ampoules 0.9 % sodium chloride
- 2 ampoules 2 % lignocaine
- 3 ampoules diazepam (Valium®) (10 mg)
- 2 ampoules midazolam (Dormicum®) (5 mg)
- 1 ampoule clonazepam (1 mg) (Rivotril®)
- 1 injection bottle thiopental sodium
- 2 ampoules etomidate (Hypnomidate®)
- 2 ampoules succinylcholine (suxamethonium chloride)

Anesthetic machine
For neuraxial anesthesia, ganglion block, i. v. regional anesthesia and plexus anesthesia, an anesthesia trolley with facilities for intubation is also required (Fig. 1.4).

Monitoring
- Electrocardiogram (ECG)
- Pulse oximeter (Fig. 1.5)
- Temperature sensor, touch-free miniature infrared skin thermometer (e. g., M.U.S.S. Medical, Hamburg, Germany) (Fig. 1.6)
- Nerve stimulator

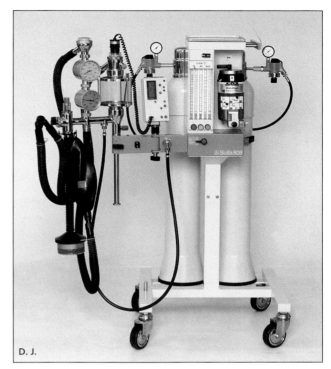

Fig. 1.4 Anesthetic machine

The treatment of side effects and severe complications – e. g., after inadvertent intravascular, epidural, or subarachnoid injection of a local anesthetic, is discussed here together with the individual block techniques.

Local anesthetics for pain therapy

Local anesthetics are substances that inhibit the flow of sodium through the cell membrane and thereby cause a local and reversible block of stimulus conduction.

Chemical structure and physicochemical properties [7]
All local anesthetics in common clinical use have three characteristic molecular sections in their chemical structure:

An aromatic residue, which basically determines the lipophilic properties of the agent. Substitution in the aromatic group allows the pK_a and lipid solubility of the substance to be influenced.

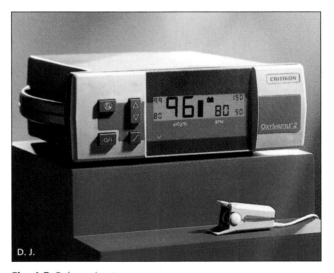

Fig. 1.5 Pulse oximeter

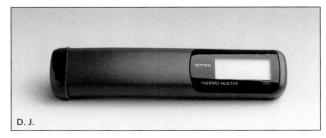

Fig. 1.6 Temperature sensor

An intermediate chain, which in local anesthetics of the ester type (Table 1.1) contains a relatively unstable ester bond that can be broken down hydrolytically by pseudocholinesterases (CO–O). Local anesthetics of the amide type (Table 1.2) are much more stable, since the amide bond (NH–CO) in their intermediate chain cannot be broken down in plasma. The length of the chain between the aromatic residue and the substituted amino group has an influence on the intensity of effect of the local anesthetic. The agent's protein-binding capacity and lipid solubility can be altered by substitution in the intermediate chain.

A substituted amino group, the protonization of which determines the ratio of the cationic to the basic form. Only the free base is capable of penetrating lipoprotein membranes. However, to be able to affect the nerve membrane, the local anesthetic must be available as a cation. The type of amino group substitution affects the distribution coefficient, the plasma protein bond and the intensity and duration of the drug's action.

Clinical significance of the physicochemical properties

Local anesthetics differ with regard to their molecular weight, their lipid and water solubility, pKa and protein-binding characteristics. These factors in turn have a substantial influence on the potency of the drug's local anesthetic effect, on the onset of the effect and on its duration (Table 1.3a, 1.3b).

The local anesthetic potency can be influenced both by lipid solubility and by the protein-binding capacity of the agent [3]. From the site of the injection to the nerve, the local anesthetic has to penetrate a series of lipoprotein membranes. The greater its lipid solubility (which can be measured *in vitro* as a lipid-water distribution coefficient), the easier it is for it to reach the site at which it is to act, and the easier it is to quickly establish relatively high concentrations of the agent in the nerve. The agent's protein-binding capacity also appears to be decisive for binding the local anesthetic to the lipoprotein membrane in the nerve.

However, the clinical distinction that is made in local anesthetics between those of mild potency (procaine), medium potency (lignocaine, prilocaine, mepivacaine), and high potency (bupivacaine, etidocaine, ropivacaine) does not confirm these correlations in all respects.

The onset of effect in the isolated nerve, at physiological pH, depends on the pKa value of the local anesthetic. The lower this value is, the more local anesthetic base can diffuse toward the membrane receptors, and the shorter the time will be to the onset of the nerve block. Higher concentrations of local anesthetic accelerate the onset of effect.

The duration of effect depends on the dosage and concentration of the local anesthetic, its binding to the membrane receptors (protein-binding capacity), and its reabsorption from the tissue into the blood.

Equipotent concentrations

Medium-duration local anesthetics have more or less the same clinical potency (except perhaps for lignocaine (lidocaine) – due to stronger vasodilation, this local anesthetic is resorbed more powerfully from the location of action, and this can affect the duration and intensity of the block).

Equipotent concentrations of long-acting local anesthetics cannot be demonstrated in the same way, since the three local anesthetics mentioned have completely different block profiles: etidocaine (highest lipophilic capacity) produces a mainly motor block, ropivacaine has a mainly sensory effect, and bupivacaine has both motor and sensory effects. Anesthetic concentrations of bupivacaine and ropivacaine are equipotent (1 to 1).

Table 1.1 Local anesthetics with an ester bond

Block profile (Table 1.4)

The block profile shows the relation between sensory and motor block. Physicochemical properties determine the block profile. At high anesthetic concentrations – so far as these are toxicologically permissible – the excess quantity of the agent can also block fibers not primarily affected (motor and sensory fibers). On the other hand, the block profile is not altered by low concentrations. A reduced motor block is obtained at the cost of reduced analgesic quality, and this is why opioid supplementation can be necessary with lower concentrations of local anesthetic.

Side effects and systemic effects

(Tables 1.5 and 1.6)

When assessing the safety and tolerability of a local anesthetic, account needs to be taken not only of its central nervous and cardiovascular effects, but also of its allergenic potential and of possibly toxic degradation products that may form as it is metabolized.

▨ *Systemic effects*

Adverse systemic effects of local anesthetics can occur when their plasma concentration is high enough to affect organs with membranes that can be irritated.
Toxic plasma levels can be reached as a result of:
– Inadvertent intravascular or intrathecal injection;
– Overdosing, particularly in areas with good blood perfusion and correspondingly high resorption;
– Unadjusted dosage in patients with hepatic or renal disease.

The severity of the reaction depends on the absolute plasma level, as well as on the speed at which it is reached. The anesthetic effect of the agents most commonly administered more or less correlates with their systemic toxicity: bupivacaine > etidocaine > ropivacaine > lignocaine > mepivacaine > prilocaine > procaine.

At significant plasma levels local anesthetics develop their greatest toxic effect in the central nervous system (CNS) and cardiovascular system (CVS).

CNS toxicity: Central reactions predominate in terms of frequency and clinical significance. The symptoms of these are listed in Table 1.6 in order of severity and toxicity. For speedy and appropriate treatment, it is important to observe and react immediately when even the preconvulsive signs of CNS intoxication are seen – particularly numbness in the tongue and perioral region. Since the symptoms of CNS toxicity occur either immediately after injection of the local anesthetic (intravascular injection) or within the first half hour (overdose), constant verbal contact must be maintained with the patient during this period.

Table 1.2 Local anesthetics with an amide bond

Aromatic residue	Intermediate chain	Substitued amino group	Year introduced
		Lignocaine	1944
		Mepivacaine	1957
		Prilocaine	1960
		Bupivacaine	1963
		Etidocaine	1972
		Carticaine	1974
		Ropivacaine	1996

Cardiovascular toxicity: toxic effects on the cardiovascular system usually occur after administration of very high doses. They are seen in the form of conduction disturbances in the autonomic cardiac and vascular nerve fibers, depression of cardiac function, and peripheral vasodilation (Tables 1.5 and 1.6).

Table 1.3 a Physicochemical and pharmacological parameters

Agent	Molecular weight	pK$_a$ (25°)	Distribution coefficient (lipid/water)	Protein binding (%)	Potency in vitro (isolated nerve)
Procaine	236	8.9	0.02	5.8	1
Lignocaine	220	7.7	2.9	64–70	4
Mepivacaine	234	7.7	0.9	77–80	3–4
Prilocaine	246	7.6	0.8	55	3–4
Bupivacaine	288	8.1	27.5	95	16
Etidocaine	276	7.7	141	95	16
Ropivacaine	274	8.1	9	95	16

Table 1.3 b Local anesthetic potency and duration of effect

Immediate treatment measures in cases of CNS and CVS intoxication are described in detail in the section on complications in Chap. 4.

Substance-specific side effects

When lignocaine and etidocaine are metabolized, one of the metabolites produced is 2,6-xylidine. At extremely high doses, this is mutagenic, and there is evidence from animal experiments that it has a carcinogenic effect. This is of dubious clinical relevance. Plasma levels after regional anesthesia with prilocaine are significantly lower than those with mepivacaine and lignocaine. The fastest metabolic processes here allow the highest dosages. On the other hand, during degradation of prilocaine, ortho-toluidine is produced – a methemoglobin precursor and carcinogen. In addition, hydroxylation of the aromatic ring can produce aminophenol, a powerful cell toxin [8]. Ortho-toluidine and its products oxidize hemoglobin into methemoglobin. Clinically, cyanosis, headaches, cardiac palpitation, and vertigo can occur at a low methemoglobin level of 10–20 %; from a level of 60 % upward there is loss of consciousness, shock, and death. In severe methemoglobinemia, breakdown into functioning hemoglobin can be accelerated by i. v. injection of a redox pigment such as toluidine blue, provided there is no genetic enzyme damage (e. g., glucose-6-phosphate dehydrogenase deficiency) or toxic enzyme damage (e. g., chlorate poisoning). It is only at dosages much higher than 600 mg prilocaine that individual cases of clinically relevant methemoglobinemia can occur. In normal circumstances, methemoglobin production is not clinically significant, but the drug should not be used in patients with heart disease, anemic patients, or in obstetrics.

Allergenic potential

There is no reliable data regarding the frequency of allergic reactions after the administration of local anesthetics. There is no doubt that these are extremely rare, although the symptoms can range from allergic dermatitis to anaphylactic shock. Occasional cases of allergic reactions to ester local anesthetics have been reported, and the preservative substances which the various preparations contain (e. g., parabens), and the antioxidant sodium bisulfide in epinephrine-containing solutions, are also under discussion as potential causes of these. In patients with suspected intolerance of local anesthetics, intracutaneous testing with 20 µl of the agent can be carried out. When the result is positive, subcutaneous provocation tests at increasing dosages (0.1 ml each diluted at 1 : 10 000, 1 : 1000, and 1 : 10; undiluted at 0.1 ml, 0.5 ml, 1 ml) can be considered. When these tests are being carried out, it is vital to prepare all the necessary safety measures in case of a severe reaction.

Selection of suitable substances for regional block

When surgical interventions are being carried out under regional anesthesia, priority must go to shutting off the sensory and motor systems, and knowledge of the expected length of the operation is vital to the choice of anesthetic. The onset of effect and the toxicity of the drug used play an important part, but not a decisive one. In the context of pain therapy, in which the fast-conducting A delta fibers and the slow-conducting C fibers (Table 1.7) are the target of the block, toxicity is much more important compared with the duration of the effect. In diagnostic and therapeutic blocks,

Table 1.4 Relative block profile of local anesthetics with long-term effects

Table 1.5 Toxicity of clinical dosages of local anesthetics

Local anesthetic	Central nervous system	Heart
Lignocaine	++	+
Mepivacaine	++	+
Prilocaine	+	+/−
Bupivacaine	+++	++++++ [*]
Ropivacaine	++(+)	+++

[*] Clinical dosage can be equivalent to lethal dosage when incorrectly administered.

in which there is a risk of intravascular injection – e. g., in a stellate ganglion block or superior cervical ganglion block – prilocaine should be selected, as it is the medium-term local anesthetic with the lowest toxicity (mepivacaine or lignocaine are alternatives) (Table 1.8).

Table 1.6 Symptoms of local anesthetic intoxication

Central nervous system	Cardiovascular system
Excitation phase, low toxicity	
Tingling on lips, tongue paresthesias, perioral numbness, ringing in the ears, metallic taste, anxiety, restlessness, trembling, muscle twitching, vomiting	Cardiac palpitation, hypertonia, tachycardia, tachypnea, dry mouth
Excitation phase, moderate toxicity	
Speech disturbance, dazed state, sleepiness, confusion, tremor, choreoid movements, tonic–clonic cramp, mydriasis, vomiting, tachypnea	Tachycardia, arrhythmia, cyanosis and pallor, nausea and vomiting
Paralytic phase, severe toxicity	
Stupor, coma, irregular breathing, respiratory arrest, seizure, flaccidity, vomiting with aspiration, sphincter paralysis, death	Severe cyanosis, bradycardia, drop in blood pressure, primary heart failure, ventricular fibrillation, asystole

Table 1.7 Functional distinctions between nerve fibers

Fiber type	Function
A_α	Motor, touch, pressure, depth sensation
A_β	Motor, touch, pressure, depth sensation
A_γ	Regulation of muscle tone
A_δ	Pain, temperature, touch
B	Preganglionic sympathetic function
C	Pain, temperature, touch, postganglionic sympathetic function

Table 1.8 Overview of drugs

Drug	Potency	Duration of effect	Toxicity	Half-life (min)	Vdiss
Lignocaine	1 (ref.)	2 h	1 (ref.)	96'	91
Mepivacaine	1	2–3 h	1.2	114'	84
Prilocaine	1	2–3 h	0.5	93'	261

Recommended maximum doses without epinephrine, according to specialist information:

Lignocaine	Mepivacaine	Prilocaine
200 mg	300 mg	400 mg

Bupivacaine has an important role for regional blocks, being a longer-term local anesthetic that provides high-quality analgesia and easily controlled motor block. Its anesthetic potency is about four times greater than that of local anesthetics with medium-term effects (such as prilocaine). When the lower dosage required in pain therapy in comparison with regional anesthesia is taken into account, bupivacaine can be used for practically all pain therapy procedures, in spite of its high relative toxicity.

Ropivacaine is the most recent long-term local anesthetic in the amino amide series. The differential block is even more marked than with bupivacaine, and the drug is associated with much lower CNS toxicity and cardiac toxicity. These characteristics make it particularly suitable for regional anesthesia procedures in which higher dosages or concentrations are required. Ropivacaine provides good analgesic quality while largely maintaining the motor system (up to 80 % of patients have no measurable motor block on the Bromage scale). At a dosage of 2 mg/ml, the drug is therefore the local anesthetic of choice for epidural obstetric analgesia and for postoperative analgesia (Table 1.4). With its pharmacological profile, ropivacaine is the first local anesthetic with primarily analgesic effects, and it is therefore particularly suitable for pain therapy indications.

Every anesthetist and pain therapy physician who uses anesthetic methods for temporary interruption of stimulus conduction in a ganglion, nerve, or neural plexus should be familiar with the properties and potential applications of the following agents:

Procaine (Novocaine®)

Class of drug: Local anesthetic of the ester type.
Single threshold dose: 500 mg without epinephrine in adults.
LD$_{50}$ (mouse): 52.2–60.0 mg/kg body weight i. v.
Plasma half-life: < 0.14 h.
Latency: medium.
Duration of effect: 0.5–1 h, depending on the area of application and the concentration used.
Metabolism: Procaine is broken down in plasma by pseudocholinesterase into p-aminobenzoic acid – a naturally occurring component of folic acid synthesis – and into diethylaminoethanol. The metabolites are excreted in the urine or broken down in the liver.
Tolerability and control: Procaine is one of the local anesthetics that have the lowest toxicity. Due to its short half-life, procaine is easily controlled.
Clinical uses: It is not so much its local anesthetic potency that predominates in procaine, but rather its muscle-relaxing properties and vasodilatory effect, which are at the forefront in infiltration therapy and trigger-point treatment. In the therapeutic field, very good results can be obtained with superior cervical ganglion block. However, procaine's high allergenic potency in comparison with amide local anesthetics argues against its use.
Dosage: Procaine is administered at concentrations of 0.5–2 %. Precise dosages are described in the relevant sections of this book.

Lignocaine (Xylocaine®, lidocaine)
(Table 1.8)

Class of drug: Local anesthetic of the amide type.
Single threshold dose: 200 mg without epinephrine in adults.
LD$_{50}$ (mouse): 31.2–62.2 mg/kg body weight i. v.
Plasma half-life: ca. 1.6 h.
Latency: fast.
Duration of effect: 1–2 h, depending on the area of application and the concentration used.
Metabolism: Lignocaine is metabolized in hepatic microsomes. Only ca. 3 % of the substance is excreted unchanged from the kidney.
Tolerability and control: Lignocaine is one of the local anesthetics with moderate relative toxicity. This is characterized by a medium-term duration of effect, and good distribution characteristics.
Lignocaine causes vasodilation, which may be less than that of procaine. When the medium-duration local anes-

thetics are compared, the strength of the associated vasodilatory effect is in the following order: lignocaine > mepivacaine > prilocaine. Lignocaine is therefore often used with epinephrine.

Clinical uses: Lignocaine is widely used in clinical practice, particularly in neural and segmental therapy. It is also suitable for infiltration anesthesia, for peripheral nerve block, for epidural anesthesia, and for mucosal surface anesthesia (2 % gel, Emla®).

Dosage: Lignocaine is mainly administered as a 0.5 % or 1 (1.5) % solution. Precise dosages are described in the relevant chapters of this book.

Mepivacaine (Scandicaine®, Meaverine®) (Table 1.8)

Class of drug: Local anesthetic of the amide type.
Single threshold dose without epinephrine in adults: 200 mg in the ENT area, 300 mg in all other applications (500 mg with vasopressor), with no differentiation between regions with different resorption.
LD$_{50}$ (mouse): 40.3 ± 3.2 mg/kg body weight i. v.
Plasma half-life: ca. 1.9 h.
Latency: fast.
Duration of effect: 1–3 h, depending on the area of application and the concentration used.
Metabolism: Mepivacaine is metabolized in the hepatic microsomes.

After intravenous administration, up to 16 % of the agent is excreted unchanged from the kidney. Degradation in the liver mainly produces m-hydroxymepivacaine and p-hydroxymepivacaine. These metabolites are conjugated with glucuronic acid and excreted in the urine. Another metabolite, pipecoloxylidide, collects in bile and passes through the enterohepatic circulation with its degradation products. No 2,6-xylidine is produced when mepivacaine is metabolized, and there is no evidence that either the agent or its metabolites have mutagenic or carcinogenic properties.

Tolerability and control: Mepivacaine is another of the local anesthetics with moderate relative toxicity. It is characterized by a medium-term duration of effect, with good distribution properties and some vasodilatory effect.

Clinical uses: Mepivacaine is the local anesthetic of choice when a medium-term effect is required for use in diagnostic and therapeutic blocks in pain therapy – particularly in outpatients. It is suitable for infiltration anesthesia, intravenous regional anesthesia, peripheral nerve block and ganglion block, and for epidural anesthesia.

Dosage: Mepivacaine is mainly used as a 1 % or 0.5 % solution. Precise dosages are described in the relevant chapters of this book.

Prilocaine (Xylonest®) (Table 1.8)

Class of drug: Local anesthetic of the amide type.
Single threshold dose: 400 mg (600 mg with vasopressor).
LD$_{50}$ (mouse): 62 mg/kg b. w. i. v.
Plasma half-life: ca. 1.5 h.
Latency: fast.
Duration of effect: 2–3 h, depending on the area of application and the concentration used.
Metabolism: Prilocaine is primarily metabolized in hepatic microsomes, but also in the kidney and lungs. During degradation, the metabolite ortho-toluidine is produced. At dosages higher than 600 mg, the body's reduction systems may become exhausted. At dosages higher than 800 mg, noticeable methemoglobinemia can be expected (see the section on substance-specific side effects). Fast elimination from the blood leads to low systemic toxicity.

Tolerability and control: Among the amide local anesthetics, prilocaine has the best ratio between anesthetic potency and toxicity. Due to its high distribution volume and marked absorption in the lungs, plasma levels are significantly lower than those of mepivacaine and lignocaine (by a factor of 2–3). It has a medium-term duration of effect.

Clinical uses: It is suitable for peripheral nerve block, infiltration anesthesia (particularly large-volume), intravenous regional anesthesia, and diagnostic and therapeutic blocks in pain therapy. Prilocaine is particularly suitable for outpatients, but not suitable for continuous administration. The substance should not be used in anemic patients with a history of cardiac disease, or in obstetrics.

Dosage: Prilocaine is mainly used as a 0.5 % or 1 % solution. Precise dosages are described in the relevant chapters of this book.

Bupivacaine (Carbostesin®, Marcaine®)

Class of drug: Local anesthetic of the amide type.
Single threshold dose: 150 mg without epinephrine in adults.
LD$_{50}$ (mouse): 7.8 ± 0.4 mg/kg b. w. i. v.
Plasma half-life: ca. 2.7 h.
Latency: medium.
Duration of effect: 2.5–20.0 h, depending on the area of application and the concentration used. A mean duration of effect of 3–6 h can be assumed.
Metabolism: Bupivacaine is broken down in the hepatic microsomes at a high metabolic rate. The predominant metabolization involves dealkylation to pipecoloxylidide (desbutyl-bupivacaine). There is no evidence that either the agent or its metabolites have mutagenic or carcinogenic properties.

Tolerability and control: Bupivacaine is one of the local anesthetics that have a high relative toxicity. Its anesthetic potency is about four times greater than that of mepivacaine. It is characterized by a slower onset of effect and a long duration of effect.

Clinical uses: Bupivacaine is indicated as a long-term local anesthetic, particularly for regional anesthesia in the surgical field, in postoperative analgesia, and in pain therapy for various pain conditions.

It is suitable for infiltration anesthesia, peripheral nerve block, ganglion block, and plexus block, as well as all forms of neuraxial anesthesia. When dosages are strictly observed, it can be used for practically all pain therapy blocks. However, in outpatient pain therapy, the patient should be observed for an adequate period after the administration of bupivacaine.

Dosage: Depending on the indication, bupivacaine is administered as a 0.125–0.5 % solution. A 0.75 % solution is also still being marketed. Higher concentrations are not required in pain therapy. Precise dosages are described in the relevant chapters of this book.

Table 1.9 Important rules to observe when administering regional anesthesia or therapeutic nerve block

Before the block

1. **Preoperative information**
   – Explain the injection procedure
   – Mention potential side effects and complications
   – Advise the patient of what to do following the procedure
   – Document the discussion
2. **Determine the patient's neurological status** before the block – exclude neurological abnormalities
3. Exclude **contraindications**
4. Avoid **premedication** in outpatients (particularly in blocks in which there is an increased risk of intravascular injection – e. g., stellate ganglion or superior cervical ganglion)
5. Ensure **optimal positioning** of the patient
6. Secure **intravenous access**
7. **Added vasopressors** are usually **contraindicated** in pain therapy
8. With rarely used blocks, the **anatomical** and **technical** aspects of the procedure should always be studied again beforehand

During the injection

1. Carry out an **aspiration test** before and during the injection
2. Administration of a **test dose** is necessary in most blocks
3. Always inject local anesthetics in **incremental** doses **(several test doses)**
4. Maintain **verbal contact** with the patient
5. Keep careful **notes** of the block

Ropivacaine (Naropin®)

Class of drug: Local anesthetic of the amide type, pure S-enantiomer.

Single threshold dose: highest documented dose: epidural: 250 mg (25 ml, 10 mg/ml).

Peripheral nerve block: axillary plexus block 300 mg (40 ml, 7.5 mg/ml), inguinal femoral perivascular block ("three-in-one" block) 500 mg (50 ml, 10 mg/ml).

LD_{50} (mouse): ca. 11.0–12.0 mg/kg b. w. i. v.

Plasma half-life: ca. 1.8 h.

Duration of effect: Epidural anesthesia ca. 7 h (analgesia); ca. 4 h (motor block), 10 mg/ml.

Plexus anesthesia (brachial plexus, lumbosacral plexus): 9–17 h, 7.5 mg/ml.

Infiltration anesthesia: postoperative analgesia after inguinal herniectomy > 7 h (5–23 h), 7.5 mg/ml. Peripheral nerve blocks in pain therapy: 2–6 h (0.2–0.375 mg/ml).

Latency: medium (declining latency at increasing concentrations).

Metabolism: Ropivacaine is metabolized in the liver, mainly through aromatic hydroxylation. Only ca. 1 % of the substance is excreted unchanged in the urine. The main metabolite is 3-hydroxyropivacaine.

Tolerability: Ropivacaine provides relatively low toxicity for a long-term local anesthetic. Compared with bupivacaine, it has a lower arrhythmogenic potential, and the margin between convulsive and lethal doses is wider. Ropivacaine has more favorable receptor kinetics ("fast in – medium out") in cardiac sodium channels, and in comparison with bupivacaine has only slight depressant effects on the energy metabolism of the mitochondria and cardiac muscle cells.

Clinical uses: The first clinical tests were carried out in 1988. Its relatively low toxicity means that effective dosages can be administered (e. g., 10 mg/ml solution for epidural anesthesia) – providing more intensive motor block, a higher success rate, and better analgesic quality than 0.5 % bupivacaine, for example. At lower concentrations (2 mg/ml), only a slight motor block is observed even with several days of epidural infusion (Table 1.4). This offers a wider spectrum of possible uses of the drug in postoperative pain therapy in connection with patient mobilization.

Dosage: Ropivacaine is administered at concentrations of 2 mg/ml (0.2 %), 7.5 mg/ml (0.75 %), and 10 mg/ml (1 %). Continuous epidural infusion has official approval. Cumulative daily dosages of up to 675 mg (see specialist information) are well tolerated in adults. Precise information on dosages is given in the following chapters.

Examination and patient preparation

Before regional anesthesia, the same type of examination of the patient should be carried out as for general anesthesia. Contraindications must be excluded, as well as neurological abnormalities, and when there are relative contraindications – e. g., hemorrhagic diathesis, stable systemic neural disease or local nerve damage, a careful assessment of the risk–benefit ratio needs to be made.

Particular attention needs to be given to anatomical relationships, palpation of the landmarks, and precise localization and marking of the puncture point.

To ensure cooperation, the patient should be given detailed information on the aim of the block, its technical implementation and possible or probable paresthesias and their significance. The patient should also be informed about potential adverse effects and complications of the block, and outpatients in particular should be familiarized with guidelines on behavior after the procedure. The patient information session should be documented using a consent form signed by the patient.

In general, premedication and the administration of sedatives or analgesics should be avoided, particularly in outpatient pain therapy. Constant verbal contact should be maintained with the patient during the block, so that potential side effects or complications can be recognized immediately. In addition, any sedation that is not adjusted individually can lead to respiratory and circulatory reactions, which may be mistaken for early symptoms of local anesthetic intoxication.

Documentation of treatment

The patient history, including investigations at other centers, and diagnostic results should be documented just as carefully as the preparation, implementation, and success of the block. In particular, anatomical abnormalities, instrumentation problems, injection pains, blood aspiration, paresthesias and complications must be recorded in detail. The checklists and record forms used in our outpatient pain department have been adapted for each individual block technique, and are included in the following chapters.

2 Occipital nerves
Greater occipital nerve
Lesser occipital nerve

Anatomy

After exiting from the lower edge of the obliquus capitis inferior muscle, the second cervical spinal nerve divides into anterior and posterior branches.

The anterior branches of the first four cervical spinal nerves form the cervical plexus, which is covered by the sternocleidomastoid muscle. The superficial branches of the cervical plexus, which penetrate the cervical fascia and pass to the skin, include the sensory **lesser occipital nerve** (anterior branch from C2 and C3). This emerges at the posterior edge of the sternocleidomastoid muscle, above the center. It ascends steeply along the splenius capitis muscle and divides into several branches (Fig. 2.1). The areas it supplies include the skin on the upper exterior side of the neck, the upper part of the auricle and the adjoining skin of the scalp.

The posterior branch of the second cervical spinal nerve passes in a dorsal direction around the obliquus capitis inferior muscle and runs between the occipitovertebral muscles and the semispinalis capitis muscle. Here it divides into three branches: an ascending branch, which supplies the longissimus capitis muscle; a descending branch, which anastomoses with the posterior branch of C3 (the third occipital nerve); and the medial greater occipital nerve (posterior branch of C2). The sensory **greater occipital nerve** passes in a cranial direction, goes through the semispinalis capitis muscle and trapezius muscle and reaches the skin about 2–3 cm away from the median line in the area of the superior nuchal line. It gives off several branches toward the top of the head and extends laterally as far as the ear. The course of its branches follows the branches of the occipital artery.

Blocks of the greater and lesser occipital nerves

Indications
Blocks of the **greater** and **lesser occipital nerves** are carried out for prognostic, diagnostic and therapeutic purposes in patients with painful conditions in the region of the back of the head.

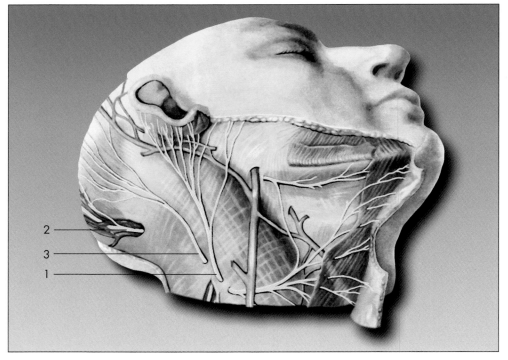

Fig. 2.1 Nerves supplying the surface of the back of the head:
(1) great auricular nerve,
(2) greater occipital nerve and occipital artery,
(3) lesser occipital nerve

Diagnostic
- Differential diagnosis to clarify pain at the back of the head – e. g., in suspected tumors of the posterior cranial fossa.

Therapeutic
- Occipital neuralgia characterized by pain in the suboccipital area and back of the head [5].

Neuralgia of the occipital nerves caused by compression is anatomically almost impossible. The origin of the neuralgia has to be clarified under all circumstances. The cause is often degenerative change – e. g., in the vertebral column, or muscle tension with irritation of the nerve roots. There may also be articular disease or tumors in the second and third cervical dorsal roots.
In whiplash injuries, consideration can be given to activation of the numerous myofascial trigger points – e. g., in the area of the cervical musculature, masticatory muscles and sternocleidomastoid, trapezius, occipitofrontal and suboccipital muscles – and simultaneous treatment of these is possible [6].

Genuine occipital neuralgia is extremely rare.

Specific contraindications
None.

Procedure

Preparations
Check that the emergency equipment is complete and in working order. Sterile precautions, skin prep.

Materials
Syringes (2 ml), fine 26-G needles (2.5 cm), disinfectant, swabs for compression (Fig. 2.2).

Patient positioning
Sitting, with head tilted forward slightly.

Landmarks
Occipital artery, inferior nuchal line: one-third of the distance between the external occipital protuberance and the foramen magnum.

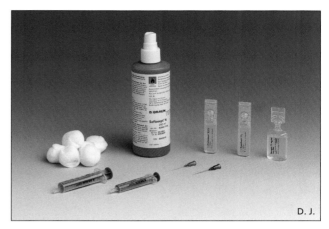

Fig. 2.2 Materials

Injection techniques
Greater occipital nerve
The needle is inserted about 2.5 cm from the midline, directly medial to the easily palpable occipital artery. It is advanced at a slightly cranial angle (Fig. 2.3) between the insertions of the trapezius and semispinalis muscles until bone contact is made. After minimal withdrawal and aspiration, the local anesthetic is injected.

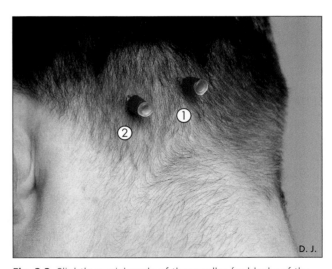

Fig. 2.3 Slightly cranial angle of the needles for blocks of the greater occipital nerve (1) and lesser occipital nerve (2)

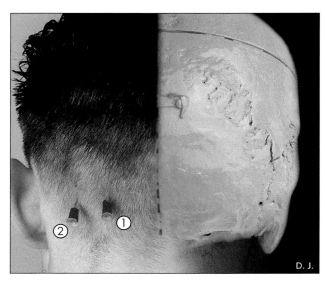

Fig. 2.4 Puncture points: (1) greater occipital nerve and (2) lesser occipital nerve

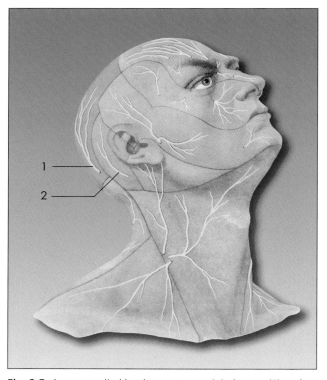

Fig. 2.5 Areas supplied by the greater occipital nerve (1) and lesser occipital nerve (2)

Lesser occipital nerve
The injection is carried out 2.5 cm lateral to the puncture point described above (Fig. 2.4). Bone contact is also sought at a slightly cranial angle and the needle is withdrawn a little, followed by aspiration and injection.

Spread of the blocks
The areas supplied are illustrated in Figure 2.5.

> There are close anatomical connections both with the trigeminal nerve and with the third occipital nerve. The third occipital nerve in particular is often anesthetized as well.

Dosage
Diagnostic
0.5–1 ml local anesthetic – e. g., 0.5–1% prilocaine, mepivacaine, or lidocaine.

Therapeutic
1–1.5 ml local anesthetic – e. g., 0.75 % ropivacaine, 0.5% bupivacaine, often with 1–2 mg dexamethasone added.

> Higher doses should be avoided due to the high vascular perfusion and resultant resorption.

Block series
When there is evidence of improvement in the symptoms, 8–12 blocks are indicated.

Complications
Inadvertent intra-arterial injection may occur, extremely rarely.

Treatment measures
See Chap. 4, p. 42.

3 Trigeminal nerve

Anatomy

The trigeminal nerve, the largest of the cranial nerves, exits from the pons with a small motor root (the portio minor) and a large sensory root (portio major).

In the semilunar cave of the dura mater, the sensory root swells to become the trigeminal ganglion (semilunar ganglion). The motor root runs along the medial side of the ganglion to the mandibular nerve.

The trigeminal ganglion lies on the dorsal surface of the petrous bone. The three main branches originate from its anterior margin (Fig. 3.1): the **ophthalmic nerve, maxillary nerve and mandibular nerve.**

Ophthalmic nerve

The optic branch is purely sensory and passes lateral to the cavernous sinus and abducent nerve to the superior orbital fissure. It draws sympathetic fibers from the internal carotid plexus and in turn gives off sensory fibers to the oculomotor nerve, trochlear nerve and abducent nerve. Before entering the fissure, the ophthalmic nerve branches into the lacrimal nerve, nasociliary nerve and frontal nerve. The **frontal nerve** runs along the levator palpebrae superioris muscle to behind the centre of the orbital cavity. There it divides into the **supraorbital nerve,** which passes to the supraorbital notch and the **supratrochlear nerve,** which runs in a medial direction toward the trochlea.

The branches of the supratrochlear nerve supply the upper eyelid, the root of the nose and the adjoining skin of the forehead (upper end branch), as well as the skin and conjunctiva of the medial canthus (lower end branch).

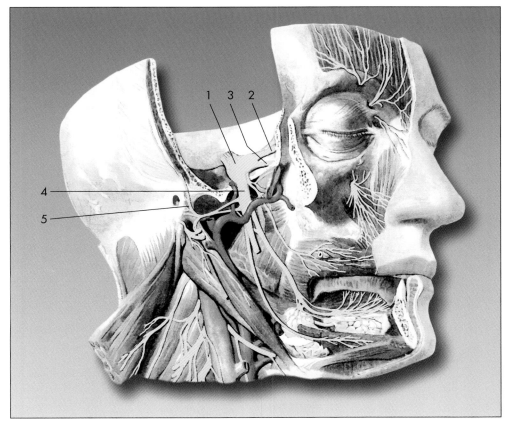

Fig. 3.1 Sensory supply of the face.
(1) Trigeminal ganglion,
(2) ophthalmic nerve,
(3) maxillary nerve,
(4) mandibular nerve and
(5) auriculotemporal nerve

Maxillary nerve

The second branch of the trigeminal nerve is also purely sensory. It emerges from the skull through the round foramen and enters the pterygopalatine fossa. From here, it gives off the zygomatic nerve to the orbit and the pterygopalatine nerves – two very short nerves – which connect with the **pterygopalatine (sphenopalatine) ganglion.**

As a continuation of its trunk, the infraorbital nerve penetrates through the inferior orbital fissure to the base of the orbit, to the infraorbital groove and infraorbital canal. After passing through the infraorbital foramen, it reaches the facial surface of the maxilla. Here it divides into three groups of branches, which supply the wing of the nose, the lower eyelid and the upper lip.

Mandibular nerve

The largest branch of the trigeminal nerve, the mandibular nerve contains the sensory and motor fibers.

After passing through the oval foramen, the mandibular nerve forms a short, thick nerve trunk, on the medial side of which lies the **otic ganglion.** In its further course, the mandibular nerve divides into an anterior trunk, with mainly motor fibers and a posterior trunk of primarily sensory fibers. The most important nerves and areas of supply in the posterior trunk are:

- **Mental nerve** (skin and mucosa of the lower lip and chin),
- **Inferior alveolar nerve** (molar and premolar teeth of the mandible),
- **Lingual nerve** (floor of the mouth, mucosa of the anterior two-thirds of the tongue),
- **Auriculotemporal nerve** (ear, skin and fascia of the temple).

The sensory branch of the anterior trunk, the **buccal nerve,** supplies the skin and mucosa in the area of the buccinator muscle.

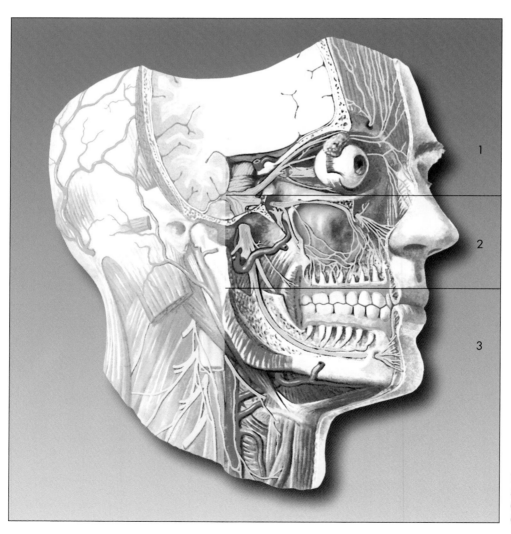

Fig. 3.2 (1) Supraorbital and supratrochlear nerves, (2) infraorbital nerve, (3) mental nerve

Blocks of the supraorbital and supratrochlear nerves

The end branches of these two nerves provide the sensory supply for the skin of the forehead, root of the nose and the skin and conjunctiva of the medial canthus (Fig. 3.2).

Indications
Diagnostic
- Differential diagnosis of hyperalgesic zones – e. g., the frontal part of the occipitofrontalis muscle.

Therapeutic
- Trigeminal neuralgia of the first branch and post-herpetic neuralgia;
- Postoperative and posttraumatic pain;
- Minor surgical interventions (note higher dosages) along the surface of the innervated area – e. g., removal of cysts and atheromas, wound care.

Specific contraindications
None.

Procedure

Preparations
Check that the emergency equipment is complete and in working order. Sterile precautions, skin prep.

Materials
2-ml syringes, fine 26-G needles (2.5 cm), disinfectant, swabs for compression (Fig. 3.3).

Skin prep
For all blocks.

Patient positioning
Supine.

Landmarks (Fig. 3.4)
Supraorbital foramen, upper angle of the orbit.
Supraorbital nerve: palpation of the supraorbital foramen at the edge of the orbit.
Supratrochlear nerve: palpation of the upper angle of the orbit on the medial side of the root of the nose.

Injection techniques
Supraorbital nerve
After palpation of the supraorbital foramen, a swab is laid on the eyelid to prevent uncontrolled spread of the local anesthetic. The needle is introduced as far as the supraorbital foramen (bone contact), slightly withdrawn

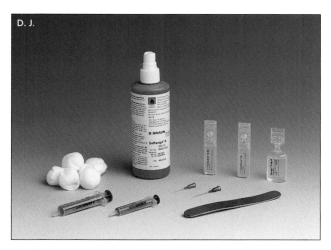

Fig. 3.3 Materials

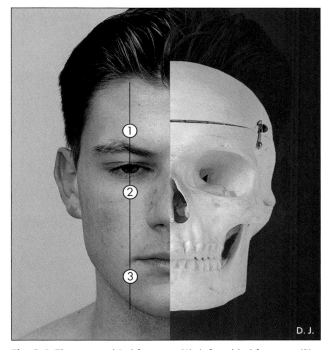

Fig. 3.4 The supraorbital foramen (1), infraorbital foramen (2) and mental foramen (3) lie on a single line running about 2.5 cm lateral to the midfacial line and passing through the pupil

and after aspiration, the injection is carried out slowly (Fig. 3.5).

Supratrochlear nerve
After palpation of the upper angle of the orbit, a swab is laid on the eyelid to prevent uncontrolled spread of the local anesthetic. The needle is introduced at the upper internal angle of the orbit (Fig. 3.6) and minimally withdrawn after bone contact. Slow injection of the local anesthetic follows after careful aspiration.

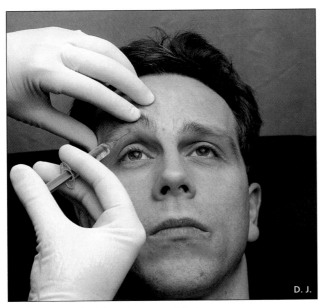

Fig. 3.5 Anesthetizing the supraorbital nerve

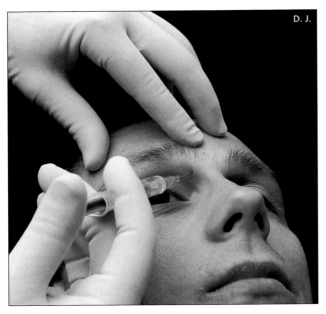

Fig. 3.6 Anesthetizing the supratrochlear nerve

> It is not necessary to elicit paresthesias. Look for bone contact, withdraw the needle slightly, aspirate and only then inject.

Dosage
Diagnostic
0.5–1 ml local anesthetic – e. g., 0.5–1 % prilocaine, mepivacaine, lidocaine.

Therapeutic
0.5–1 ml local anesthetic – e. g., 0.5–0.75 % ropivacaine, 0.25–0.5 % bupivacaine.

Surgical
Up to 5 ml local anesthetic.
Shorter procedures: e. g., 1 % prilocaine or 1 % mepivacaine.
Longer procedures: 0.75 % ropivacaine, 0.5 % bupivacaine.

Side effects
Possible hematoma formation (prophylactic compression).

> After the injection, carry out thorough compression (massaging in), to prevent hematoma formation and to encourage the local anesthetic to spread.

Complications
Risk of vascular and neural lesions in injections into the foramina and bone channels.

> **Caution**
> No injections should be made into the supraorbital foramen, due to the risk of neural injury.

Blocks of the infraorbital nerve

The infraorbital nerve, the end branch of the maxillary nerve, emerges about 1 cm below the middle of the lower orbital margin through the infraorbital foramen (Figs. 3.2, 3.31).

Indications
Diagnostic
- Differential diagnosis of trigger zones.

Therapeutic
- Trigeminal neuralgia in the second branch and postherpetic pain;
- Facial pain in the innervation area of the infraorbital nerve, posttraumatic pain and pain after dental extraction;
- Minor surgical procedures on the surface of the area of distribution (note higher dosages).

Specific contraindications
None.

Procedure

Preparation and materials (Fig. 3.3)

Skin prep
For all blocks.

Patient positioning
Supine.

Landmarks
Infraorbital foramen, orbital margin (cf. Figs. 3.2 and 3.4).

Extraoral injection
Palpation of the infraorbital foramen, about 1 cm below the middle of the lower orbital margin.

Intraoral injection
Palpation of the lower orbital margin.

Injection techniques
Extraoral injection
After palpating the infraorbital foramen, the needle is introduced cranially just below the palpation point until bone contact is made (Fig. 3.7) and then withdrawn slightly.

Intraoral injection
The center of the lower orbital margin is palpated and marked with the middle finger. The upper lip is raised with a spatula or with the thumb and index finger. The needle is introduced above the second premolar towards the infraorbital foramen, until bone contact is made and then withdrawn slightly (Fig. 3.8).

> For both of these techniques, it is important that slow injection of the local anesthetic should only be carried out after careful aspiration. Afterwards, thorough compression should be carried out to prevent hematoma formation and to obtain better distribution of the local anesthetic.

> **Caution**
> No injections should be made into the infraorbital canal, due to the risk of neural injury.

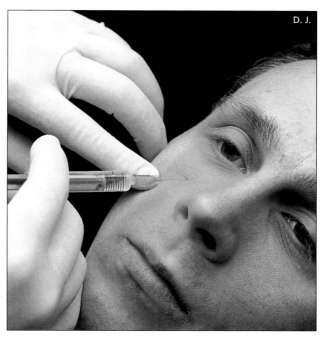

Fig. 3.7 Extraoral technique for blockading the infraorbital nerve

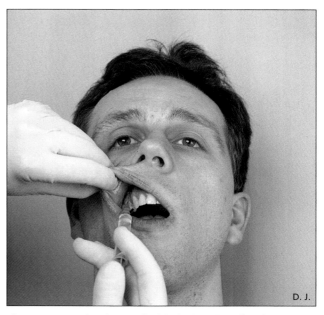

Fig. 3.8 Intraoral technique for blockading the infraorbital nerve

Dosages
Diagnostic
0.5–1 ml local anesthetic – e. g., 0.5–1 % prilocaine, mepivacaine, lidocaine.

Therapeutic (extraoral technique)
0.5–1 ml local anesthetic – e. g., 0.5–0.75 % ropivacaine, 0.5 % bupivacaine.

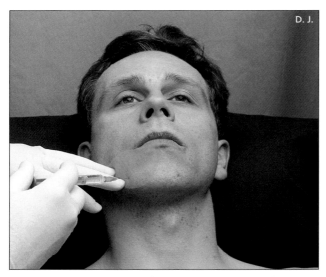

Fig. 3.9 Extraoral technique for blockading the mental nerve

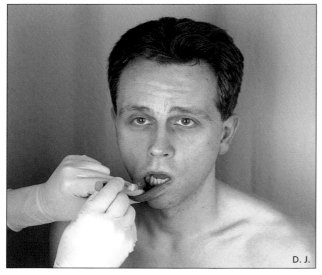

Fig. 3.10 Intraoral technique for blockading the mental nerve

Surgical
Up to 5 ml local anesthetic extraorally.
Shorter procedures: 1 % prilocaine or 1 % mepivacaine.
Longer procedures: 0.75 % ropivacaine, 0.5 % bupivacaine.
Intraorally: 2–3 ml local anesthetic.

Side effects
Potential hematoma formation (prophylactic compression).
If the needle is advanced too far, penetration of the orbit can occur.
Symptom: temporary double vision.

Complications
Injection into the bone canal carries a risk of neural lesions.

Blocks of the mental nerve

The mental nerve, the sensory end branch of the mandibular nerve, emerges from the mental foramen at the level of the second premolar (Fig. 3.2).
It provides the sensory supply of the skin and mucosa of the lower lip and chin (Fig. 3.33).

Indications
Diagnostic
▨ Differential diagnosis of trigger points and hyperalgesic zones.

Therapeutic
▨ Trigeminal neuralgia of the third branch;
▨ Posttraumatic pain and pain in the innervation area of the mental nerve;
▨ Treatment of canine tooth, first premolars and incisors of the lower jaw;
▨ Post-extraction pain (intraoral technique);
▨ Surgical procedures on the surface of the lower lip (note higher dosages).

Specific contraindications
None.

Procedure

Preparation and materials (Fig. 3.3)

Skin prep
In all blocks.

Patient positioning
Supine.

Landmarks
Mental foramen (cf. Figs. 3.2 and 3.4).

Extraoral and intraoral injection
Palpation of the mental foramen at the level of the second premolar.

Injection techniques
Extraoral injection
After palpation of the mental foramen, the needle is inserted about 2.5 cm lateral to the midline (Fig. 3.9) until bone contact is made.

Intraoral injection
After palpation of the mental foramen, the lower lip is pressed downward using a spatula. The needle is inserted between the first and second premolars, into the lower reflection of the oral vestibule, in the direction of the neurovascular bundle (Fig. 3.10).

For both of these techniques, it is important that slow injection should only be carried out after careful aspiration. Afterwards, thorough compression should be carried out to prevent hematoma formation and to obtain better distribution of the local anesthetic.

Dosage
Diagnostic
0.5–1 ml local anesthetic – e. g., 0.5–1 % prilocaine, mepivacaine, lidocaine.

Therapeutic (extraoral technique)
0.5–1 ml local anesthetic – e. g., 0.5–0.75 % ropivacaine, 0.5 % bupivacaine.

Surgical
Up to 5 ml local anesthetic extraorally.
Shorter procedures: 1 % prilocaine or 1 % mepivacaine.

Longer procedures: 0.75 % ropivacaine, 0.5 % bupivacaine.
Intraorally: 2–3 ml local anesthetic.

Side effects
Potential hematoma formation (prophylactic compression).

Complications
Injection into the bone canal carries a risk of neural lesions.

> **Caution**
> Injections should never be made into the mental canal, due to the risk of neural injury.

Blocks of the maxillary nerve and pterygopalatine ganglion

The maxillary nerve emerges from the skull through the round foramen. It connects with the pterygopalatine (sphenopalatine) ganglion in the pterygopalatine fossa (Fig. 3.11). The nerve and ganglion are responsible for sensory and autonomic supply to the central area of the face and head.

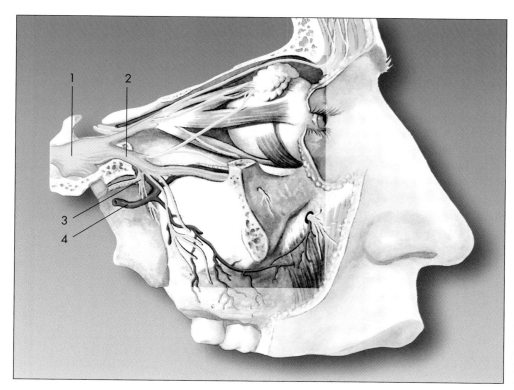

Fig. 3.11 (1) Trigeminal ganglion (gasserian ganglion) and (2) pterygopalatine fossa with the maxillary nerve, pterygopalatine ganglion (3) and maxillary artery (4)

Indications

Diagnostic
- Differential diagnosis of facial pain.

Therapeutic
- Trigeminal neuralgia in the second branch, post-herpetic neuralgia;
- Cluster headache [6], histamine headache, Sluder's neuralgia [19];
- Facial pain in the area of supply;
- Pain in the eye region (iritis, keratitis, corneal ulcer), root of the nose, upper jaw and gums;
- Postoperative pain in the area of the maxillary sinus and teeth;
- Pain after dental extraction.

Neural therapy
- Hay fever, vasomotor rhinitis;
- Diseases of the oral mucosa;
- Localized paresthesias.

Specific contraindications
Bleeding diathesis, anticoagulation treatment.

Procedure

These blocks should only be carried out with appropriate experience!

Preparations
Check that the emergency equipment is complete and in working order. Sterile precautions. Intravenous access.

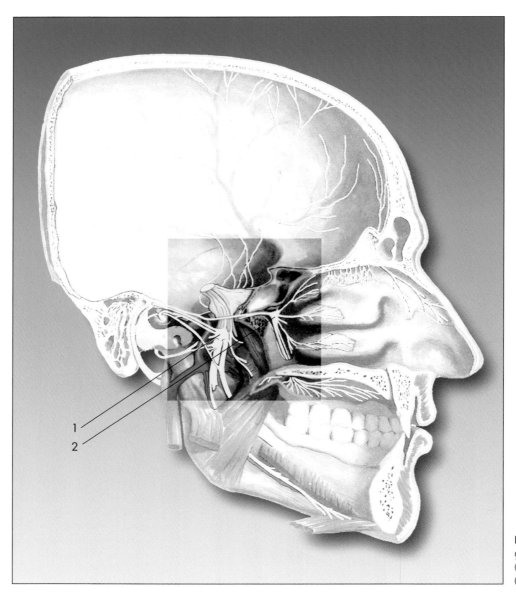

Fig. 3.12 Nerves and ganglia in the vicinity: (1) otic ganglion, (2) pterygopalatine ganglion

Materials
2-ml syringe, 22-G needle (4 cm) for the intraoral technique, 5-ml and 10-ml syringe, 23-G needle (6 cm) for the extraoral technique. Disinfectant, spatula for the intraoral technique, compresses, cooling element available, emergency drugs (Fig. 3.13).

Skin prep
In all blocks.

Intraoral technique

Patient positioning
The patient should be sitting, leaning back slightly and with the head tilted back.

Landmarks
Posterior edge of the seventh upper tooth (second maxillary molar) (Fig. 3.14).

Injection technique
Using a 22-G needle (4 cm), the puncture is made medial to the posterior edge of the seventh upper tooth (second maxillary molar) through the greater palatine foramen. The needle is introduced at an angle of about 60°. The vicinity of the ganglion is reached at a depth of 3.5–4 cm. The greater palatine canal is about 3.4 cm long in adults.
After careful aspiration at various levels, the local anesthetic is injected (Fig. 3.15).

> Intraoral access is associated with fewer complications.

Dosage
Therapeutic
Intraorally: 1–2 ml local anesthetic – e. g., 0.75 % ropivacaine, 0.5 % bupivacaine.

Extraoral technique

Above the zygomatic arch

> Injection above the zygomatic arch is much more elegant and more comfortable for the patient.

Patent positioning
Sitting, with face in profile and with the mouth slightly opened. Alternative: supine.

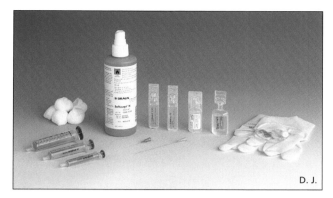

Fig. 3.13 Materials

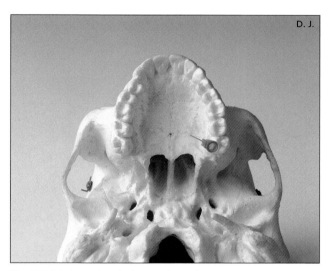

Fig. 3.14 Intraoral technique: orientation

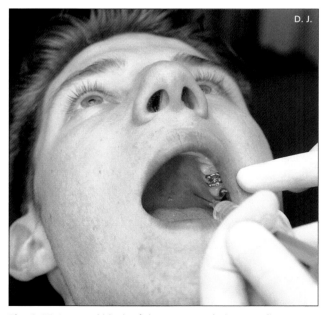

Fig. 3.15 Intraoral block of the pterygopalatine ganglion

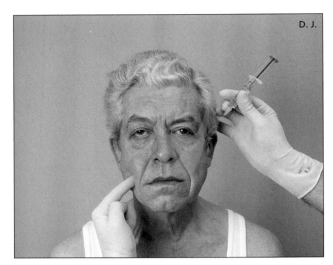

Fig. 3.16 Orientation for injections above the zygomatic arch

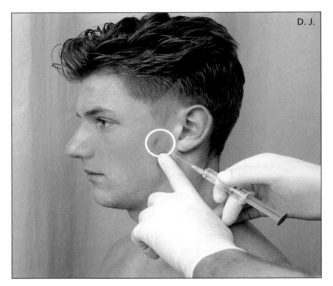

Fig. 3.17 Extraoral technique beneath the zygomatic arch (mandibular fossa)

Landmarks
Center of the upper margin of the zygomatic arch.

Injection technique
A skin injection is made directly above the middle of the zygomatic arch. A 6-cm long needle is introduced at an angle of ca. 45° in the direction of the pterygopalatine fossa (contralateral molar teeth) (Fig. 3.16).
After paresthesias have been elicited in the area of the nostril, the upper lip and the cheek, the needle is minimally withdrawn and aspirated carefully at various levels and the local anesthetic is administered slowly in several small doses. Repeated aspiration at various levels must be carried out during this procedure.

It is not really possible to block the maxillary nerve and pterygopalatine ganglion separately using this method.

Below the zygomatic arch

Patient positioning
Supine or sitting, face in profile with the mouth slightly open.

Landmarks
Mandibular fossa.

Injection technique
The most important requirement for carrying out this block successfully is accurate location of the mandibular fossa between the condylar and coronoid processes of the mandible.
It is helpful here for the patient to open and close the mouth. After skin infiltration, a 6-cm needle is introduced at an angle of 45° in the direction of the dorsal part of the eyeball (Fig. 3.17).
After ca. 4–4.5 cm, the lateral part of the pterygoid process is reached and the needle is withdrawn slightly and lowered into the pterygopalatine fossa (about 0.5 cm medial to the pterygoid). After the paresthesias described above have developed and after careful aspiration at various levels, the local anesthetic is carefully injected in several small doses.
If pain occurs in the region of the orbit, the procedure should be stopped.

Dosage
Diagnostic
Up to 5 ml local anesthetic – e. g., 0.5 % prilocaine, mepivacaine, lidocaine.

Therapeutic
Extraorally: 5–10 ml local anesthetic – e. g., 0.5 % ropivacaine, 0.25 % bupivacaine.
In acute conditions, with 1–2 mg dexamethasone added.

Surgical
Extraorally: 5–10 ml local anesthetic – e. g., 0.75 % ropivacaine, 0.5 % bupivacaine, 1 % prilocaine, 1 % mepivacaine.

Block series
A sequence of six to eight blocks is recommended for the extraoral technique.

Side effects

- Transient amblyopia (extremely rare);
- Horner's syndrome, extremely rare and mainly with high doses. There are contacts with the superior cervical ganglion via the pterygoid canal, deep petrosal nerve and greater superficial petrosal nerve.
- Hematoma in the cheek or orbital cavity due to vascular puncture (Figs. 3.18 and 3.19).
- Immediate outpatient treatment: alternating ice-pack and heparin ointment, depending on the spread of the hematoma, for ca. 1 hour. This can be continued at home, with the patient also taking Reparil® coated tablets if appropriate. Resorption of the hematoma, which is harmless but visually uncomfortable for the patient, occurs within two weeks at the most.

Complications

- Intravascular injection (maxillary artery and maxillary vein, see Fig. 3.27).
- Epidural or subarachnoid injection (see Fig. 3.28).

Both of these complications are extremely rare. Immediate treatment: see Chap. 4, p. 42.

> **Caution**
> The maxillary artery and vein lie in the immediate vicinity.

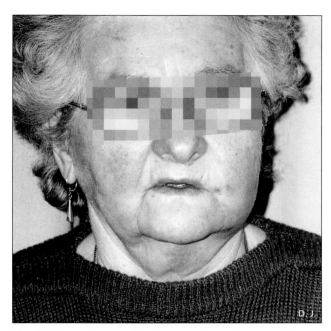

Fig. 3.18 Hematoma in the cheek: status on the second day after injection and immediate treatment

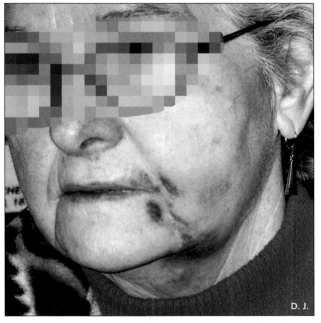

Fig. 3.19 Hematoma in the cheek: seven days after injection

Record and checklist

Maxillary nerve and pterygopalatine ganglion

Block no. _____ ☐ Right ☐ Left

Name: _____ Date: _____

Diagnosis: _____

Premedication: ☐ No ☐ Yes _____

Purpose of block:		☐ *Diagnosis*	☐ *Treatment*
Needle:	☐ *22 G*	☐ *40 mm long*	☐ *60 mm long*
i. v. access:		☐ *Yes*	☐ *No*
Monitoring:		☐ *ECG*	☐ *Pulse oximetry*
Ventilation facilities:		☐ *Yes (equipment checked)*	
Emergency equipment *(drugs)*		☐ *checked*	
Patient:		☐ *Informed*	☐ *Consent*

Position:	☐ *Supine*	☐ *Sitting*	
Approach:	☐ *Above the zygomatic arch*		☐ *Intraoral*
	☐ *Below the zygomatic arch (mandibular fossa)*		

Local anesthetic: _____ *ml* _____ % _____
Test dose: _____ *ml*

Addition to
injection solution: ☐ *No* ☐ *Yes* _____

Patient's remarks during injection:
☐ *None*   ☐ *Pain*   ☐ *Paresthesias*   ☐ *Warmth*
Neural area   _____   _____   _____

Objective block effect after 15 min:
☐ *Cold test*   ☐ *Temperature measurement right* _____°C *left* _____°C
☐ *Numbness (V2)*

Monitoring after block: ☐ *< 1 h* ☐ *> 1 h*
     Time of discharge: _____

Complications: ☐ *None*
              ☐ *Yes (hematoma, intravascular injection, other)*
_____

Subjective effects of block: *Duration:* _____
☐ *None*   ☐ *Increased pain*
☐ *Reduced pain*   ☐ *No pain*

VISUAL ANALOG SCALE

0	10	20	30	40	50	60	70	80	90	100

Special notes: _____

_____
_____
_____
_____
_____

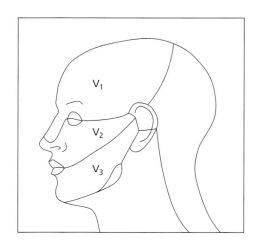

Nasal block of the pterygopalatine ganglion

The pterygopalatine (sphenopalatine) ganglion, which lies in the pterygopalatine fossa (sphenomaxillary fossa), is triangular in shape; extending to ca. 5 mm, it is the largest neuronal conglomerate outside of the brain. The ganglion has three types of nerve fiber and it is connected to the trigeminal nerve via sensory fibers. It is linked to the facial nerve, internal carotid plexus and superior cervical ganglion via sympathetic fibers; the motor fibers have parasympathetic (visceromotor) connections. There is also direct contact between the anterior horn of the spinal cord and the neurohumoral axis (adenohypophysis) [15, 21].

Indications

Greenfield Sluder [19] drew attention to the significance of this ganglion as long ago as 1903. In 1918, he described a number of symptoms capable of being treated by injection or local application of a local anesthetic or cocaine administration, with the associated anesthesia of the pterygopalatine ganglion: headache; pain in the eyes, mouth, or ears; lumbosacral pain, arthritis, glaucoma and hypertension.

Similar observations were reported by Ruskin [17], Byrd and Byrd [5] and Amster [1]. More recent studies [3, 8,14,16] have shown that nasal local anesthesia of the ganglion can be used with good success rates in the treatment of:

- Acute migraine.
- Acute or chronic cluster headache.
- Various types of facial neuralgia.
- Tumor pain in the nasal and pharyngeal area.

Specific contraindications

None.

Procedure

Materials (Fig. 3.20)
2-ml syringe, plastic part of a plastic indwelling catheter (for self-administration in tumor pain), nasal speculum, applicators (cotton buds).

Patient positioning
Supine or sitting, with head tilted back.

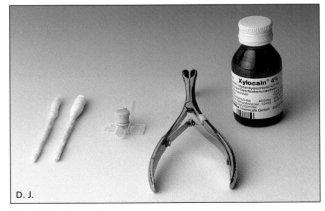

Fig. 3.20 Materials

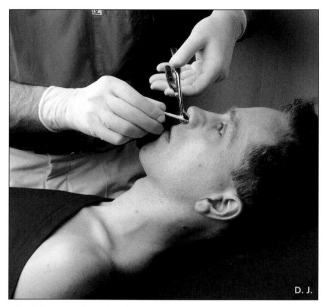

Fig. 3.21 Nasal application

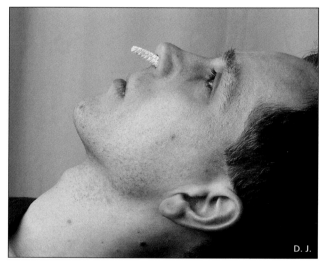

Fig. 3.22 The anesthetic should be allowed 20–30 minutes to take effect

Application
An applicator soaked in local anesthetic – e. g., 2 % lidocaine gel or a 4 % aqueous lidocaine solution – preferably a cotton bud – is carefully advanced along the inferior nasal concha as far as the posterior wall of the nasopharynx (Fig. 3.21) and left in place there for 20–30 minutes (Fig. 3.22).

In patients with cancer pain, the plastic part of a plastic indwelling catheter can be advanced as far as possible into the nasal cavity and the local anesthetic – e. g., 0.5 % bupivacaine – can be instilled with a 2-ml syringe. The block can be carried out bilaterally.

> To prevent trauma, the applicator should not be advanced forcefully if resistance is encountered.

Dosage
Local anesthetics: 2 % lidocaine gel, 1.5–2 ml 4 % lidocaine (aqueous solution) or 1.5–2 ml bupivacaine. Disadvantage: the onset of effect is slightly slower.
10 % cocaine: at a dosage of 0.2–0.4 ml, there is no reason to fear adverse CNS effects [3]. Advantage: very fast onset of effect.
If the dosages are observed, there is no difference between these substances with regard to effectiveness and resorption.

Block series
In acute pain, one or two applications are recommended. In chronic conditions, one to three applications per day can be given over a period of up to three weeks. In cancer pain, applications may be indicated three times per day over a longer period.

Side effects
The method is not very invasive and has no side effects to speak of. Effects that may occur include: a sense of pressure in the nose, sneezing, short-term lacrimation due to irritation of branches of the lacrimal gland, a bitter taste and slight numbness in the oral and pharyngeal cavity.

Complications
Extremely rarely, toxic effects are possible as a result of resorption of the local anesthetic into very well vascularized tumor tissue. In long-term treatments, erosions may sometimes lead to spinal resorption of the local anesthetic. To prevent this, periodic rinsing with a physiological NaCl solution can be carried out.

Block of the mandibular nerve and otic ganglion

After passing through the oval foramen, the mandibular nerve forms a short, thick nerve trunk, with the otic ganglion lying on the medial side of it. Its most important branches (Fig. 3.23) are the buccal nerve, lingual nerve, inferior alveolar nerve, mental nerve and auriculotemporal nerve.

Indications

Diagnostic
- Differential diagnosis of trigeminal neuralgia (anterior two-thirds of the tongue) and glossopharyngeal neuralgia (posterior third of the tongue).

Therapeutic
- Tinnitus (the otic ganglion has connections with the chorda tympani, the nerves of the pterygoid canal and the medial pterygoid nerve);
- Trigeminal neuralgia in the third branch;
- Trismus after dental extraction;

- Dental surgery and maxillary surgery (higher dosages required);
- Temporomandibular joint dysfunction syndrome (in collaboration with an orthodontist), if infiltration of the trigger points of the temporalis muscle, lateral pterygoid muscle and masseter muscle is unsuccessful.

Specific contraindications
Bleeding diathesis, anticoagulation treatment.

Procedure

This block should only be carried out with appropriate experience.

Preparation and materials (see p. 25, Fig. 3.13)

Skin prep
In all blocks.

Patient positioning
Supine, with face in profile.

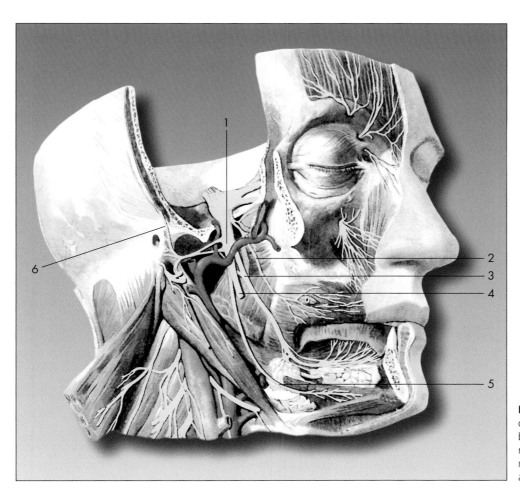

Fig. 3.23 Distribution areas of the mandibular nerve (1): buccal nerve (2); lingual nerve (3); inferior alveolar nerve (4); mental nerve (5); auriculotemporal nerve (6)

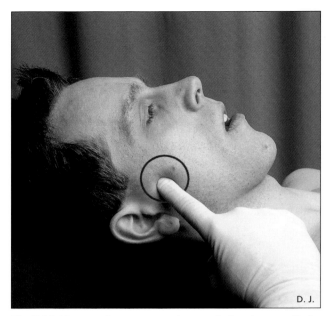

Fig. 3.24 The most important requirement is that the mandibular fossa should be identified precisely. It lies between the condylar process and the coronoid process of the mandible and is easiest to localize when the patient opens and closes his or her mouth

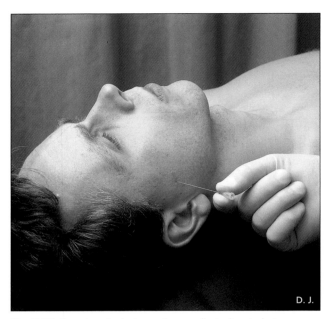

Fig. 3.25 Puncture technique: the needle is directed at an angle of 90°

Landmarks
Mandibular fossa, zygomatic arch, tragus (the puncture point lies ca. 2 cm laterally, Fig. 3.24).

Injection technique
After skin infiltration, a 6-cm long needle is introduced into the skin perpendicularly (Fig. 3.25).
Paresthesias in the lower jaw region, lower lip and lower incisors occur when the needle reaches a depth of ca. 4–4.5 cm.
After paresthesias have clearly developed, the needle is withdrawn slightly, aspirated carefully at various levels and the local anesthetic is slowly injected in several small doses. Aspiration should be repeated several times at different levels as this is done.
There is a delayed onset of the desired effect in the area of the auriculotemporal nerve.

> If contact is made with the pterygoid process when the needle is being introduced, withdraw the needle 0.5–1 cm and correct dorsally.

Distribution of the block
The area supplied by the mandibular nerve is shown in Figure 3.32.
The otic ganglion (Fig. 3.26), which lies directly under the oval foramen, is always anesthetized along with the nerve.

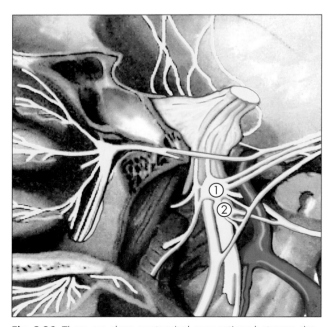

Fig. 3.26 There are close anatomical connections between the otic ganglion (1) and the mandibular nerve (2)

Mandibular nerve and otic ganglion

Block no.   ☐ Right   ☐ Left

Name: _____   Date: _____
Diagnosis: _____
Premedication: ☐ No   ☐ Yes _____

Purpose of block: ☐ Diagnosis   ☐ Treatment
Needle: ☐ 22 G   ☐ 50 mm long   ☐ 60 mm long
i. v. access: ☐ Yes   ☐ No
Monitoring: ☐ ECG   ☐ Pulse oximetry
Ventilation facilities: ☐ Yes (equipment checked)
Emergency equipment (drugs): ☐ checked
Patient: ☐ Informed   ☐ Consent

Position: ☐ Supine   ☐ Sitting
Approach: ☐ Mandibular fossa

Local anesthetic: _____ ml _____ % _____
Test dose: _____ ml
Addition to
injection solution: ☐ No   ☐ Yes _____
Patient's remarks during injection:
☐ None   ☐ Pain   ☐ Paresthesias   ☐ Warmth
Neural area   _____   _____   _____

Objective block effect after 15 min:
☐ Cold test   ☐ Temperature measurement right ____°C left ____°C
☐ Numbness (V3)
Monitoring after block: ☐ < 1 h   ☐ > 1 h
                  Time of discharge: _____

Complications: ☐ None
                 ☐ Yes (hematoma, intravascular injection, other)
                 _____
                 _____

Subjective effects of block: Duration: _____
☐ None   ☐ Increased pain
☐ Reduced pain   ☐ No pain

VISUAL ANALOG SCALE

|iiiiiiiii|iiiiiiiii|iiiiiiiii|iiiiiiiii|iiiiiiiii|iiiiiiiii|iiiiiiiii|iiiiiiiii|iiiiiiiii|iiiiiiiii|
0   10   20   30   40   50   60   70   80   90   100

Special notes: _____
_____
_____
_____
_____
_____

Record and checklist

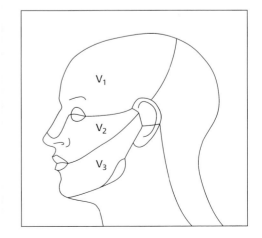

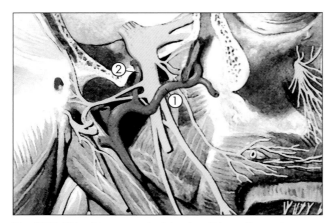

Fig. 3.27 Risk of intravascular injection: (1) maxillary artery, (2) middle meningeal artery

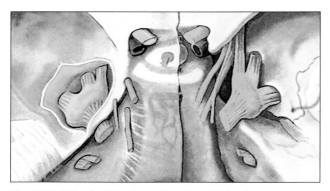

Fig. 3.28 Risk of epidural or subarachnoid injection

Dosage
Diagnostic
Up to 5 ml local anesthetic – e. g., 5 % prilocaine, mepivacaine, lidocaine.

Therapeutic
5–10 ml local anesthetic – e. g., 0.5 % ropivacaine, 0.25 % bupivacaine.
In acute conditions, with 1–2 mg dexamethasone added.

Surgical
10 ml local anesthetic – e. g., 0.75 % ropivacaine, 0.5 % bupivacaine, 1 % prilocaine, 1 % mepivacaine.

Block series
A series of six to eight blocks is recommended. When there is evidence of symptomatic improvement, further blocks can also be carried out.

Side effects
- Transient facial paralysis caused by injecting too superficially.

- Hematoma in the cheek due to vascular puncture. These harmless hematomas can take up to two weeks to resolve. Immediate treatment: see the section on blocks of the maxillary nerve and pterygopalatine ganglion, Figs. 3.18 and 3.19.

Complications
- Intravascular injection (middle meningeal artery and maxillary artery, Fig. 3.27).
- Epidural or subarachnoid injection (Fig. 3.28). Immediate treatment: see Chap. 4, pp. 43, 44.

> **Caution**
> The middle meningeal artery and maxillary artery lie in the immediate vicinity.

Trigeminal nerve: comparison of analgesia zones

Figures 3.29 to 3.33 provide schematic illustrations of the areas supplied by the individual nerves. During blocks, the anesthetic spread may overlap.

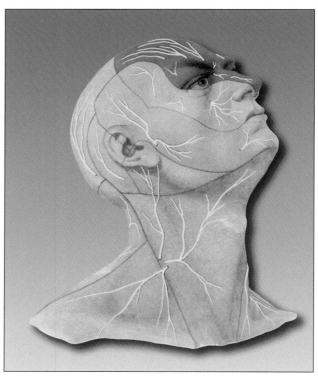

Fig. 3.29 Ophthalmic nerve

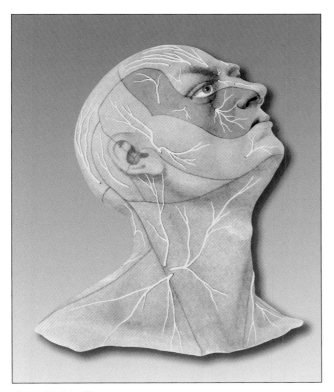

Fig. 3.30 Maxillary nerve

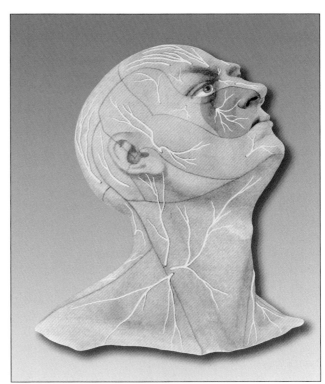

Fig. 3.31 Infraorbital nerve

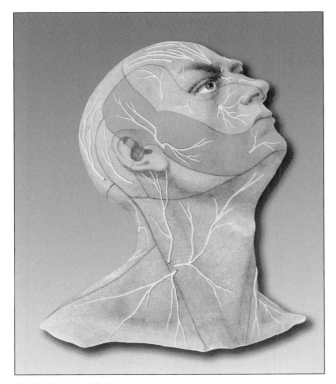

Fig. 3.32 Mandibular nerve

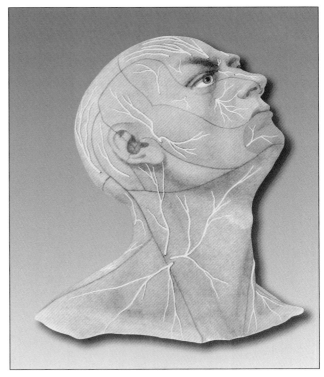

Fig. 3.33 Mental nerve

4 Cervicothoracic ganglion (stellate ganglion)

Anatomy

There are two sympathetic trunks arranged paravertebrally that belong to the peripheral autonomic nervous system. In the area of the neck, these include four sympathetic trunk ganglia on each side, serving as cholinergic switchpoints: the superior and middle cervical ganglia, the vertebral ganglion and the cervicothoracic ganglion (Fig. 4.1).

The **cervicothoracic ganglion (stellate ganglion)** at the level of C7–T1 arises from the fusion of the lowest cervical ganglion (7th and 8th cervical ganglion) with the highest thoracic ganglion (1st and/or 2nd thoracic ganglion).

The immediate vicinity of the ganglion is dominated by the first rib, the pleura and the brachial plexus. The ganglion lies ventral to the vertebral artery, medial and dorsal to the common carotid artery and the jugular vein and lateral to the esophagus and trachea. It is separated from the transverse processes of the 6th and 7th cervical vertebrae by the longus colli muscle (Fig. 4.2).

It receives afferent fibers from the white rami communicantes of the 1st and 2nd thoracic nerves and gives off gray rami communicantes to the 1st (and 2nd) thoracic nerves and the 8th (and 7th) cervical nerves.

The stellate ganglion is connected to the neighboring ganglia, the brachial plexus, the cranial intercostal nerves and the phrenic nerve and with the vagus nerve and recurrent laryngeal nerve (Fig. 4.3). Fibers from the gray rami communicantes also supply the heart and great vessels (subclavian, carotid, vertebral, inferior thyroid and intercostal arteries), the esophagus and the trachea, as well as the thymus gland (Fig. 4.4).

The size and development of the stellate ganglion are subject to considerable variation. Average sizes of between 25 mm (15–50 mm) × 3–10 mm × 5 mm have been reported (Fig. 4.5) [17, 18, 25]. This corresponds to the size of the superior cervical ganglion and it is much more voluminous than the middle cervical ganglion. On the other hand, the stellate ganglion is only developed in 80 % of patients; some authors [17,18] have only been able to identify it in 38 % of individuals studied.

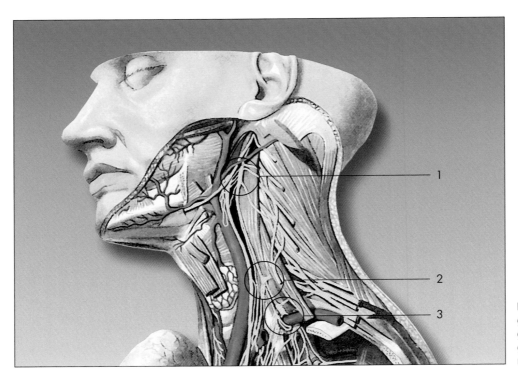

Fig. 4.1 The cervical ganglion trunk: superior cervical ganglion (1), middle cervical ganglion (2) and cervicothoracic ganglion (3)

Block of the stellate ganglion

Indications

Block of the stellate ganglion is a useful method of pain therapy in patients with perfusion disturbances in the areas of the head, neck, upper extremities and upper thoracic wall.

The following indications have been described in the literature:

- Vasospastic diseases in the areas of the face, shoulder and arm.
- Arterial dysfunctions: Raynaud-Bürger syndrome, anterior scalene syndrome, ischemic Volkmann's contracture.
- Venous dysfunctions: thrombophlebitis, postphlebitic edema.
- Combined dysfunctions – e. g., lymphedema after breast amputation.
- Head: intracranial vascular spasms, facial paralysis, vertigo, central post stroke syndrome (contralateral block!).
- Eye: central vein thrombosis, occlusion of the central retinal artery.
- Nose: vasomotor rhinitis.
- Ear: Menière's disease [10, 11, 13, 24], sudden deafness [15], tinnitus. Our own results in the treatment of tinnitus show that up to eight weeks after the start of the disease, 80 % of patients can be successfully treated using 2–10 blocks over a period of one to six weeks. Up to 12 weeks after the start of the disease, the success rate with 10–16 blocks, spread over

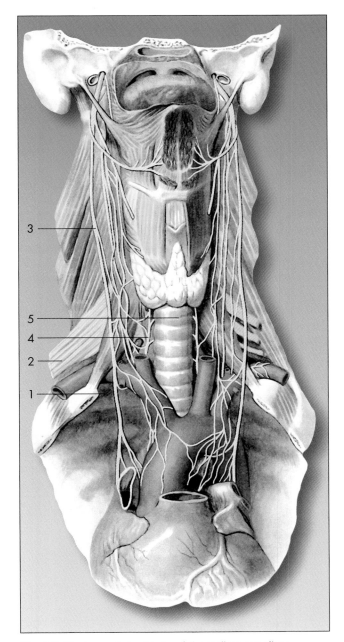

Fig. 4.2 The immediate vicinity of the stellate ganglion: (1) pleura, (2) brachial plexus, (3) vagus nerve, (4) recurrent laryngeal nerve, (5) trachea

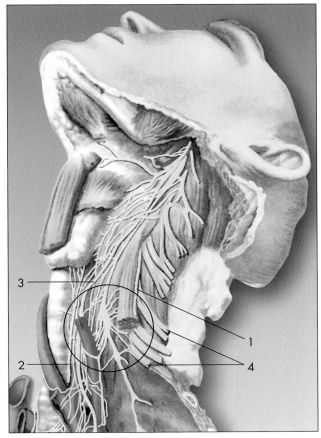

Fig. 4.3 Close anatomical connections in the ganglion trunk include those to the phrenic nerve (1), recurrent laryngeal nerve (2), vagus nerve (3) and brachial plexus (4)

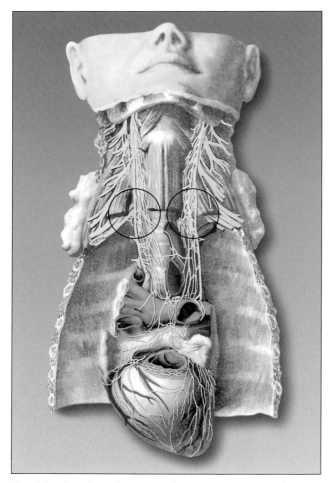

Fig. 4.4 Fibers from the gray rami communicantes supply the heart, esophagus, airways and thymus

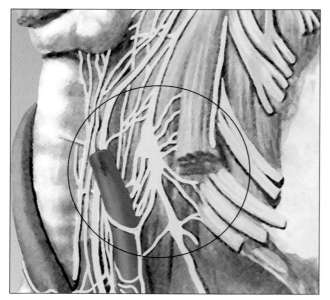

Fig. 4.5 The average size of the stellate ganglion is 25 mm (15–50 mm) × 3–10 mm × 5 mm

a period of six weeks, was only 35 %. If the condition was present for more than six months, block treatment was unsuccessful.

▨ Traumatic cerebral edema [9].
▨ Complex regional pain syndrome (CRPS) in the area of the face, neck and arm [35].
▨ Phantom pain.
▨ Hyperhidrosis.
▨ Joint stiffness.
▨ Positive effect on the immune system [21].
▨ Acute herpes zoster and zoster neuralgia in the head and neck region. A trigeminal and cervical localization is described in ca. 25 % of cases. Good to very good results are obtained with block of the stellate ganglion in acute zoster (with opioids added if necessary [8]).

In assessing the success rates reported in the literature, it should be noted whether a distinction has been made between acute and chronic herpes zoster. The 85 % success rate reported by Colding [4] when treatment was initiated within three weeks of the start of disease confirms the results of other authors [5, 29, 32, 36]. Milligan and Nash [23] regard one year after the start of disease as being the limit for useful application of the stellate ganglion block. The results of their block series – freedom from pain in 22 % of patients – are therefore not comparable.

Our own results [15] in the treatment of zoster neuralgia: up to 12 weeks after the start of disease, the success rate with 7–19 blocks, spread over a period of 3–10 weeks, was 80 %. If the disease had started six months or more previously, the results were varied and unsatisfactory.

Specific contraindications

Grade 2 atrioventricular (AV) block, contralateral pneumothorax, recent lytic therapy after myocardial infarction or pulmonary embolism, anticoagulation treatment, severe asthma/emphysema (if appropriate, priority can be given to block of the superior cervical ganglion here; see Chap. 5), paralysis of the contralateral phrenic nerve or recurrent laryngeal nerve.

In addition, blocks should never be carried out bilaterally at the same time.

Procedure

The paratracheal anterior technique is today's standard.

This block should only be carried out by experienced pain therapists.

Preparations
Check that the emergency equipment is complete and in working order. Sterile precautions, skin prep. Intravenous access, ECG monitoring, ventilation facilities, pulse oximetry.
Avoid premedication: The patient must remain responsive at all times so that any possible side effects or complications will be apparent immediately.

Materials
Fine 26-G needles 2.5 cm long for local anesthesia, 5-ml syringe, 10-ml syringe, 22-G needle (3 cm or 5 cm long, depending on the patient's anatomy) with injection tube (immobile needle), intubation kit, emergency drugs, positional cushions, disinfectant (Fig. 4.6).

Skin prep
In all blocks.

Patient positioning
Supine, with neck extended.

Landmarks
Sternocleidomastoid muscle, common carotid artery, jugular fossa, transverse processes of the 6th or 7th cervical vertebra.
1. The 6th cervical vertebra is palpated. For this purpose alone, the patient rotates the head toward the opposite side (Fig. 4.7).
2. For palpation of the site between the larynx and the sternocleidomastoid muscle, a cushion is placed under the shoulder blades and the head is tilted back. The patient must not swallow, speak, cough, or move and is asked to breathe with the mouth slightly open, in order to relax the neck muscles (Fig. 4.8).
3. The index and middle fingers are moved between the trachea and sternocleidomastoid muscle to locate the pulse in the common carotid artery. This is displaced laterally together with the medial margin of the sternocleidomastoid muscle (Fig. 4.9). The transverse process is now identified. Usually, the transverse process of C6 is easily palpated at the level of the cricoid, or the transverse process of C7 can be located using the two-finger method (Fig. 4.8).

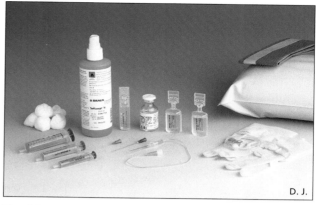
Fig. 4.6 Materials

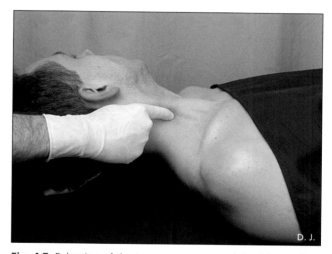
Fig. 4.7 Palpation of the transverse process of the 6th vertebra

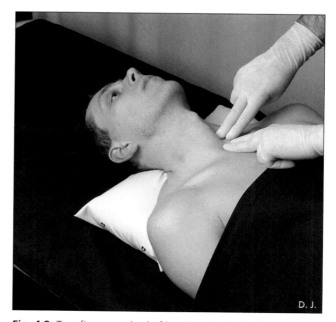
Fig. 4.8 Two-finger method of locating the level of C7

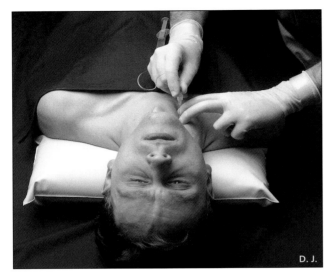

Fig. 4.9 Introducing the needle

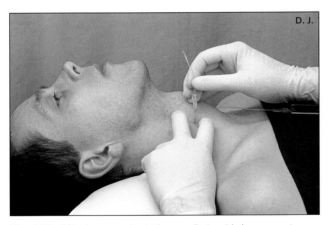

Fig. 4.10 After bone contact, the needle is withdrawn ca. 1 mm. The injection is carried out after aspiration at various levels

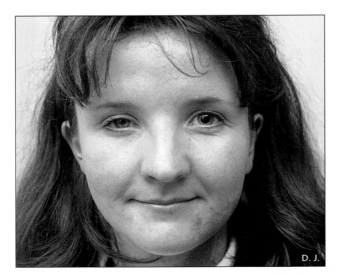

Fig. 4.11 Horner's syndrome: ptosis, miosis and enophthalmos

Injection technique

> The injection can be made at the level of C6 or C7. The transverse process of the sixth cervical vertebra is easier to palpate; the distance from the pleura is greater and there is less danger of puncturing the vertebral artery. Block at the level of C7 can extend as far as T3, with a reduced dose of the local anesthetic. However, the likelihood of injuring the pleura or puncturing the vertebral artery is greater here.

After skin infiltration, the needle is introduced vertical to the skin at this point and advanced until bone contact is made with the transverse process (Figs. 4.9 and 4.10). The transverse process is reached at a depth of 2–4 cm, depending on the anatomy.

After making bone contact, the needle is withdrawn about 1 mm and with careful aspiration at various levels, an initial test dose of 1 ml of the local anesthetic is injected.

> If there is no bone contact, or if paresthesias in the brachial plexus are elicited, the needle must be withdrawn and corrected medially. If the transverse process is still not reached, the direction of the needle should be carefully corrected caudally or cranially.

After 1 minute, slow injection of the remaining dose can be carried out.

> A single test dose by no means guarantees correct positioning of the needle. The remaining dose must never be injected quickly and carelessly. It must be administered slowly in small quantities (several test doses) with constant aspiration.

Effect of the block (Horner's syndrome)

Characteristic unilateral symptoms of a stellate block are: conjunctival injection, increased tear production, swelling of the nasal mucosa, reddening, hyperthermia and anhidrosis in the affected side of the face. At higher doses, hyperthermia and anhidrosis in the region of the shoulder and arm can occur.

Horner's syndrome is regarded as the clinical sign of a successfully conducted block. In 1869, the ophthalmologist Johann Friedrich Horner described the triad of ptosis, miosis and enophthalmos as a sequela of paralysis of the sympathetically innervated ocular muscles (Fig. 4.11).

Horner's syndrome is not automatically a sign of complete block of the stellate ganglion. Two effects of the block need to be distinguished:
■ After ca. 1–2 minutes, Horner's syndrome develops as a result of cerebral (facial) spread. This can be achieved with a low dose of the local anesthetic.
■ Complete block, including the shoulder and arm region, requires a higher dose and the local anesthetic needs to spread as far as T4.

This complete cervicothoracic sympathetic block is only obtained after ca. 15–20 minutes. Horner's syndrome occurs not only after block of the stellate ganglion, but is also characteristic of all blocks of the cervical sympathetic trunk.

Dosage
"Low dose" for indications in the head region (cerebrofacial effects) [3, 9, 15, 30]: 2–4 ml local anesthetic – e. g., 0.375–0.5 % ropivacaine, 0.25–0.5 % bupivacaine, or 1 % prilocaine, 1 % mepivacaine, 1 % lidocaine.
"Medium high dose" for indications in the shoulder and arm region [3, 6, 12, 25, 30, 33, 35]: 10–15 ml local anesthetic – e. g., 0.2–0.375 % ropivacaine, 0.25 % bupivacaine or 0.5 % prilocaine, 0.5 % mepivacaine, 0.5 % lidocaine.
In acute pain, 1–3 mg morphine, 0.0125–0.025 mg fentanyl [8, 22, 34], or 0.03 mg buprenorphine with local anesthetic, or in 0.9 % NaCl solution.

Block series
If the clinical picture being treated does not show temporary improvement after the second block, there is no point in carrying out a series of treatments. Otherwise, for all the indications mentioned, a series of 6–10 blocks can be carried out. In difficult cases (e. g., herpes zoster ophthalmicus), further blocks can also be carried out when there is a visible trend toward improvement.

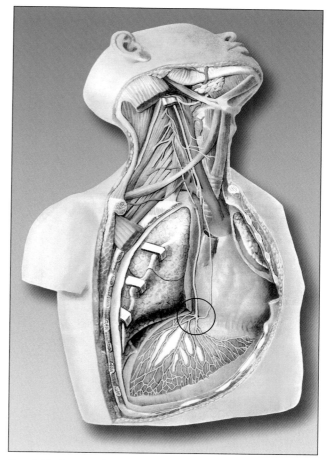

Fig. 4.12 Course of the phrenic nerve

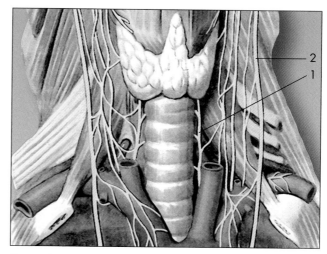

Fig. 4.13 Positions of the recurrent laryngeal nerve (1) and vagus nerve (2)

Side effects

Hematoma formation (harmless but sometimes uncomfortable and worrying).

Persistent coughing [27].

Simultaneous anesthetization of the following nerves:

- Phrenic nerve (Fig. 4.12), main symptom: dyspnea with normal auscultation findings.
- Vagus nerve (Fig. 4.13), main symptom: tachycardia, hypertension.
- Recurrent laryngeal nerve (Fig. 4.13), main symptom: foreign-body sensation in the throat, hoarseness. It should be noted here that in ca. 43 % of cases, anastomoses with the cervicothoracic ganglion are found [17, 18].
- Brachial plexus: a partial brachial plexus block may occur if the local anesthetic spreads into the area of the roots of C6–T1.

When giving consent, the patient must be clearly informed about the possibility of these adverse effects – most of which do not require any treatment other than reassurance. Nursing staff also need to be informed.

Complications

Intravascular injection

Intravascular injections are extremely rare when the correct technique is used. In particular, there is a risk of injection into the vertebral artery (the diameter of this is ca. 0.3 mm larger on the left side than on the right!); more rarely, there is a risk of puncturing the carotid artery, the inferior thyroid artery, or the first intercostal artery (Fig. 4.14).

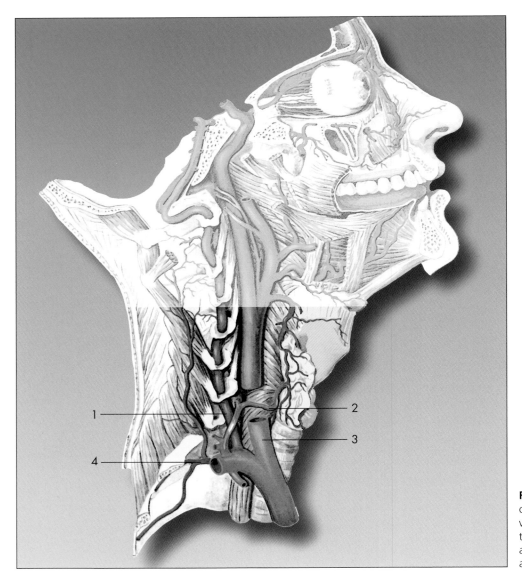

Fig. 4.14 Risk of intravascular injection into the vertebral artery (1), inferior thyroid artery (2), carotid artery (3) and first intercostal artery (4)

Most complications arise when the local anesthetic is administered without prior bone contact. Bilateral block of the stellate ganglion is contra-indicated, since bilateral paresis of the recurrent or phrenic nerves would be life threatening.

CNS intoxication

Intravascular administration (Fig. 4.15), overdosage and/or rapid vascular uptake of the local anesthetic can quickly lead to toxic CNS reactions. Symptoms include:

- Upbeating nystagmus
- Sudden vertigo, pressure in both ears and in the head.
- Brief blackouts, not usually requiring treatment (Fig. 4.16).
- Reversible "locked-in syndrome" with brief apnea and inability to move or respond to external stimuli [7]. The patient remains conscious, is hemodynamically stable and vertical eye movement is maintained.
  Treatment: constant verbal contact, oxygen administration, support for breathing (with mask ventilation if necessary), cardiovascular monitoring, diazepam if necessary (0.05 mg/kg body weight, i. v.).
- Tonic-clonic seizure: a very serious complication (Fig. 4.17). Provided that immediate and correct treatment is given, it does not lead to cerebral injury or even death.
  Treatment: thiopental (1–2 mg/kg b. w. – routinely ca. 150 mg – i. v., carefully dosed), to prevent additional cardiovascular or CNS depression.
  Sedation with diazepam (10–20 mg).
  Oxygen administration (mask), support for breathing. The airways must be kept free, if necessary with succinylcholine (60–80 mg) to make intubation easier. Vasopressor administration to support circulation. Leg elevation, fluid volume replacement. Cardiovascular monitoring; cardiopulmonary resuscitation if necessary.

Preconvulsive signs of toxic reactions are a numb sensation on the lips and tongue, vertigo, metallic taste, drowsiness, ringing in the ears, visual disturbances, slurred speech, muscle tremor, nystagmus.

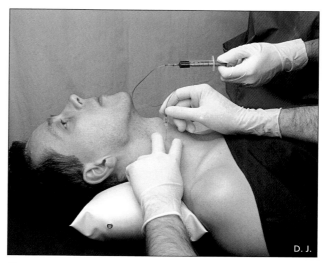

Fig. 4.15 Inadvertent intra-arterial injection must be avoided, since even small amounts of local anesthetic are sufficient to cause CNS intoxication

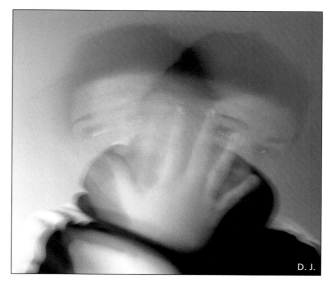

Fig. 4.16 Blackout

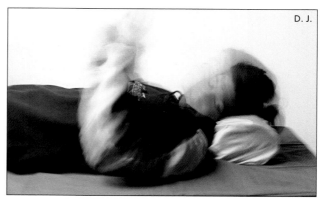

Fig. 4.17 Tonic–clonic seizure

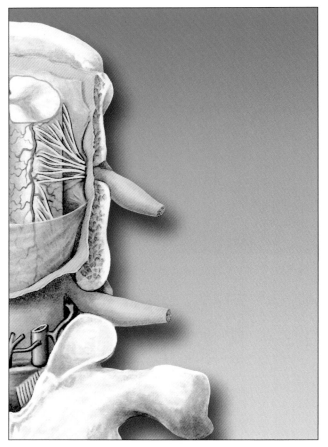

Fig. 4.18 If the puncture is too medial, there is a risk of epidural or subarachnoid injection

Effects on the cardiovascular system
Toxic effects on the cardiovascular system only occur after very high doses of local anesthetic, manifesting as a drop in blood pressure, bradycardia, circulatory collapse and cardiac arrest.
Treatment: leg elevation, fluid volume replacement, oxygen administration, vasopressor administration if needed, cardiopulmonary resuscitation if needed.

Epidural or subarachnoid injection [31]
There is a risk of perforating the dural membrane if the puncture is carried out too medially (Fig. 4.18). Cerebrospinal fluid (CSF) pressure is very low in the cervical area and it is almost impossible to aspirate CSF. The resultant high epidural anesthesia or high spinal anesthesia is extremely rare. It can lead to bradycardia, hypotension and possibly to respiratory arrest and loss of consciousness. The first signs are: heaviness in the limbs, sweating, dyspnea, apprehension and anxiety.
Treatment: immediate endotracheal intubation, ventilation with 100 % oxygen, fast volume supply, atropine i. v. in bradycardia, vasopressor administration if needed.

> After a stellate block has been carried out, the patient must be monitored for 60 minutes. In the outpatient department, medium-term local anesthetics (e. g., prilocaine, mepivacaine, or lidocaine) are preferable.

Pneumothorax
The frequency of this is extremely low when the paratracheal technique is used. If it occurs at all, it involves sheath pneumothorax with spontaneous resorption (Fig. 4.19). However, if there is a suspicion of pneumothorax, a thoracic radiograph is required after 4–6 hours.

Esophageal perforation or tracheal perforation
Extremely rare. Puncture of the esophagus (Fig. 4.19) causes a bitter taste during the injection. Immediate follow-up is indicated if there is any suspicion.

Although a relatively simple and common block, side effects can be life threatening. Only carry out in an appropriate situation, with adequate personnel available to help.

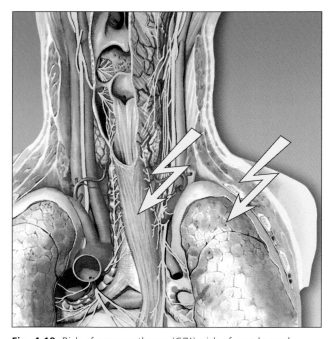

Fig. 4.19 Risk of pneumothorax (C7!); risk of esophageal perforation

Cervicothoracic ganglion (stellate ganglion)

Block no.   ☐ Right   ☐ Left

Record and checklist

Name: _____   Date: _____
Diagnosis: _____
Premedication: ☐ No   ☐ Yes _____

Purpose of block: ☐ Diagnosis   ☐ Treatment
Needle: ☐ 22 G   ☐ 40 mm long   ☐ 50 mm long
i. v. access: ☐ Yes
Monitoring: ☐ ECG   ☐ Pulse oximetry
Ventilation facilities: ☐ Yes (equipment checked)
Emergency equipment (drugs):   ☐ Checked
Patient: ☐ Informed   ☐ Consent

Position: ☐ Supine   ☐ Neck extended
Approach: ☐ Paratracheal ☐ C6   ☐ C7
               ☐ Other _____

Local anesthetic: ____ ml ____ % _____
Test dose: ____ ml
Addition to
injection solution: ☐ No   ☐ Yes _____
Patient's remarks during injection:
☐ None   ☐ Pain   ☐ Paresthesias   ☐ Warmth
Neural area   _____ _____ _____

Objective block effect after 15 min:
☐ Cold test   ☐ Temperature measurement right ___°C left ___°C
Horner's syndrome   ☐ Yes   ☐ No
Segments affected: ☐ C2 ☐ C3 ☐ C4 ☐ C5 ☐ T___
Monitoring after block: ☐ < 1 h   ☐ > 1 h
               Time of discharge: _____

Complications: ☐ None
                  ☐ Yes (hematoma, intravascular injection, other)
                  _____

Side effects: ☐ None
☐ Yes (recurrent laryngeal nerve, phrenic nerve, vagus nerve) _____

Subjective effects of block: Duration: _____
☐ None   ☐ Increased pain
☐ Reduced pain   ☐ No pain

VISUAL ANALOG SCALE

0   10   20   30   40   50   60   70   80   90   100

Special notes:
_____
_____
_____

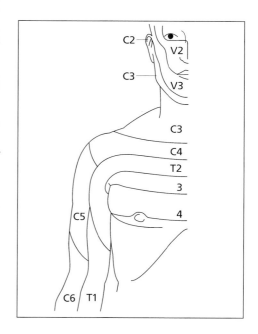

5 Superior cervical ganglion

Anatomy

The superior cervical ganglion arises from the fusion of three or four upper cervical ganglia. It lies medial to the vagus trunk, in front of the longus capitis muscle and behind the internal carotid artery, in the angle of the vertebrae and transverse processes of the second and third cervical vertebrae (Figs. 5.1 and 5.2). In the literature, its long, flat, or spindle-like extension is described as being 14–43 mm in length, 6–8 mm in breadth, and 3–5 mm in depth [4,5]. The superior cervical ganglion is thought to contain 760 000 to 1 000 000 nerve fibers in all [4, 5]. This underlines its importance as a switchpoint with numerous double or triple connections to neighboring ganglia, nerves, and vessels. The superior cervical ganglion takes its preganglionic fibers mainly from the spinal nerves coursing thoracically, with only a few being drawn from the neighboring cervical nerve roots. An unknown number of these preganglionic fibers pass through the ganglion toward the higher carotid ganglia, without switching. **Rami communicantes** connect the superior cervical ganglion with numerous organs, vessels, muscles, bones, joints, the last four cranial nerves, the vertebral plexus, and also with the phrenic nerve. It supplies the upper cervical spinal nerves with **gray rami communicantes,** and it sends off vascular fibers to the internal and external carotid arteries. **Autonomic branches** pass from the ganglion to the larynx, pharynx, heart, and – together with vascular plexuses – to the salivary and lacrimal glands, to the hypophysis, thyroid, and other glands. There are also contacts with the middle cervical ganglion and to the tympanic plexus. There are connections with the pterygopalatine ganglion via the nerve of the pterygoid canal, deep petrosal nerve, and greater superficial petrosal nerve.

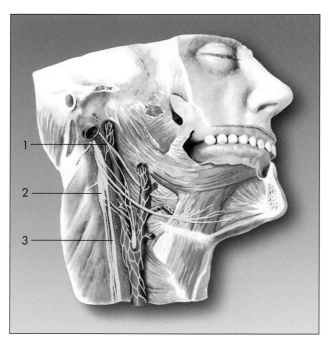

Fig. 5.1 Topographic position of the superior cervical ganglion: (1) glossopharyngeal nerve, (2) superior cervical ganglion, (3) vagus nerve. The superior cervical ganglion has an average size of: 26.6 mm (14–43 mm) × 7.2 mm × 3.4 mm

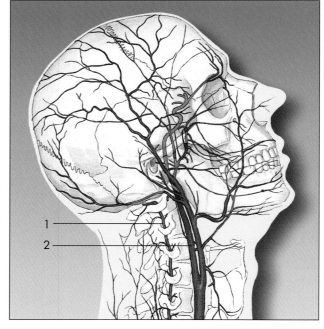

Fig. 5.2 Arteries in the immediate vicinity of the ganglion: (1) vertebral artery and (2) internal carotid artery

Blocks of the superior cervical ganglion

Indications
The areas of application are partly identical to those for the stellate block, but due to its marked cerebrofacial effects, block of the superior cervical ganglion is particularly suitable for the head and facial region – although controlled studies are still lacking here.

Therapeutic
- Migraine [2], cluster headache, headaches of cervical origin.
- Complex regional pain syndrome (CRPS) in the head region.
- Perfusion disturbances, vasospastic diseases.
- Central post stroke syndrome (contralateral block!).
- Facial pain.
- Vertigo (of vertebral origin).
- Peripheral facial paralysis.
- Trigeminal neuralgia in the 1st and 2nd branches.
- Post-herpetic neuralgias* (otic, ophthalmic).
- Sudden deafness,* tinnitus.*
- Hyperhidrosis in the head region.

* The explanations given in Chap. 4, p. 37, also apply here.

Neural therapy
- Asthma, urticaria, vasomotor rhinitis, etc.

Specific contraindications
Grade 2 atrioventricular (AV) block, recent antithrombotic therapy after myocardial infarction or pulmonary embolism, anticoagulation treatment, contralateral paresis of the phrenic nerve or recurrent laryngeal nerve. Simultaneous bilateral block.

Procedure

Lateral extraoral technique

This block should only be carried out by an experienced anesthetist.

Preparations
Check that the emergency equipment is complete and in working order. Sterile precautions. Intravenous access, ECG monitoring, pulse oximetry, ventilation facilities.

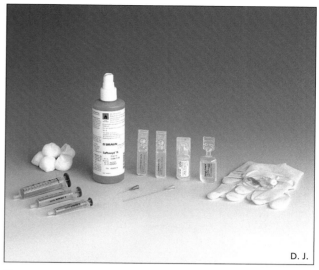

D. J.

Fig. 5.3 Materials

Materials
2-ml syringe, 5-ml syringe, 23-G needle (6 cm), intubation kit, emergency drugs, disinfectant (Fig. 5.3).

Skin prep
In all blocks.

Patient positioning
Supine, with the head turned about 30°–40° to the opposite side.

Landmarks
Mastoid process, angle of mandible, medial margin of the sternocleidomastoid muscle (Fig. 5.4). The angle of the mandible and the mastoid are marked with the index and middle finger. From the anterior margin of the mastoid process, a vertical line is drawn downward; about 1 cm above the angle of the mandible, a horizontal mark is applied. The intersection of these two lines defines the injection point (Fig. 5.5).

Injection technique
After skin infiltration, a 6-cm long needle is introduced in the direction of the contralateral mastoid at a craniodorsal angle of about 20° (Fig. 5.6). In normal anatomy, bone contact is made at about 3.5–5 cm, and careful aspiration is carried out at various levels after the needle has been minimally withdrawn. Only then can a test dose of 0.5 ml of the local anesthetic be administered.
After about 1 minute, slow injection of the remaining dose can be carried out. The patient's upper body is then raised.

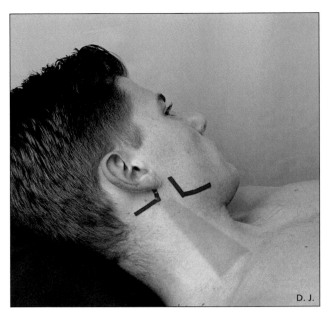

Fig. 5.4 Landmarks for locating the puncture position. Angle of the mandible, mastoid, medial margin of the sternocleido-mastoid muscle

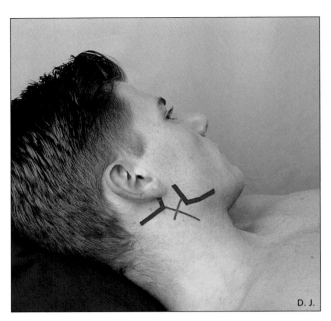

Fig. 5.5 Marking the injection position

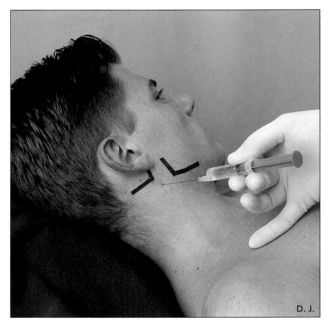

Fig. 5.6 Craniodorsal puncture in the direction of the contra-lateral mastoid

A single test dose by no means guarantees correct positioning of the needle. The remaining dose must never be injected quickly and carelessly. It must be administered slowly in small quantities (several test doses) with repeated aspiration.

If the correct direction is missed, the patient will complain of uncomfortable pain and will resist the injection. In this case, the needle must be withdrawn to the subcutaneous tissues so that its position can be corrected.

Effects of the block

Characteristic signs of a successful block are radiation and a warm sensation in the area of the back of the head, ear, eyes and corner of the mouth and the ipsilateral half of the face (Figs. 5.7 and 5.8). Conjunctival injection, increased tear production and obstruction in the ipsilateral half of the nose are equally characteristic, as is Horner's syndrome – which is by no means restricted to stellate block, but occurs in all blocks of the sympathetic cervical trunk.

Dosage

Therapeutic
5 ml local anesthetic – e. g., 0.5–1 % procaine, 0.5–1 % prilocaine, 0.5–1 % lidocaine, 0.2 % ropivacaine, 0.125 % bupivacaine.

Block series

A series of 6–10 blocks is appropriate for all indications. In difficult cases (e. g., herpes zoster), additional blocks can also be carried out when there is evidence of improvement.

Side effects

Hematoma formation (harmless).
Simultaneous anesthetization of the following nerves:
- Phrenic nerve, main symptom: dyspnea.
- Recurrent laryngeal nerve, main symptoms: foreign-body sensation in the neck and hoarseness.
- Vagus nerve, main symptoms: tachycardia, hypertension.
- Glossopharyngeal nerve, main symptoms: numbness in the posterior third of the tongue, paresis of the pharyngeal muscles.
- Partial anesthesia of the cervical plexus.
- Persistent coughing.

When giving consent, the patient must be informed about these adverse effects and prepared for them.

Complications

Caution
Most complications arise when the local anesthetic is administered without prior bone contact. Bilateral block of the superior cervical ganglion is contraindicated, since bilateral paralysis of the recurrent nerve or phrenic nerve is life-threatening.

Intravascular injection
There is a particular risk of injection into the vertebral artery (Fig. 5.9), the diameter of which is about 0.3 mm wider on the left side than on the right. Intra-arterial administration of a local anesthetic can produce toxic reactions very quickly.
On the symptoms and treatment, see Chap. 4, p. 43.

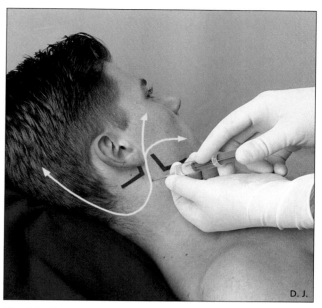

Fig. 5.7 Characteristic directions of radiation during the injection

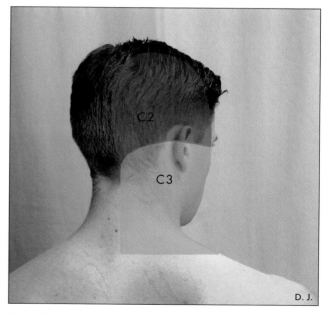

Fig. 5.8 Spread of the block

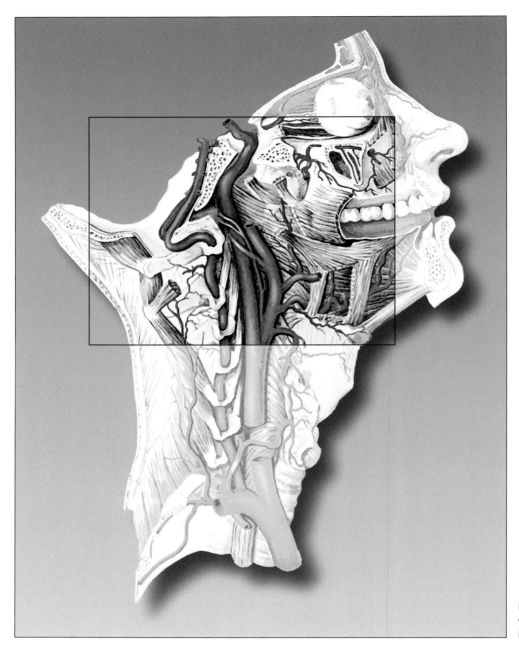

Fig. 5.9 Course of the vertebral artery and risk of intra-arterial injection

Epidural or subarachnoid injection
There is a risk of perforating the dural membrane. Cerebrospinal fluid (CSF) pressure is very low in the cervical area, and it is almost impossible to aspirate CSF. The resultant high epidural anesthesia or high spinal anesthesia can lead to bradycardia, a drop in blood pressure, and possibly to respiratory arrest and loss of consciousness.
For treatment, see Chap. 4, p. 44.

Due to the potential complications, the patient must be monitored after the block has been carried out – for at least 30 minutes after procaine administration, and for at least 60 minutes after administration of ropivacaine or bupivacaine.

Superior cervical ganglion
Block no.   ☐ Right   ☐ Left

Record and checklist

Name: _____   Date: _____
Diagnosis: _____
Premedication: ☐ No   ☐ Yes _____

Purpose of block: ☐ *Diagnosis*   ☐ *Treatment*
Needle: ☐ *23 G*   ☐ *50 mm*   ☐ *60 mm*   ☐ _____
i. v. access: ☐ *Yes*
Monitoring: ☐ *ECG*   ☐ *Pulse oximetry*
Ventilation facilities: ☐ *Yes (equipment checked)*
Emergency equipment *(drugs):*   ☐ *Checked*
Patient: ☐ *Informed*   ☐ *Consent*

Position: ☐ *Supine*   ☐ *Head turned to opposite side*
Approach: ☐ *Extraoral (towards C2 vertebra)*

Local anesthetic: _____ ml _____ % _____
Test dose: _____ ml
Addition to
injection solution: ☐ *No*   ☐ *Yes* _____
Patient's remarks during injection:
☐ *None*   ☐ *Pain*   ☐ *Paresthesias*   ☐ *Warmth*
Neural area   _____   _____   _____

Objective block effect after 15 min:
☐ *Cold test*   ☐ *Temperature measurement right* _____°C *left* _____°C
Horner's syndrome   ☐ *Yes*   ☐ *No*
Segments affected: ☐ *C2*   ☐ *C3*   ☐ *C4*   ☐ *C5 (numbness, warmth)*
Monitoring after block: ☐ *< 1 h*   ☐ *> 1 h*
                    Time of discharge: _____

Complications:
☐ *None*   ☐ *Yes (hematoma, intravascular injection, other)*
_____

Side effects:
☐ *None*   ☐ *Yes (recurrent laryngeal nerve, phrenic nerve, vagus*
                nerve, glossopharyngeal nerve...) _____

Subjective effects of block: Duration: _____
☐ *None*   ☐ *Increased pain*
☐ *Reduced pain*   ☐ *No pain*
VISUAL ANALOG SCALE

|||||||||||||||||||||||||||||||||||||||||||||||||||||||||||||||||||||||||||||||||||||
0   10   20   30   40   50   60   70   80   90   100

Special notes: _____
_____
_____

	1. h			2. h		
	15	30	45	15	30	45
220						
200						
180						
160						
140						
120						
100						
80						
60						
40						
20						

mm Hg

O₂

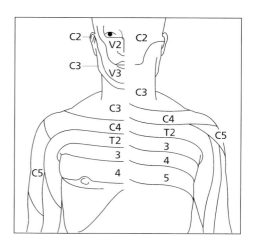

6 Deep (and superficial) cervical plexus

Anatomy

The anterior branches of the four upper cervical spinal nerves (C1 to C4) form the **cervical plexus** (Fig. 6.1), which is covered by the sternocleidomastoid muscle. The branches of the cervical plexus carry motor, sensory, proprioceptive and autonomous fibers and divide into cutaneous branches penetrating the cervical fascia and deeper muscular branches that mainly innervate the joints and muscles.

The **cutaneous branches** of the cervical plexus are the lesser occipital nerve, great auricular nerve, transverse cervical (colli) nerve and the supraclavicular nerves (Fig. 6.2). The **lesser occipital nerve** (from C2 and C3) passes on the splenius capitis muscle to its insertion area, where it fans out into several branches and supplies the skin on the upper side of the neck and the upper part of the auricle and the adjoining skin of the scalp. The largest plexus branch is usually the **great auricular nerve** (from C2 and C3), which passes upwards behind the external jugular vein and divides into a posterior and an anterior

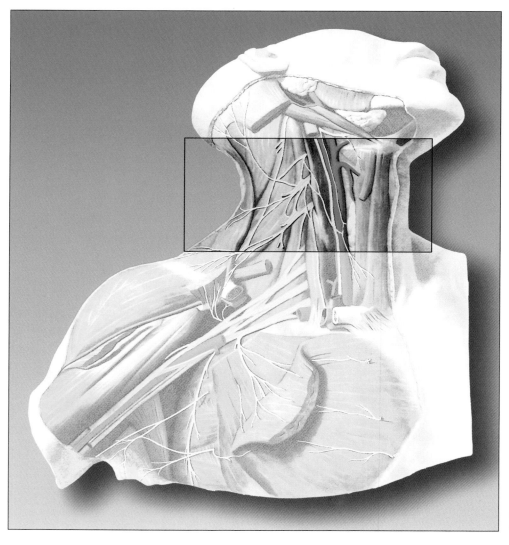

Fig. 6.1 Anatomy of the deep cervical plexus

end branch. The posterior branch supplies the skin lying behind the ear and the medial and lateral surfaces of the lower part of the auricle. The anterior branch supplies the skin in the lower posterior part of the face and the concave surface of the auricle. The **transverse cervical nerve** (from C2 and C3) passes almost horizontally over the external surface of the sternocleidomastoid muscle in an anterior direction toward the hyoid bone, divides into superior and inferior branches and supplies the skin over the anterolateral side of the neck between the mandible and the sternum. The common trunk of the **supraclavicular nerves** (from C3 and C4) appears at the posterior edge of the sternocleidomastoid muscle, just

below the transverse cervical nerve, passes downwards and divides into anterior, medial and posterior supraclavicular nerve branches. The areas supplied by the supraclavicular nerves include the skin over the caudal part of the neck and the skin above the shoulders and the lateral upper chest, as well as the skin covering the anterior part of the deltoid muscle and occupying the acromial region.

The **muscular branches** of the cervical plexus include segmentally arranged nerve branches supplying the deeper anterior neck muscles (the rectus capitis anterior and lateralis, longus colli, longus capitis and intertransverse, scalenus anterior and medius and levator scapulae), as

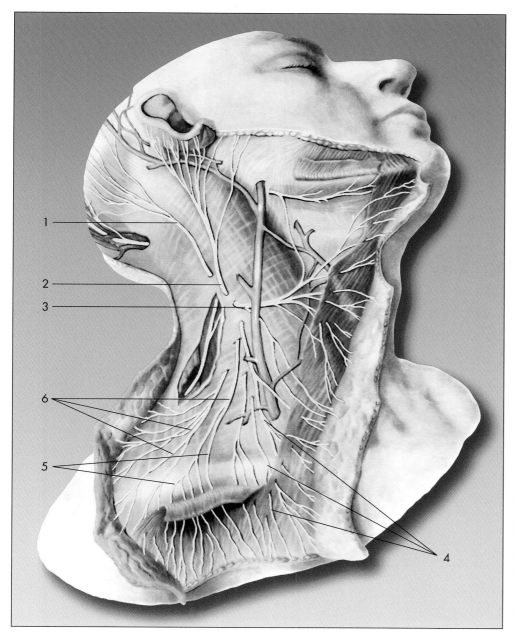

Fig. 6.2 Anatomy of the superficial cervical plexus: (1) lesser occipital nerve, (2) great auricular nerve, (3) transverse cervical (colli) nerve, (4) medial supraclavicular nerves, (5) intermediate supraclavicular nerves, (6) lateral supraclavicular nerves

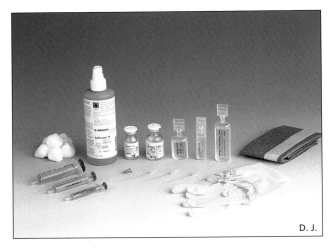

Fig. 6.3 Materials

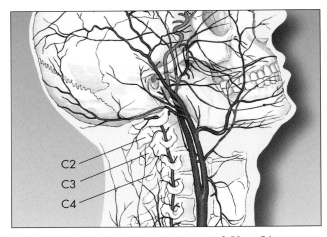

Fig. 6.4 Landmarks: transverse processes of C2 to C4

well as the inferior descending cervical nerve, the trapezius branch and the phrenic nerve. The **inferior descending cervical nerve** (from C2 and C4) gives off several fibers to the carotid and jugular neural plexus and joins with the superior descending cervical nerve to form the ansa cervicalis. The area supplied includes the sternothyroid muscle, sternocleidomastoid muscle, thyrohyoid muscle, geniohyoid muscle and omohyoid muscle.

The **trapezius branch** appears at the surface just below the accessory nerve and passes to the trapezius muscle. The **phrenic nerve** (from C4 and C3/5) is the motor nerve for the diaphragm, but it also contains sensory and sympathetic fibers that supply the fibrous pericardium, mediastinal pleura and the central part of the diaphragmatic pleura as the nerve courses through the thorax. Connections have been described between the phrenic nerve (left or right branch) or the phrenic plexus and the following structures: inferior and middle cervi-

cal ganglion, subclavian plexus, pulmonary plexus, inferior vena cava, esophagogastric junction, cardiac end of the stomach, hepatic portal, suprarenal cortex, etc.

Block of the deep cervical plexus

Indications
Diagnostic
- Localization and differentiation of various types of neuralgia.

Therapeutic
- Post-herpetic neuralgia.
- Occipital and cervicogenic head pain.
- Torticollis.

Surgical
In combination with a block of the superficial cervical plexus:
- Carotid endarterectomy [1, 2].
- Extirpation of cervical lymph nodes.
- Plastic surgery in the innervation area.

Specific contraindications
Grade 2 atrioventricular (AV) block, anticoagulant treatment, contralateral paresis of the phrenic nerve or recurrent laryngeal nerve.
Simultaneous bilateral blocks.

Procedure

This block should only be carried out by experienced anesthetists.

Preparations
Check that the emergency equipment is complete and in working order. Sterile precautions. Intravenous access, ECG monitoring, pulse oximetry, ventilation facilities.

Materials
2-ml syringes, 5-ml syringes, 10-ml syringes, three fine 22-G needles (5 cm), intubation kit, emergency drugs, disinfectant (Fig. 6.3).

Skin prep
In all blocks.

Patient positioning
Supine, with the head tilted slightly backward and turned about 45° to the opposite side.

Landmarks

Posterior edge of the sternocleidomastoid muscle, caudal part of the mastoid process, Chassaignac's tubercle (C6), transverse processes of C2, C3, C4 and C5 (Figs. 6.4 and 6.6).

The patient is asked to turn the head toward the opposite side and raise it slightly, making the posterior edge of the sternocleidomastoid apparent.

The transverse process of C6 and the caudal tip of the mastoid process are located. A line is drawn from the mastoid process along the posterior edge of the sternocleidomastoid muscle to the level of C6 (Figs. 6.5 and 6.6). The transverse process of C2 is palpated and marked on the skin. This lies about 1.5 cm caudal to the mastoid process and about 0.5–1 cm dorsal to the marked line. The transverse processes of C3, C4 and C5 are also palpated and marked. The distances between them are each ca. 1.5 cm and like C2 they lie about 0.5–1 cm dorsal to the marked line.

Injection technique

The aim is to block the anterior branches of the cervical plexus in the groove of the transverse process.

After thorough skin prep, skin infiltration is carried out at the marked areas of C2, C3 and C4 and the needles are introduced (Fig. 6.6). To do this, the therapist stands at the patient's head. In the sequence C2 to C4, the needles are directed perpendicular to the skin and advanced slightly caudal (ca. 30°) to the transverse process. In normal anatomy, the distance from the transverse processes to the skin varies between 1.5 and 3.5 cm. After clear bone contact and minimal withdrawal of the needle, careful aspiration needs to be carried out at various levels.

> The tip of the needle must reach the transverse process in order to ensure good anesthesia.

Only then may the local anesthetic be injected in several small doses, with repeated aspiration (Fig. 6.7).

> An injection should never be carried out without definite bone contact. The local anesthetic must be slowly administered in small amounts (several test doses) and with repeated aspiration.

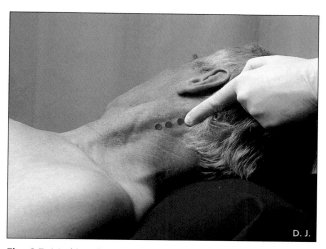

Fig. 6.5 Marking the guiding lines

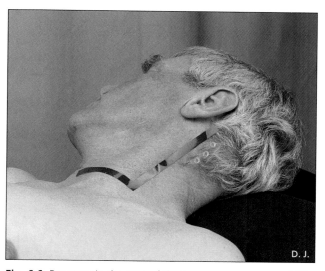

Fig. 6.6 Puncture in the area of the transverse processes of C2, C3 and C4

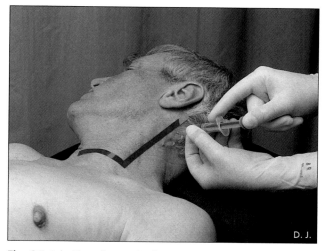

Fig. 6.7 Injection after aspiration

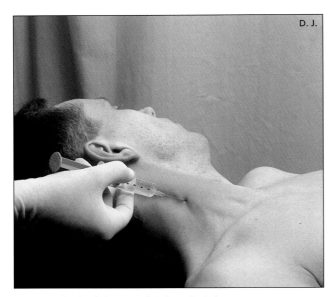

D. J.

Fig. 6.8 Block of the superficial cervical plexus

> **Caution**
> If the needle slips along the transverse process and enters an intervertebral foramen, there is a risk of dural puncture.

Effects of the block
If the local anesthetic spreads in the direction of the superior cervical ganglion and/or the cervicothoracic ganglion, Horner's syndrome may develop (see Chap. 4, p. 40).

Block series
If there is improvement after two treatment sessions, a series of 8–12 therapeutic blocks is indicated.

Dosage
Diagnostic
2 ml local anesthetic per segment, e. g. 1 % prilocaine, mepivacaine, lidocaine.

Therapeutic
3 ml local anesthetic per segment, e. g. 0.2–0.375 % ropivacaine, 0.125–0.25 % bupivacaine.

Surgical
30 ml local anesthetic:
e. g. 0.75 % ropivacaine or 0.25–0.5 % bupivacaine in mixture with 1 % prilocaine or 1 % mepivacaine.
Of this: 10 ml for fan-like injection into the superficial cervical plexus (center of the posterior edge of the sternocleidomastoid muscle, Figs. 6.2 and 6.8) and 20 ml for anesthesia of the deep cervical plexus.

Side effects
Simultaneous anesthetization of the following nerves:
- Phrenic nerve, main symptom: unilateral paralysis of diaphragmatic movement.
- Recurrent laryngeal nerve, main symptoms: hoarseness and foreign-body sensation in the throat.
- Glossopharyngeal nerve, main symptoms: numbness in the final third of the tongue, paralysis of the pharyngeal muscles.
- Vagus nerve, main symptoms: tachycardia, hypertension.
- Partial anesthetization of the upper part of the brachial plexus.

> When giving consent, the patient must be informed about these adverse effects and prepared for them.
> The patients must be monitored for 60 minutes after the block has been performed.

Complications
Intravascular injection
There is always a risk of intravascular injection due to the rich vascular supply in this area. Particular attention should be given to avoiding puncture of the vertebral artery. Toxic reactions may occur after intravascular administration of local anesthetics, and the symptoms and treatment of these are outlined in Chap. 4, p. 42.

Epidural or subarachnoid injection
When the needle slides along the transverse process and enters an intervertebral foramen, there is a risk of dural puncture and subarachnoid injection of local anesthetic. This can lead to a high spinal or high epidural block. The clinical picture and management of this is covered in Chap. 4, p. 44.

Deep cervical plexus
Block no.
☐ Right   ☐ Left

Name: _____   Date: _____
Diagnosis: _____
Premedication: ☐ No   ☐ Yes _____
Neurological abnormalities: ☐ No
               ☐ Yes (which?) _____

Purpose of block: ☐ Diagnosis   ☐ Treatment
Needle: ☐ 22 G   ☐ 40 mm   ☐ 50 mm   ☐ 60 mm
i. v. access: ☐ Yes
Monitoring: ☐ ECG   ☐ Pulse oximetry
Ventilation facilities: ☐ Yes (equipment checked)
Emergency equipment (drugs):   ☐ Checked
Patient: ☐ Informed   ☐ Consent

Position: ☐ Supine   ☐ Head turned to opposite side
Puncture technique: 3-needle technique (C2, C3, C4)

Local anesthetic: _____ ml _____ % _____ per Segment
Addition to injection: ☐ No ☐ Yes _____
Patient's remarks during injection:
☐ None   ☐ Pain   ☐ Paresthesias   ☐ Warmth
Neural area   _____ _____ _____

Objective block effect after 15 min:
☐ Cold test   ☐ Temperature measurement right ____°C   left ____°C
☐ Sensory (C2, C3, C4, C5)   ☐ Motor
Segments affected: _____ (numbness, warm sensation)
Monitoring after block: ☐ < 1 h   ☐ > 1 h
               Time of discharge: _____

Complications:
☐ None   ☐ Yes (intravascular, epidural, subarachnoid injection)
Side effects:
☐ None   ☐ Yes (Horner's syndrome, phrenic nerve, recurrent laryn-
               geal nerve, brachial plexus...) _____

Subjective effects of block: Duration: _____
☐ None   ☐ Increased pain
☐ Reduced pain   ☐ No pain
VISUAL ANALOG SCALE

|‖‖‖‖‖|‖‖‖‖‖|‖‖‖‖‖|‖‖‖‖‖|‖‖‖‖‖|‖‖‖‖‖|‖‖‖‖‖|‖‖‖‖‖|‖‖‖‖‖|‖‖‖‖‖|
0   10   20   30   40   50   60   70   80   90   100

Special notes: _____
_____
_____

Record and checklist

	1. h			2. h		
	15	30	45	15	30	45
220						
200						
180						
160						
140						
120						
100						
80						
60						
40						
20						

mm Hg

O₂

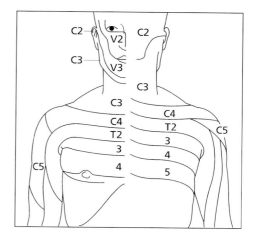

7 Brachial plexus
Interscalene block
Supraclavicular perivascular (subclavian perivascular) block
Axillary block

Anatomy

The brachial plexus arises from the union of the spinal nerve roots of C5, C6, C7, C8 and T1 and it often also contains fine fibers from the fourth cervical nerve and second thoracic nerve.

After they have left their intervertebral foramina, the roots of the plexus appear in the interscalene groove between the scalenus anterior and scalenus medius muscles and they join together there to form the primary cords or **trunks** (Fig. 7.1). The upper roots (C5, C6) form the **superior trunk,** the roots of C7 continue as the **middle trunk** and the **inferior trunk** arises from the roots of C8 and T1. After passing through the interscalene groove, the primary cords of the plexus, lying close together, move towards the first rib. The suprascapular nerve and subclavian nerve already branch off from the superior trunk here, in the posterior triangle of the neck above the clavicle. When crossing the first rib, the trunks of the plexus lie dorsal to the subclavian artery and are enclosed along with the artery by a con-

nective tissue sheath. The plexus runs through under the middle of the clavicle, following the course of the subclavian artery, into the tip of the axilla. As it does so, each of the primary cords divides into the **anterior (ventral) divisions and posterior (dorsal) divisions.** These supply the ventral flexor muscles and the dorsal extensor muscles of the upper extremity.

In the axilla itself, the nerve cords regroup and separate into the individual nerves (Fig. 7.2).

The ventral branches of the superior and middle trunk combine to form the **lateral cord** (fasciculus lateralis, C5, C6, C7).

The following nerves emerge from this:

- Musculocutaneous nerve
- Median nerve (lateral root)
- Lateral pectoral nerve

All of the dorsal branches of the three trunks form the **posterior cord** (fasciculus posterior, C5–8, T1). The end branches of this are the:

- Radial nerve
- Axillary nerve
- Thoracodorsal nerve
- Inferior subscapular nerve
- Superior subscapular nerve

The ventral branches of the inferior trunk continue as the **medial cord** (fasciculus medialis, C8, T1). The following nerves emerge from this:

- Ulnar nerve
- Median nerve (medial root)
- Medial pectoral nerve
- Medial antebrachial cutaneous nerve
- Medial brachial cutaneous nerve

Introduction

The classical blocks of the brachial plexus using Hirschel's [18] (axillary approach) and Kulenkampff's [21] (supraclavicular block) anesthesia have been continuously developed and supplemented with additional access routes (Fig. 7.4). As representative techniques for a multitude of clinical procedures for plexus anesthesia, the axillary perivascular block [3, 17, 58], subclavian peri-

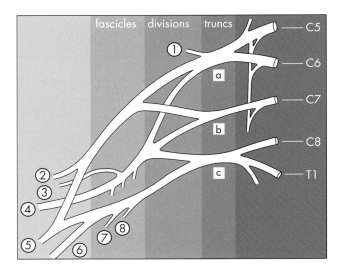

Fig. 7.1 Trunks: (a) superior trunk, (b) medial trunk, (c) inferior trunk, divisions and cords of the brachial plexus. (1) Suprascapular nerve, (2) musculocutaneous nerve, (3) axillary nerve, (4) radial nerve, (5) median nerve, (6) ulnar nerve, (7) medial antebrachial cutaneous nerve, (8) medial brachial cutaneous nerve

vascular block using the Winnie and Collins technique [57], Winnie's interscalene block [54, 58] and Raj's infraclavicular approach [34] may be mentioned. All of the blocks of the brachial plexus are based on the concept that the neural plexus lies within a perivascular and perineural space in its course from the transverse processes to the axilla. Like the epidural space, this space limits the spread of the local anesthetic and conducts it to the various trunks and roots. Within the connective tissue sheath, the concentration and volume of the local anesthetic used determine the extent of the block's spread.

Apart from technical aspects, the main differences between the various block procedures are that the injection is made into the interscalene space, the subclavian space or the axillary space – leading to different focuses for the block.

In this chapter, three techniques that are among the standard methods for plexus anesthesia will be described: the interscalene, subclavian perivascular and axillary blocks of the brachial plexus.

All three procedures have well-known advantages in contrast with general anesthesia:

▨ They can be used on an outpatient basis.
▨ Use in patients with a full stomach, high-risk and emergency patients and patients who are anxious about general anesthesia.
▨ Absence of side effects such as nausea and vomiting.
▨ Absence of postoperative pulmonary complications.
▨ Excellent postoperative pain control, particularly with the use of long-term local anesthetics.
▨ Sympathetic block with vasodilation, better perfusion and faster recovery of traumatized extremities.

Certain points should always be observed when preparing for this procedure:

▨ Contraindications must be excluded.
▨ The anatomic relationships in each patient must be precisely studied and studied again for repeated blocks.
▨ Neurological abnormalities must be excluded.
▨ The procedure must be explained to the patient in detail in order to ensure cooperation.
▨ The patient must be placed in a comfortable position during the intervention.
▨ All patients should be informed of possible side effects and complications; they must also be advised of what they should and should not do after their treatment.

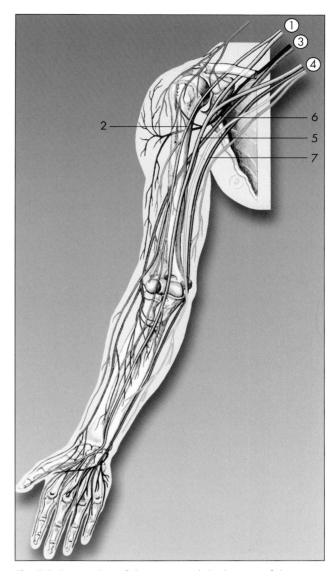

Fig. 7.2 Regrouping of the nerve cords in the area of the axilla and their distal distribution. (1) Lateral cord, (2) musculocutaneous nerve, (3) posterior cord, (4) medial cord, (5) median nerve, (6) radial nerve, (7) ulnar nerve

Interscalene block

Indications

Therapeutic

▨ Shoulder and upper arm pain ("frozen shoulder"): humeroscapular periarthritis, muscles of the rotator cuff, post-stroke pain (ca. 70 % of patients have severe shoulder pain). The aim of the block is to allow pain-free and adequate physiotherapy.
▨ Mobilization of the shoulder.
▨ Shoulder arthrosis.

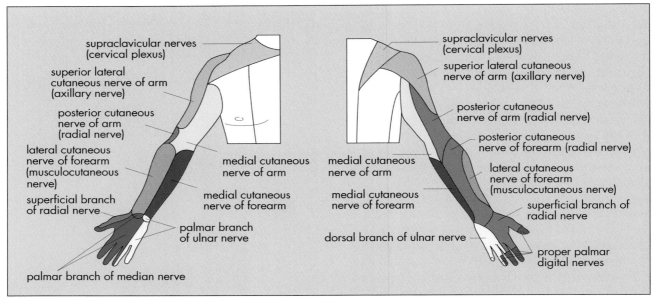

Fig. 7.3 Brachial plexus, cutaneous innervation

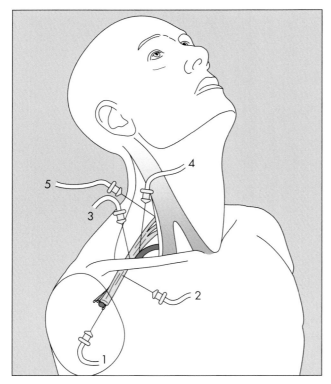

Fig. 7.4 Various access routes for blockading the brachial plexus: (1) axillary block, (2) infraclavicular block, (3) Kulen-kampff supraclavicular block, (4) Winnie and Collins subclavian perivascular block, (5) Winnie interscalene block

▨ Post-herpetic neuralgia in the innervation area.

▨ Lymphedema after breast amputation.

▨ Vascular diseases and injuries, with continuous block in the acute stage.

▨ Complex regional pain syndrome (CRPS) type I (sympathetic reflex dystrophy) and type II (causalgia): If abduction of the arm is possible, an axillary block is preferable here (see p. 70).

▨ Postamputation pain, e. g. after exarticulation.

▨ Tumor-related pain: Continuous administration (e. g., in Pancoast tumor) is an alternative to repeated single applications here. The therapeutic effect of additional opioid administration is variously evaluated in the literature [20, 50]. The period of treatment is limited. It can provide support for oral opioid administration, but it cannot replace it.

Surgical

▨ Clavicle, shoulder, upper arm [1, 45] (the exception is the inner side):

As a single-administration or continuous regional anesthesia [16, 31, 49] or in combination with basic general anesthesia.

In combination with basic general anesthesia, the administration of 20–25 ml 0.75 % ropivacaine or 20 ml 0.5 % bupivacaine allows a marked reduction in the dosage of the general anesthetic and, in our own experience, leads to excellent postoperative pain control.

▨ Repositioning of shoulder luxation.

Contraindications

Specific

- Infection or malignant disease in the neck and nuchal region.
- Pyoderma of the skin in the puncture area.
- Contralateral paresis of the phrenic or recurrent laryngeal nerves.
- Anticoagulation treatment.
- Distorted anatomy, e. g. due to prior surgical interventions or trauma in the neck and nuchal region.

Relative

The decision should be taken after carefully weighing up the risks and benefits:

- Hemorrhagic diathesis.
- Stable systemic neural diseases.
- Local neural injury (caution when there is unclear responsibility between surgery and anesthesia).
- Asthma.

Procedure

This block should only be carried out by experienced anesthetists or under their supervision.

Preparations

Check that the emergency equipment is complete and in working order. Sterile precautions. Intravenous access, ECG monitoring, pulse oximetry, intubation kit, emergency medication, ventilation facilities.

Materials (Figs. 7.5. and 7.6)

- Stimuplex HNS 11 nerve stimulator (B. Braun Melsungen).
  3.5–4 cm long atraumatic 22-G (30°) needle with "immobile needle" injection lead, e.g. Stimuplex D (B. Braun Melsungen).
- 2.5–3.8(5) cm long Plexufix 24-G (45°) needle with "immobile needle" injection lead, syringes: 2, 10 and 20 ml.
  Local anesthetics, disinfectant, swabs, compresses, sterile gloves and drape.

Skin prep

In all blocks.

Patient positioning

Supine, with the head turned to the opposite side.

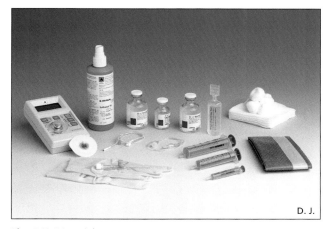

Fig. 7.5 Materials

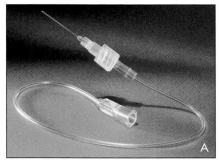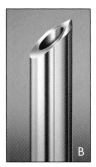

Fig. 7.6 A, B 24-G needle with short-beveled tip

Landmarks

Sternocleidomastoid muscle, interscalene groove between the scalenus anterior and scalenus medius muscles (Fig. 7.7), transverse process (C6), external jugular vein.

Location of the puncture site

To locate the injection site, the patient's arm is drawn in the direction of the knee (Fig. 7.8). The patient is asked to turn the head to the opposite side and raise it slightly (ca. 20°), so that the posterior edge of the sternocleidomastoid muscle clearly emerges (Fig. 7.9). The transverse process (C6) is palpated at the lateral edge of the sternocleidomastoid muscle. For confirmation (pleura) and guidance, the pulsation of the subclavian artery (at the lower end of the interscalene groove) and the upper edge of the clavicle can also be palpated and their distance from the injection site can be estimated (Fig. 7.10).

Dorsal to the sternocleidomastoid muscle, the scalenus anterior muscle is palpated. The interscalene groove between the scalenus anterior and scalenus medius muscles, after being moistened, is felt with "rolling fingers" and located (Fig. 7.11).

The injection site in the interscalene groove lies at the level of the cricoid, opposite the transverse process of C6 (Chassaignac's tubercle). The external jugular vein often crosses the level of the cricoid process here (Fig. 7.12).

When there are anatomical difficulties, it is helpful for the patient to inhale deeply or to try and blow out the cheeks. The scalene muscles then tense up and the interscalene groove becomes clearly palpable.

Injection technique

After disinfecting the puncture area, draping and skin infiltration, the injection site is delimited cranially and caudally using the index and middle fingers. The injection needle is advanced between the fingers in the direction of the transverse process (C6). The direction of insertion runs inward and ca. 30–40° caudally, as well as slightly dorsally (Fig. 7.13). The index and middle finger continue to palpate the interscalene groove.

Even when the needle is positioned superficially, paresthesias often occur in the area of the elbow, index finger and thumb. Paresthesias in the shoulder region also frequently occur. These result from stimulation of the suprascapular nerve, which is often located in the connective tissue sheath [3].

> When the anatomy is normal and no paresthesias are elicited after ca. 2–2.5 cm, the needle position needs to be corrected.

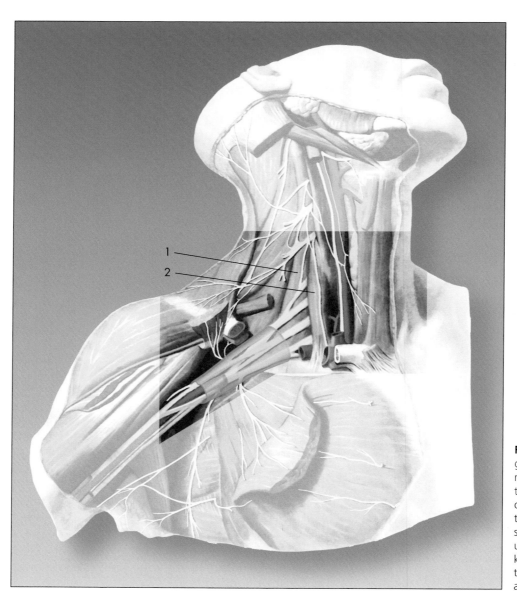

Fig. 7.7 The interscalene groove. Scalenus medius muscle (1) and scalenus anterior muscle (2). Injection of the local anesthetic into the proximal neurovascular sheath of the brachial plexus. The plexus is located in a kind of "sandwich" between the scalenus anterior muscle and scalenus medius muscle

Once the paresthesias have been elicited, the correct positioning of the needle is checked by aspirating at various levels and quickly injecting an initial dose of the local anesthetic (2–3 ml). The patient will experience a brief pain (pressure paresthesia) due to expansion of the perivascular space. During further injection of the local anesthetic, aspiration at various levels has to be repeated after every 4–5 ml. Pressure from the index and middle finger allows the direction of spread of the local anesthetic to be guided during the injection. After successful injection, the entire area is massaged in order to ensure even distribution of the local anesthetic. This also serves for hematoma prophylaxis.

> The patient must be informed about the expected paresthesias and the significance of them.

Electrostimulation

Stimulant current of 1–2 mA and 2 Hz is selected for a stimulation period of 0.1 ms.

The injection needle is advanced in the direction of the transverse process (C6). After the motor response from the relevant musculature (elbow, index finger and thumb), the stimulant current is reduced to 0.2–0.3 mA. Slight twitching suggests that the stimulation needle is in the immediate vicinity of the nerve. After aspiration, incremental injection of a local anesthetic is carried out. During the injection, the twitching slowly disappears.

Dosage

Therapeutic

Unilateral administration (block series):

10 ml local anesthetic, e. g. 0.2 % ropivacaine or 0.125–0.25 % bupivacaine in shoulder and upper arm pain, shoulder arthrosis, postapoplectic pain, lymphedema after breast amputation.

10–20 ml local anesthetic, e. g. 0.2–0.375 % ropivacaine or 0.25 % bupivacaine in post-herpetic neuralgia, vascular diseases and injuries, complex regional pain syndrome (CRPS) types I and II, post-amputation pain.

25 ml local anesthetic, e. g. 1 % prilocaine or 1 % mepivacaine in combination with 5–10 ml diazepam i. v. to mobilize the shoulder.

Locating the interscalene groove

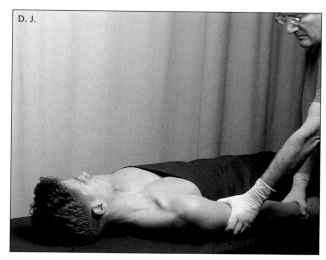

Fig. 7.8 1. Drawing the arm towards the knee

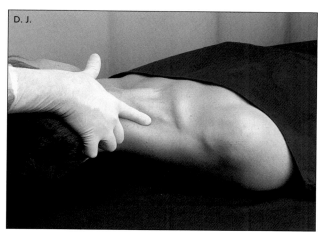

Fig. 7.9 2. Turning the head to the opposite side and raising it slightly

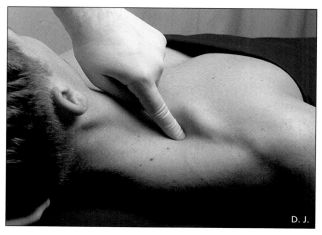

Fig. 7.10 3. Palpating the clavicle and subclavian artery

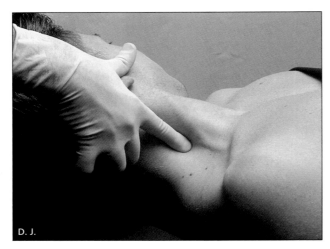

Fig. 7.11 4. Palpating the interscalene groove with "rolling" fingers

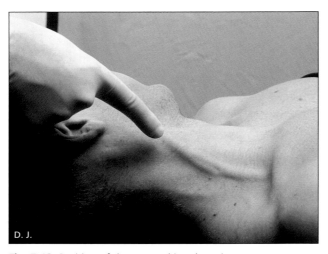

Fig. 7.12 Position of the external jugular vein

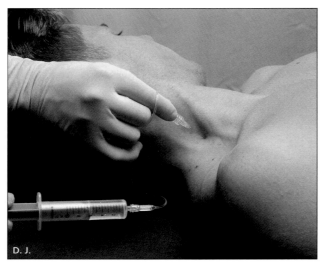

Fig. 7.13 Injection in the direction of the transverse process of C6

Surgical

Single techniques and block series

40 ml local anesthetic is sufficient for an adequate block of the brachial plexus and caudal part of the cervical plexus. In the literature [13, 23, 38, 49, 54], the doses administered vary from 30 ml to 50 ml. A mixture of 20 ml 0.75 % ropivacaine (0.5 % bupivacaine) with 20 ml 1 % prilocaine (1 % mepivacaine) has proved its value very well in practice (in our own experience). This leads to a fast onset and long duration of effect.

25 ml local anesthetic, e. g. 1 % prilocaine (1 % mepivacaine), in combination with 5–10 mg diazepam i. v. for repositioning shoulder luxation.

20–25 ml local anesthetic, e. g. 0.75 % ropivacaine or 0.5 % bupivacaine, in combination with basic general anesthesia, for surgical interventions in the area of the shoulder and clavicle. This leads to very good postoperative pain control.

20 ml local anesthetic is sufficient to block the lower part of the cervical plexus and the upper part of the brachial plexus. The brachial plexus is only incompletely anesthetized with this amount and block of the area supplied by the ulnar nerve is often absent.

Continuous administration

40 ml local anesthetic (see above) to carry out the intervention.

As the subsequent 24-hour infusion for postoperative analgesia:

- 0.2 % ropivacaine **6–14 ml/h**
- 0.25 % bupivacaine [16] **0.25 mg/kg b.w./h**
- 0.125 % bupivacaine **0.125 mg/kg b.w./h,** in combination with opioids if appropriate [31].

> **Caution**
> Individual adjustment of the dosage and period of treatment is absolutely necessary. The following information is therefore only intended to provide guidance.

Distribution of the blocks

The complete distribution of the anesthesia is shown in Figure 7.14.

Block series

When there is evidence of improvement in the symptoms, a series of 8–12 blocks can be carried out.

Side effects

Simultaneous anesthesia of the following nerves and ganglia (Fig. 7.15):

- Vagus nerve, main symptoms: tachycardia, hypertension.
- Recurrent laryngeal nerve, main symptoms: hoarseness and foreign-body sensation in the throat.
- Phrenic nerve, main symptoms: unilateral paralysis of diaphragmatic movement and simulation of pneumothorax, particularly with continuous blocks [13, 31].
- Cervicothoracic (stellate) ganglion, with Horner's syndrome.

The patient must be prepared for these adverse effects during the patient information procedure.

Complications

Neural injuries
Traumatic neural injuries are an extremely rare complication of this technique [2, 49].
Prophylaxis: Only needles with short-beveled tips should be used. Intraneural positioning should be excluded. Vasopressor additives should be avoided. For details, see p. 76 in the section on axillary blocks.

Intravascular injection [11]
There is a particular risk of intravascular injection into the vertebral artery (Fig. 7.15) or other cervical vessels. This can very quickly lead to toxic reactions. On the symptoms and treatment, see Chap. 4, pp. 42, 43.

Epidural or subarachnoid injection [22, 35, 46]
Epidural injection of the local anesthetic can lead to high epidural block and subarachnoid administration can lead to total spinal block. Both complications are severe and life-threatening and require immediate treatment (see Chap. 4, p. 44).
Prophylaxis: injection with short needles and introduction of the needle in a caudal direction.

CNS intoxication
Overdosage and/or intravascular diffusion of the local anesthetic can, in extremely rare cases, lead to CNS intoxication (see Chap. 4, p. 43).

Pneumothorax
When the technique is carried out correctly, this complication is unlikely. The needle is advanced at a safe distance from the pleural cupula.

Pressure on the carotid artery
Extremely rare and transient. Caused by the volume of the injection [41].

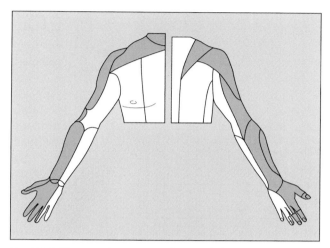

Fig. 7.14 The neural areas most frequently blocked 15 minutes after administration of the block with bupivacaine [19]

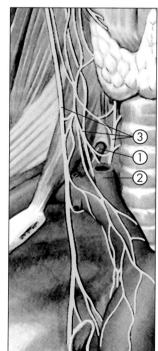

Fig. 7.15 The most important nerves and vessels in the injection area: (1) vertebral artery, (2) carotid artery, (3) laryngeal, vagus and phrenic nerves

Record and checklist

Interscalene block of the brachial plexus

Block no.   ☐ Right   ☐ Left

Name: _____ Date: _____
Diagnosis: _____
Premedication: ☐ No   ☐ Yes _____

Neurological abnormalities: ☐ No
                                   ☐ Yes (which?) _____

Purpose of block: ☐ Diagnosis   ☐ Treatment
Position: ☐ Supine   ☐ Head turned to opposite
Needle type: ☐ 24 G, Plexufix, short-beveled tip 45°
                    ☐ 0.55 × 25 mm   ☐ 0.55 × _____
                    ☐ Other _____
i. v. access: ☐ Yes
Monitoring: ☐ ECG   ☐ Pulse oximetry
Ventilation facilities: ☐ Yes (equipment checked)
Emergency equipment (drugs):   ☐ Checked
Patient: ☐ Informed   ☐ Consent

Puncture technique: ☐ interscalene groove located   ☐ Level C6
                    ☐ Paresthesias   ☐ Electrostimulation
Neural area   _____

Local anesthetic: _____ ml _____ % _____
(incremental)
Addition: ☐ Yes _____   ☐ No
Patient's remarks during injection:
☐ None   ☐ Paresthesias   ☐ Warmth
☐ Pain caused (intraneural positioning?) _____
Neural area _____

Objective block effect after 15 min:
☐ Cold test   ☐ Temperature measurement right ____ C° left ____ C°
☐ Sensory   ☐ Motor
Monitoring after block: ☐ < 1 h   ☐ > 1 h
                    Time of discharge: _____

Complications:
☐ None   ☐ Intravascular   ☐ Epidural/subarachnoid   ☐ Pneumothorax
Side effects:
☐ None ☐ Hematoma ☐ Phrenic nerve ☐ Recurrent laryngeal nerve ☐ Horner's

Subjective effects of block: Duration: _____
☐ None   ☐ Increased pain   ☐ Reduced pain   ☐ No pain
VISUAL ANALOG SCALE

|︙︙︙︙︙︙︙︙︙︙︙︙︙︙︙︙︙︙︙︙︙︙︙︙︙︙︙︙︙︙︙︙︙︙︙︙︙︙|
0   10   20   30   40   50   60   70   80   90   100

Special notes:
_____
_____

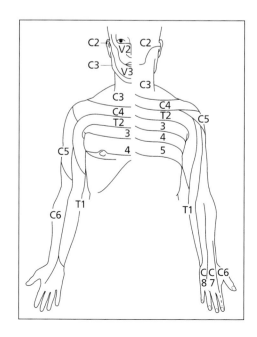

Supraclavicular perivascular (subclavian perivascular) block

Definition
Injection of a local anesthetic into the area of the brachial plexus trunks in the caudal part of the interscalene groove, in its most compact part above the clavicle. This technique was first described by Winnie and Collins [57].

Indications
Surgical
Operations in the upper arm, forearm and hand.

Therapeutic
None.

Contraindications
Specific
- Infections or malignant diseases in the area of the throat.
- Pyoderma of the skin in the injection area.
- Contralateral paresis of the phrenic nerve or recurrent laryngeal nerve.
- Anticoagulant treatment.
- Distorted anatomy, e. g. due to prior surgical interventions or trauma in the area of the throat and nape.
- Severe chronic obstructive pulmonary disease.
- Contralateral pneumothorax.

Relative
The decision should be taken after carefully weighing up the risks and benefits:
- Hemorrhagic diathesis.
- Stable systemic neural diseases.
- Local nerve injury (caution when there is unclear responsibility between surgery and anesthesia).

Procedure

This block should only be carried out by experienced anesthetists or under their supervision.
Preparations and materials (see the section on the interscalene block, p. 61, Figs. 7.5 and 7.6)

Technique
Locating the injection site
The most important landmarks are:
- The interscalene groove, with its caudal part in the supraclavicular fossa (see the section on the interscalene block, steps for location, pp. 63, 64, Figs. 7.8–7.12). The process of locating the site is often difficult when the caudal part of the interscalene groove is covered by the omohyoid muscle. During the injection, particular attention should be given to the course of the scalenus medius muscle (Fig. 7.16).

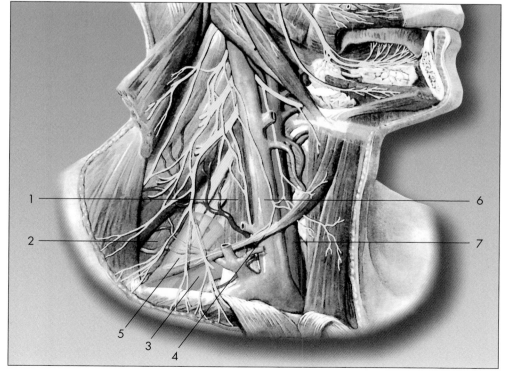

Fig. 7.16 Interscalene groove, with the brachial plexus.
(1) Scalenus anterior muscle,
(2) scalenus medius muscle,
(3) subclavian artery,
(4) omohyoid muscle,
(5) neurovascular sheath,
(6) internal jugular vein,
(7) common carotid artery

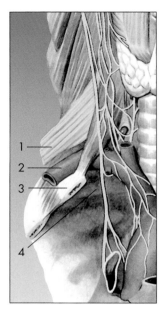

Fig. 7.17 (1) Brachial plexus, (2) subclavian artery, (3) first rib, (4) pleural cupula

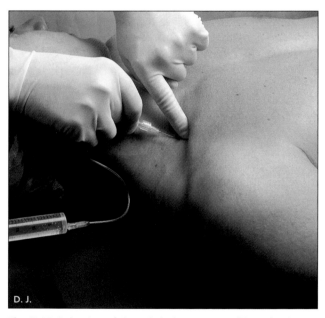

Fig. 7.18 Palpation of the subclavian artery and introduction of the needle

- The subclavian artery, which is located in the immediate vicinity of the plexus trunks. The arterial pulses are the most important mark for the injection.
- The midpoint of the clavicle. The injection point is located ca. 1.5–2 cm lateral to the clavicular head of the sternocleidomastoid muscle and 2 cm above the clavicle.
- The course of the external jugular vein as far as the supraclavicular fossa.

Caution
The close anatomical relationships in this block are characterized by the trunks of the brachial plexus, the subclavian artery, the first rib and the pleural cupula (Fig. 7.17) (see Chap. 4, Fig. 4.2).

Injection technique
- After palpation of the subclavian artery, the tip of the left index finger is laid directly above the pulsations.
- The cone of an injection needle with a short-beveled tip is fixed between the index finger and the thumb of the right hand (Fig. 7.18).
- The needle is introduced in a caudal direction along the long axis of the body, near the scalenus medius muscle. The cone of the needle almost touches the skin surface of the throat, with its shaft lying parallel to the skin surface.

Caution
The pleural cupula is located immediately medial to the first rib. It is therefore absolutely essential to avoid a dorsomedial injection, due to the risk of pneumothorax.

- Perforation of the fascia is confirmed by "fascial click", and it is accompanied by paresthesias. The patient is asked to say "now" when paresthesias are experienced and to describe the location of spread precisely. Paresthesias elicited below the shoulder, particularly in the innervation area of the median nerve, are important here. Paresthesias in the shoulder area indicate stimulation of the suprascapular nerve and are less important, since this nerve often lies outside the neurovascular sheath.

After paresthesias have been elicited, correct positioning of the needle is checked by aspiration at various levels and an initial dose of local anesthetic (2–3 ml) is quickly injected. The extension of the perivascular space which this causes creates a sensation of sudden pain for the patient (known as pressure paresthesia). During the further injection of local anesthetic, aspiration at various levels must be repeated after each 4–5 ml. The index finger of the left hand should apply pressure above the needle in order to prevent local anesthetic from spreading cranially (Fig. 7.20).

After successful injection, the entire area is massaged to ensure even distribution of local anesthetic. This also serves for hematoma prophylaxis.

> **Caution**
>
> The patient must be informed about the expected paresthesias and their significance. If severe pain occurs during the injection (intraneural location), the injection should be interrupted immediately and the position of the needle should be corrected.

Electrostimulation

Stimulant current of 1–2 mA and 2 Hz is selected for a stimulation period of 0.1 ms, and the needle is advanced in the direction of the brachial plexus trunks (Fig. 7.19). After the motor response from the relevant musculature, the stimulant current is reduced to 0.2–0.3 mA (Fig. 7.20). Slight twitching suggests that the stimulation needle is in the immediate vicinity of the nerve. After aspiration, incremental injection of a local anesthetic is carried out. During the injection, the twitching slowly disappears.

Problem situations

If the needle is positioned too far anteriorly in the vicinity of the scalenus anterior muscle, the subclavian artery may be punctured. This is definite evidence that the needle is located in the perivascular space. The needle is withdrawn subcutaneously and then introduced dorsolaterally, in the vicinity of the scalenus medius muscle, until paresthesias are elicited.

If no paresthesias are elicited, then the needle has missed all three trunks of the brachial plexus lying at the vertical level and it will come into contact with the first rib (protective function, preventing pleural puncture).

The needle is withdrawn as far as the subcutis and its direction is corrected by about 1 cm dorsally, closer to the scalenus medius muscle.

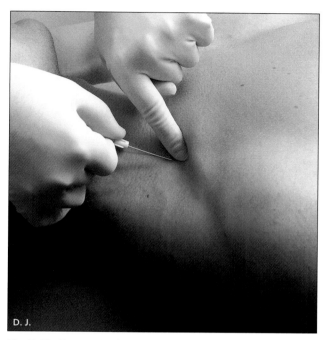

Fig. 7.19 Electrostimulation. Advancing the needle

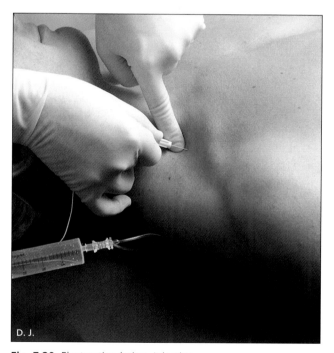

Fig. 7.20 Electrostimulation. Injection

When a tourniquet is applied, an additional block of the intercostobrachial nerve (T2) and medial brachial cutaneous nerve is sometimes required. For this purpose, the arm is abducted about 90° and 5 ml of local anesthetic is injected directly above the pulsations of the axillary artery.

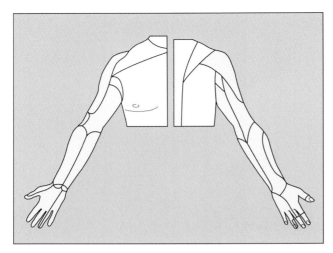

Fig. 7.21 Distribution of the block. The most frequently blocked nerve areas 15 minutes after initiating a block with bupivacaine [19]

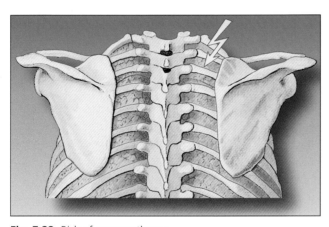

Fig. 7.22 Risk of pneumothorax

Dosage
Surgical
40 ml local anesthetic
0.75 % ropivacaine
0.5 % bupivacaine
1 % prilocaine
1 % mepivacaine

Distribution of the block
The complete distribution of the anesthesia is illustrated in Figure 7.21.

Side effects
Concomitant anesthetization of the following nerves and ganglia:
- Vagus nerve, recurrent laryngeal nerve, phrenic nerve.
- Stellate ganglion (see section on interscalene block, p. 65).

> **Caution**
> The patient must be prepared for these adverse effects during the patient information procedure.

Complications
- Pneumothorax (0.5–6 %) (Fig. 7.22).
- Neural injury (see section on axillary block, p. 76).
- Intravascular injection (see Chap. 4, section on stellate ganglion, p. 42).
- CNS intoxication (see Chap. 4, p. 43).

Axillary block

Single techniques and block series

Indications
Diagnostic
- Postamputation pain.
- Complex regional pain syndrome (CRPS) types I and II.
- Checking (confirmation) of surgical sympathectomy.
- Differential diagnosis of peripheral and central pain.

Prophylactic
- As an alternative to cervicothoracic ganglion block, when a stellate block is contraindicated or cannot be carried out for technical reasons.

Therapeutic
- Following peripheral nerve injury, with causalgia development (see case 3, p. 84).
- Following surgical neurolysis, to improve postoperative reinnervation.
- Severe arteriospasm, e. g. after accidental intra-arterial injection of thiopental (or as a continuous block).
- Complex regional pain syndrome (CRPS) types I and II (see cases 1 and 2, pp. 82, 83).
- Rheumatic diseases.
- Wrist arthrosis.
- Neuropathies, e. g. due to diabetes.
- Post-herpetic neuralgia.
- Post-amputation pain (block series in chronic pain conditions).
- Postoperative pain (in most cases, a preoperative block with a long-term local anesthetic is sufficient).

Surgical
As a single-dose or continuous block [24, 36, 37, 44]. This is the method of choice for all general, vascular, neurosurgical or orthopedic interventions and manipulations in the arm below the elbow and in the hand region.

Contraindications
Specific
▨ Infections (e. g., lymphangitis) or malignant diseases in the arm region.
▨ Anticoagulation treatment.
▨ Upper arm fractures or other conditions preventing abduction of the arm.
▨ Patient's refusal.

Relative
The decision should be taken after carefully weighing up the risks and benefits:
▨ Hemorrhagic diathesis.
▨ Stable systemic neural diseases.
▨ Local neural injury (caution when there is unclear responsibility between surgery and anesthesia).

Procedure

This block should only be carried out by experienced anesthetists or under their supervision.
Preparations and materials (see section on interscalene block, p. 61; see Figs. 7.5 and 7.6)

Skin prep
In all blocks.

Patient positioning
Supine, with the upper arm abducted (90–100°), forearm flexed (90°) and rotated outward (Fig. 7.24). Hyperabduction must be avoided. It obliterates the arterial pulsation, making palpation of the artery difficult and affecting the optimal distribution of the local anesthetic.

Landmarks
Axillary artery, deltoid muscle, pectoralis major muscle, biceps muscle, coracobrachialis muscle. The axillary fossa is delimited by the deltoid muscle and pectoralis major muscle above and by the biceps and coracobrachialis muscles below (Fig. 7.25). The axillary artery lies together with the ulnar nerve, median nerve and radial nerve, as well as the brachial and medial antebrachial cutaneous nerves in the neurovascular sheath. The sheath normally encloses the axillary vein as well, but not always.

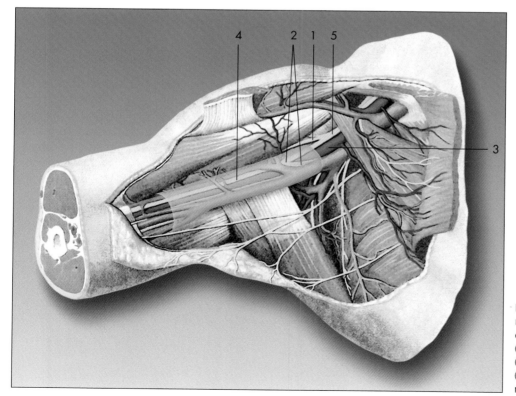

Fig. 7.23 Distal (axillary) neurovascular sheath of the brachial plexus. (1) Musculocutaneous nerve, (2) median nerve, (3) axillary artery, (4) ulnar nerve, (5) lateral cord

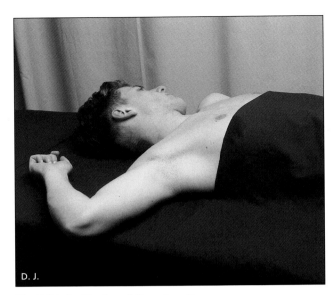

Fig. 7.24 Positioning of the extremity

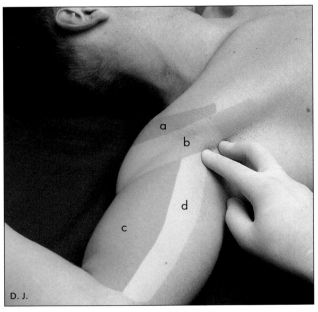

Fig. 7.25 Palpation of the axillary artery. (a) Deltoid muscle, (b) pectoralis major muscle, (c) biceps muscle, (d) coracobrachialis muscle

Location of the injection site
The axillary artery is palpated as high proximally as possible under the lateral edge of the pectoralis major muscle and fixed with the index and middle fingers (Fig. 7.25).

> The high proximal palpation and fixing of the axillary artery increases the likelihood of reaching the musculocutaneous nerve as well. This nerve leaves the axillary fossa together with the axillary nerve at the level of the coracoid process.

Injection technique
After skin prep of the entire axilla and draping, the skin is infiltrated immediately above the fixed artery. The skin at the injection site is incised with a hemostylet to make introduction of the needle easier. Winnie [53] recommends the use of an "immobile needle." This is slowly advanced proximally at an angle of ca. 15–30° in the direction of the neurovascular sheath (Fig. 7.26 A, B).

Needle position
Before the injection, it must be confirmed that the neurovascular sheath has been reached and the needle is securely positioned in the fascial compartment. The following techniques are suitable for this:

"Fascial clicks"
Entry of the needle into the neurovascular sheath is confirmed by what are termed "fascial clicks." When needles with short-beveled tips are used, perforation of the connective tissue is easily felt and is often also audible.

Pulsations (pulse-synchronous) in the needle
Positioning of the needle tip in the immediate vicinity of the artery can be confirmed by pulse-synchronous oscillation of the needle, although this does not guarantee secure positioning in the neurovascular sheath and does not provide reliable evidence on its own.

Electrical neurostimulation (Fig. 7.27)
Muscular twitching is the motor response of the relevant musculature to neural stimulation. This allows individual nerves to be targeted and located with ease and neural lesions are practically excluded. Cooperation by the patient is not required.

Technique

Stimulant current of 1–2 mA and 2 Hz is selected for a stimulation period of 0.1 ms. After the motor response from the relevant musculature, the stimulant current is reduced to 0.2–0.3 mA. Slight twitching suggests that the stimulation needle is located in the immediate vicinity of the nerve. After aspiration, incremental injection of a local anesthetic is carried out. During the injection, the muscle twitching slowly disappears. However, the success rate with this procedure is slightly lower than with other techniques [56].

Paresthesias

It is not obligatory to produce paresthesias with this block technique. Due to the potential risk of neural injury – Selander reports post-block neuropathies in 2.8 % of cases [38, 40], while other authors only report occasional complications [51, 52] – paresthesias should be avoided if possible. On the other hand, it should be emphasized that in ca. 40 % of cases, paresthesias are produced involuntarily [38, 40, 42] and these are a definite sign of correct positioning of the needle. The patient must be informed about these and must be able to report the occurrence of paresthesias immediately and describe their spread.

Arterial puncture technique

Aspiration of blood indicates that the needle is located in the axillary artery and therefore within the neurovascular sheath.

Injection

When the needle is securely located in the neurovascular sheath, aspiration is carried out at various levels and the local anesthetic is injected slowly. A certain amount of pressure is needed for this, since the fascial cover creates resistance to the injection.

Aspiration at various levels must be repeated after each injection of 4–5 ml – no matter which technique is used.

Perivascular technique

In the perivascular technique [3, 17], all of the local anesthetic is distributed in the neurovascular sheath around the artery (perivascular).

Transarterial injection

This technique is being increasingly used due to its high success rate (89–99 %) [6, 42, 56] and low complication rate and its value has been demonstrated with obese patients as well. After targeted puncture of the artery and blood aspiration (Fig. 7.28), the needle is withdrawn until no more blood can be aspirated.

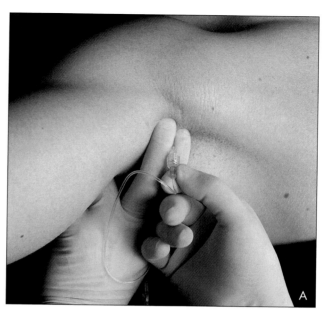

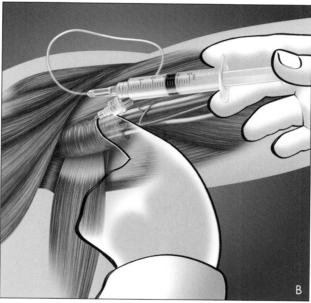

Fig. 7.26 A, B Puncturing the neurovascular sheath

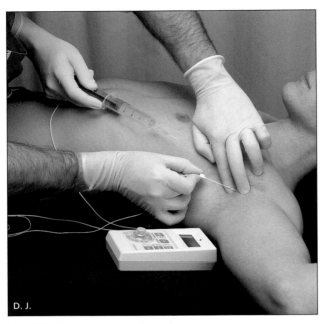

Fig. 7.27 Electrical neurostimulation

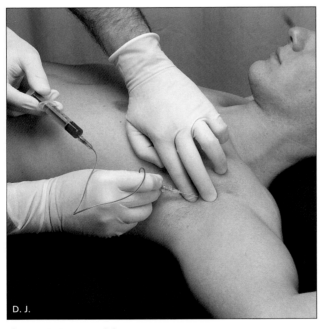

D. J.

Fig. 7.28 Transarterial access

Without creating paresthesias, 20 ml of local anesthetic is injected initially. The needle is then advanced to the opposite side of the artery and after careful aspiration, the remaining dose (20 ml) is administered [49]. The following are variants of this procedure:

Single injection into a single compartment [6]
The entire dose of the local anesthetic is deposited behind the artery (posterior).

Multiple injections into multiple compartments [42]
Half of the dose is injected behind the artery (posterior) and the other half is distributed according to the area to be operated on: in the ulnar and median nerve region (in front of the artery), radial nerve region (behind the artery) (Fig. 7.23).
Potential disadvantages of the transarterial technique are that persistent bleeding may reduce the quality of the anesthesia by diluting the local anesthetic or that a hematoma may compress neighboring nerves and shield the local anesthetic. As with all procedures, intravascular injection – into the axillary vein as well – is theoretically possible with this technique [14].

Distribution of the local anesthetic
To ensure optimal distribution of the local anesthetic, during the injection the neurovascular sheath is compressed with the fingers, distal to the needle. Applying a tourniquet distal to the injection site is ineffective, since the muscle mass is barely affected by this [55, 58]. After removal of the needle, compressing the axilla (3–5 min) (Fig. 7.29) and simultaneous massaging encourages improved distribution of the local anesthetic. It also serves for hematoma prophylaxis.

- The axillary artery should be palpated as high as possible, fixed between the index and middle fingers and punctured in a cranial direction.
- Only needles with short-beveled tips should be used, preferably an "immobile needle" with a short injection lead.
- Correct positioning of the needle in the neurovascular sheath should be checked before the injection.
- Before and during the injection (after each 4–5 ml), aspiration should be carried out at various levels.
- When severe pain occurs during the injection (intraneural position), the injection should be interrupted at once and the position of the needle should be corrected.
- After the injection, compression massage of the axillary fossa should be carried out for 3–5 minutes.
- Avoid supplementation. An incomplete plexus block should not be supplemented with other additional peripheral nerve blocks, since this would mean paresthesias would not be available as warning signals [42, 56].
- Avoid paresthesias if possible.

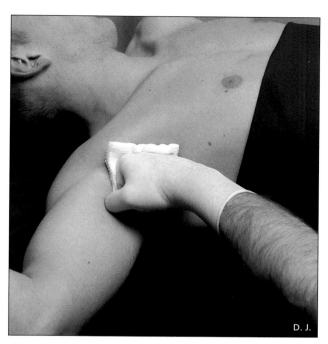

Fig. 7.29 Obligatory compression massage of the axilla

Dosage

Diagnostic
20 ml local anesthetic, e. g. 0.2 % ropivacaine, 0.125–0.25 % bupivacaine, 0.5 % prilocaine, 0.5 % mepivacaine.

Prophylactic
10–20 ml local anesthetic, e. g. 0.2–0.375 % ropivacaine, 0.125–0.25 % bupivacaine.

Therapeutic
10 ml local anesthetic, e. g. 0.2–0.375 % ropivacaine or 0.125–0.25 % bupivacaine, in diabetic and other neuropathies and in rheumatic diseases.
10–15 ml local anesthetic, e. g. 0.2 % ropivacaine or 0.125 % bupivacaine, in wrist arthrosis.
10–20 ml local anesthetic, e. g. 0.375 % ropivacaine or 0.25 % bupivacaine, in post-amputation pain, in status after surgical neurolysis and in post-herpetic neuralgia.
20 ml local anesthetic, e. g. 0.2–0.375 % ropivacaine or 0.25–0.375 % bupivacaine, in complex regional pain syndrome (CRPS) types I and II.
20 ml local anesthetic, e. g. 0.75 % ropivacaine or 0.5 % bupivacaine, in severe arteriospasm, e. g. after accidental intra-arterial injection of thiopental.

Surgical
40 ml local anesthetic, e. g. 0.75 % ropivacaine or 0.5 % bupivacaine.
A combination of 0.75 % ropivacaine or 0.5 % bupivacaine with 1 % prilocaine or 1 % mepivacaine has proved its value in practice (in our own experience).
According to De Jong [8, 9, 10], **42 ml** local anesthetic is required to reach the musculocutaneous and axillary nerves as well. Other authors report the use of 30–50 ml. There are various views regarding the additional administration of opioids [12, 20].

Distribution of the block
After onset of the full effect – the latency period can be up to 30 minutes in the axillary block – the anesthesia completely covers the arm below the elbow and the hand, as well as considerable parts of the upper arm (Fig. 7.30).

Block series
A series of blocks usually comprises 8–12 treatments. When there is noticeable improvement in the symptoms, further blocks can also be carried out (see case reports, pp. 82–85).

Side effects
- Hematoma formation due to puncture of the axillary artery. Note the obligatory prophylactic compression.

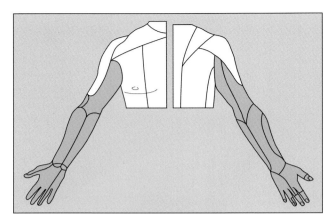

Fig. 7.30 The most frequently blocked nerve areas after axillary access, 15 minutes after initiating the block with bupivacaine [19]

> The patient must be prepared for these adverse effects during the patient information procedure.

Complications

Neural injury

Traumatic neural injury is a rare complication. It can be caused by the use of sharp needles (lesions due to nerve puncture), by intraneural or microvascular injury (hematoma and its sequelae), prolonged ischemia or by toxic effects of intraneurally injected local anesthetics [25, 38]. If functional neurological disturbances occur after surgical interventions, the following causes should be considered:

- Incorrect positioning of the arm during the operation (pressure, extension, rough manipulation).
- Direct surgical trauma.
- Injury due to ischemia (blockage), manifesting as postoperative myalgia [42].
- Inadequate attention during postoperative care, particularly with regard to the positioning of the anesthetized arm. After the administration of long-term local anesthetics, paresthesias have been described with poor postoperative positioning [49]. Patients must be given the relevant information, especially in outpatient procedures.

From the anesthesiological point of view, the following points should be taken into account:

Prophylaxis

- Only needles with short-beveled tips should be used. During the injection, the needle should be introduced parallel to the nerve.
- Intraneural positioning of the needle should be excluded. If the patient reports severe pain during the injection, it should be interrupted at once and the needle should be withdrawn.
- Vasopressor additives should be avoided. They are rarely indicated – and are even contraindicated for pain therapy – and may cause prolonged ischemia. They are also contraindicated in hypertonia, hyperthyroidism and arrhythmia [39, 40].
  In particular, reactions to epinephrine (restlessness, tachycardia, arrhythmia) may be confused with signs of overdosage of local anesthetic.
- Avoid supplementation. An incomplete plexus block should not be supplemented with other additional peripheral nerve blocks, since this would mean paresthesias would not be available as warning signals [42, 56].

Immediate documentation

In every nerve block, the following should be documented:

- Approach.
- Needle type.
- Local anesthetic used and additives, if any.
- Description of the paresthesias elicited.
- Any vascular puncture or injection pain.
- Hematoma formation.
- Any supplementation.
- Episodes of ischemia.

Diagnosis and treatment

When there is the slightest suspicion of neurological injury, a detailed examination should be carried out and the diagnosis should be made by a neurologist. In the axillary plexus block, the median and ulnar nerves are the ones most often affected. The prognosis is generally very good here. With neurological treatment and physiotherapy, restoration of function takes a few days up to a maximum of one year ("tincture of time") [38, 42, 49, 51, 52].

Intravascular injection

There is a particular risk of injection into the axillary artery or axillary vein [14]. For symptoms and treatment, see Chap. 4, pp. 42, 43.

Prophylaxis: During slow injection, aspiration should be repeated after each 4–5 ml.

CNS intoxication
In very rare cases, overdosage of local anesthetic, fast resorption of it at the injection site or inadvertent intravascular injection can lead to toxic reactions. These develop in the course of ca. 20 minutes after the injection or much more quickly with intravascular administration.

░ Early symptoms include a numb sensation on the lips and tongue, a metallic taste, sleepiness, vertigo, ringing in the ears, auditory disturbances, visual disturbances, slurred speech, muscular trembling and nystagmus.

░ Generalized tonic-clonic seizures are the most dangerous cerebral complication, but these do not lead to brain damage or death of the patient provided immediate and correct treatment is given. For therapeutic procedure in CNS intoxication, see Chap. 4, p. 43.

Pseudoaneurysm
░ Formation of a pseudoaneurysm of the axillary artery [15, 30, 59], accompanied by postoperative paresthesias and plexus paralysis.

Continuous axillary block

Indications
Prophylactic
░ Postoperative analgesia.
░ Prevention or reduction of post-amputation pain. It is recommended to start the continuous block two to three days before the planned intervention, if possible.

Therapeutic
░ After reimplantation.
░ Poor perfusion of the upper extremity.
░ Arterial occlusive disease.
░ Edema after radiotherapy (with additional corticoids).
░ Post-amputation pain (in acute pain).
░ Pain caused by trauma.

Surgical
░ This is the method of choice as a continuous [24, 36, 37, 44] or single block in all general, vascular, neurosurgical or orthopedic interventions and manipulations in the arm below the elbow and in the hand region.

Specific and relative contraindications
The contraindications correspond to those for the single block.

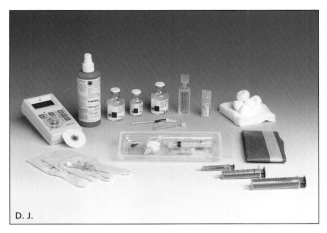
Fig. 7.31 Materials

Procedure

This block should only be carried out by experienced anesthetists.

> Continuous administration requires continuous monitoring, daily checking of the catheter position, daily exchange of the bacterial filter and dressing, as well as an obligatory test dose before every subsequent injection.

Preparations
(See the section on the interscalene block, p. 61)

Materials (Fig. 7.31)
Stimuplex HNS 11 nerve stimulator (B. Braun Melsungen). Syringes (2 ml, 10 ml, 20 ml), catheter set (e. g. Contiplex D, plastic indwelling catheter 1.3 × 55 mm (15°), e. g. B. Braun Melsungen), drape, hemostylet, disinfectant, bacterial filters, cooled physiological saline.

Skin prep
In all blocks.

Patient positioning
As for the single block.

Landmarks and location of the injection site
The anatomical orientation, with high proximal palpation and fixing of the axillary artery, are as for the single block.

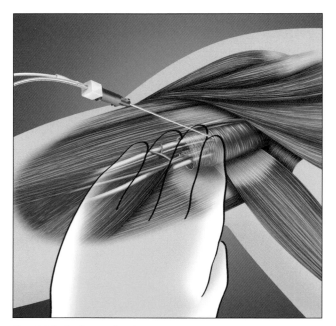

Fig. 7.32 Outlet angle of 30°

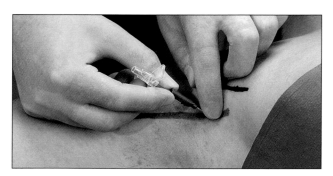

Fig. 7.33 Reaching the neurovascular sheath

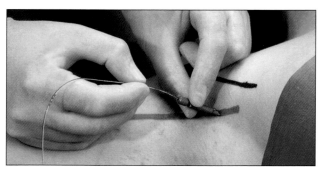

Fig. 7.34 Introducing the catheter

Injection technique
After careful skin prep of the axilla and draping, the skin is infiltrated immediately above the fixed artery. The skin is incised at the infiltration site and the needle is introduced at an outlet angle of ca. 30° proximally in the direction of the neurovascular sheath. To avoid vascular and neural injury, the needle should be advanced as slowly as possible and its cut angle should be turned towards the axillary artery (Fig. 7.32).

Needle position
"Fascial clicks" and the loss of resistance technique [26] or electrical neurostimulation [33] can be used to confirm that the neurovascular sheath has been reached and that the needle is positioned within the fascial compartment.

Introducing the catheter
When the injection needle is securely positioned in the neurovascular sheath, the metal stylet is fixed and the teflon capillary is advanced over the stylet as far as the mark. For this purpose the needle is lowered to ca. 10–20°, to allow it to be advanced parallel to the artery as much as possible (Fig. 7.33).
After removal of the stylet and aspiration at various levels, 5 ml of cold physiological saline is injected via the teflon cannula. Any paresthesia and low resistance during the injection in particular, will confirm correct positioning in the neurovascular sheath.
The catheter is introduced through the existing cannula as far as the 10-cm mark if possible (mark II), so as to avoid possible later dislocation (Fig. 7.34).

Injection of the local anesthetic
After removal of the plastic indwelling catheter, fixation of the catheter and placement of a bacterial filter and after careful aspiration and injection of a test dose, bolus administration of the local anesthetic is carried out.

Dosage [5, 24, 36, 44]
The choice and dosage of the local anesthetic depend on the goal of treatment:
- Anesthesia for surgery with subsequent pain therapy.
- Analgesia for mobilization treatment.
- Sympatholytic treatment in peripheral perfusion disturbances.

Initial bolus administration
Test dose: 3–5 ml local anesthetic, e. g. 0.375–0.75 % ropivacaine or 0.25–0.5 % bupivacaine.
Bolus administration: 20–40 ml local anesthetic, e. g. 0.375–0.75 % ropivacaine or 0.25–0.5 % bupivacaine.

Maintenance dose

Individual adjustment of the dosage and period of treatment is absolutely necessary. The following information therefore only serves for general guidance.

Intermittent administration
Every five to six hours, 5–10 ml local anesthetic, e. g. 0.5–0.75 % ropivacaine or 0.25–0.5 % bupivacaine, after a prior test dose. Reduction of the dosage and/or dosage intervals depending on the clinical picture.

Continuous infusion
Infusion of the local anesthetic via the plexus catheter should be started ca. one hour after the bolus administration. A test dose is obligatory. The following dosages have proved their value:
6–14 ml/h 0.2 % ropivacaine,
8–18 ml/h (usually 10–14 ml) 0.125 % bupivacaine or:
4–16 ml/h (usually 8–10 ml) 0.25 % bupivacaine.

If necessary, the infusion can be supplemented with bolus doses of 5–10 ml 0.5–0.75 % ropivacaine or 0.25–0.5 % bupivacaine.

Side effects and complications

- Hematoma formation due to puncture of the axillary artery.
- Formation of a pseudoaneurysm on the axillary artery [15, 30, 59], accompanied by postoperative paresthesias and plexus paralysis.
- Traumatic neural injury (extremely rare).
- Intravascular injection into the axillary artery or axillary vein [14] (extremely rare).
- CNS intoxication (very rare) due to overdosage of the local anesthetic, fast resorption of it at the injection site or inadvertent intravascular injection.
- Bacterial colonization of the catheter, with or without local or systemic infection. Prophylaxis: daily exchange of the bacterial filter, limitation of the period of catheter placement [24, 44].
- Catheter dislocation.
- Catheter leakage, particularly at infusion speeds of more than 15 ml/h.

Record and checklist

Axillary block of the brachial plexus

Block no.   ☐ Right   ☐ Left

Name: _____ Date: _____

Diagnosis: _____

Premedication: ☐ No   ☐ Yes _____

Neurological abnormalities: ☐ No

                ☐ Yes (which?) _____

Purpose of block: ☐ *Diagnosis*   ☐ *Treatment*

Needle: ☐ *24 G, short-beveled tip 45°*   ☐ *0.55 × 25 mm*   ☐ *0.55 × 50 mm*

                                          ☐ *Other:* _____

i. v. access: ☐ *Yes*

Monitoring: ☐ *ECG*   ☐ *Pulse oximetry*

Ventilation facilities: ☐ *Yes (equipment checked)*

Emergency equipment *(drugs):*   ☐ *Checked*

Patient: ☐ *Informed*   ☐ *Consent*

Position: ☐ *Supine*   ☐ *Upper arm abducted (90–100°)*

Puncture technique: ☐ *Perivascular*   ☐ *Paresthesias*

                      ☐ *Transarterial*   ☐ *Electrostimulation*

Local anesthetic: _____ *ml* _____ % _____

(incremental)

Addition to

injected solution: ☐ *No*   ☐ *Yes* _____

Patient's remarks during injection:

☐ *None*   ☐ *Paresthesias*   ☐ *Warmth*

☐ *Pain caused (intraneural positioning?)* _____

Neural area _____

Objective block effect after 15 min:

☐ *Cold test*   ☐ *Temperature measurement right* ____ °C *left* ____ °C

☐ *Sensory*   ☐ *Motor*

Monitoring after block: ☐ *< 1 h*   ☐ *> 1 h*

                       Time of discharge: _____

Complications: ☐ *None*   ☐ *Toxic signs*

☐ *Hematoma*   ☐ *Neurological injury (median, ulnar, radial nerve)*

Subjective effects of block: *Duration:* _____

☐ *None*   ☐ *Increased pain*

☐ *Reduced pain*   ☐ *No pain*

VISUAL ANALOG SCALE

| 0 | 10 | 20 | 30 | 40 | 50 | 60 | 70 | 80 | 90 | 100 |

Special notes:

_____

_____

_____

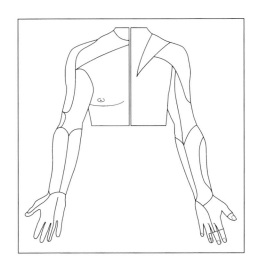

Plexus catheter in outpatients?

The catheter technique also allows plexus anesthesia to be used in operations lasting longer than the usual period of effect of local anesthetics. Independently of the surgical technique, postoperative blood perfusion disturbances almost always occur, particularly after microsurgical interventions – partly due to the body's reaction to the invasive procedure.

With continuous sympatholysis, the catheter technique allows substantial improvement in the perfusion of the operated arm. Continuous administration of local anesthetics and the consequent postoperative analgesia allow adequate physiotherapy and therefore speedy mobilization of the operated arm.

In *in-patients,* continuous plexus block for appropriate indications is also an excellent anesthesiological procedure in the context of acute analgesic therapy and sympatholysis. However, here in particular the continuous method requires constant monitoring and checking that the technique is successful. This includes in particular:

- Daily checking of the catheter position, to ensure early recognition of intravascular dislocation or dislocation of the catheter from the neurovascular sheath.
- Daily exchanging of the bacterial filter and dressing, to keep the risk of bacterial colonization of the catheter and the associated risk of infection as low as possible.
- The need for continuous monitoring of the effectiveness of the block and for adjustment of the local anesthetic dosage if necessary, makes self-administration by the patient impossible.

In *outpatient* pain therapy, the use of a catheter for continuous plexus anesthesia is therefore rare and it is only possible with very cooperative patients.

Additional reasons why the present author has for many years preferred single injections in the context of block series are as follows:

- At the beginning of the therapy, the period of treatment that will be needed is often difficult to estimate and may extend (as the cases described on the following pages show) for two or three months. The frequency of treatment necessary during this period is more easily determined using single injections.
- Although complication-free catheter placement for two to three weeks (or up to seven weeks in individual cases) has been reported in the literature [26], this is not sufficient and is associated with too many risks in outpatients.
- The goal of pain-therapy blocks, e. g. in complex regional pain syndrome, is to allow physiotherapy and intensive exercise at home for the patient.

Many patients find the catheter disturbing (with irritation and a foreign-body sensation) or even obstructive and there is a risk of inadvertent dislocation.

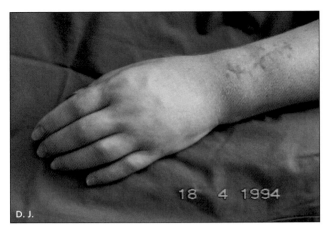

Fig. 7.35 Condition at admission on 18 April 1994

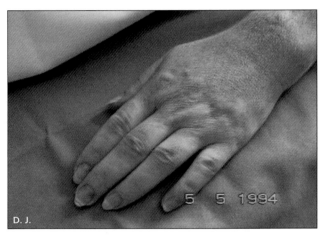

Fig. 7.36 Condition after 10 axillary blocks, physiotherapy and intensive home exercise

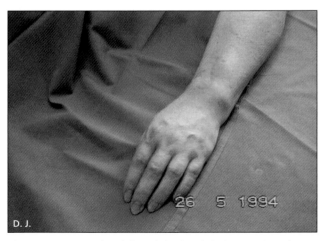

Fig. 7.37 Improved mobility of the hand during continued treatment

Example cases of axillary block of the brachial plexus

Case 1

Total number of blocks: 17.

Patient W.M., a 44-year-old woman
Post forearm osteosynthesis. After two months of unsuccessful treatment, including calcitonin therapy, the patient was referred to our outpatient pain department.

Findings on admission, 18 April 1994
Development of puffy edema (hand and distal part of the forearm), extreme pain when moving the hand, physiotherapy impossible (Fig. 7.35).

Therapy
Starting on the day of presentation, a three-week series of 10 axillary plexus blocks in all (each dosage 20 ml 0.25 % bupivacaine). After the blocks, the patient received physiotherapy and carried out intensive exercise at home [32, 48].
Due to marked improvement in the symptoms (Fig. 7.36), treatment was continued. During the subsequent three weeks, the patient received four blocks at a reduced dosage (10 ml 0.25 % bupivacaine), with the physiotherapy and home exercises continuing. The mobility of the hand was significantly improved with these measures (Fig. 7.37).
Treatment was concluded with three blocks, again at a reduced dosage (10 ml 0.125 % bupivacaine).

Final findings, 6 July 1994
Complete disappearance of symptoms.

Case 2
Total number of blocks: 23.

Patient G.H., a 46-year-old woman
Radius fracture in the right arm on 16 January 1994; removal of the external fixation on 17 March 1994, with incorrect hand position and development of puffy edema (hand and distal part of the forearm). After three months of unsuccessful treatment, the patient was referred to our outpatient pain department as therapy-resistant.

Findings on admission, 18 April 1994
Development of puffy edema, extreme pain, movement of the hand impossible, physiotherapy impossible (Fig. 7.38).

Therapy
Starting on the day of presentation, a three-week series of 10 axillary plexus blocks (each dosage 20 ml 0.25 % bupivacaine). Following the blocks, the patient received physiotherapy and carried out intensive exercises at home [32, 48].
Due to marked improvement in the mobility of the hand (Fig. 7.39) and a 60 % reduction in pain, the treatment was continued after 5 May 1994. During the subsequent three weeks, the patient received five blocks at a reduced dosage (10 ml 0.25 % bupivacaine). Physiotherapy and home exercise were continued and the pain reduction was increased up to 80 % (Fig. 7.40).
Treatment was concluded with a further eight blocks (with reduction of the dosage to 10 ml 0.125 % bupivacaine).

Final findings, 11 July 1994
Complete resolution of the edema, reduced pain and improvement in the mobility of the hand by more than 80 % (Fig. 7.41). Partial contractions in the area of the little finger and ring finger. The patient was able to return to work.

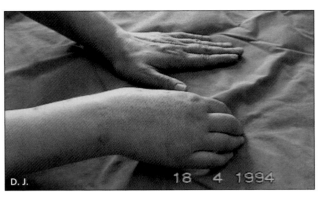

Fig. 7.38 Patient G.H. at admission

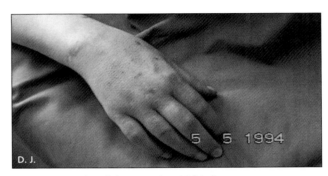

Fig. 7.39 Results of therapy after 10 blocks

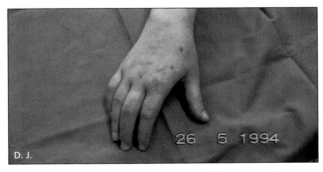

Fig. 7.40 Condition after a further five axillary plexus blocks

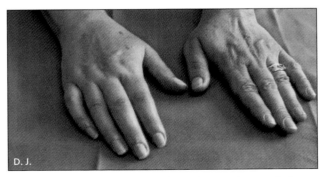

Fig. 7.41 Final findings on 11 July 1994: complete resolution of the edema. Pain reduction and increased mobility of the hand by more than 80 %

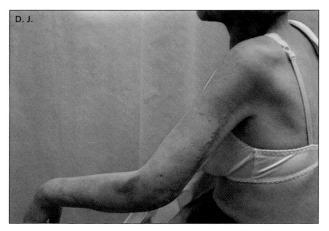

Fig. 7.42 Admission on 16 January 1995

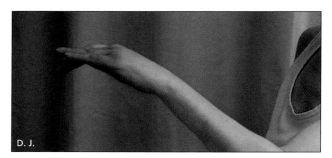

Fig. 7.43 Condition after six axillary blocks on 6 March 1995: resolution of the edema, partial mobility of the wrist

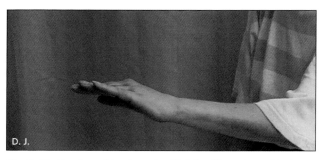

Fig. 7.44 Continued treatment with 15 axillary plexus blocks and continuing improvement in symptoms

Case 3

Total number of blocks: 29 (including four stellate blocks and four cervicobrachial plexus blocks).

Patient S.G., a 47-year-old woman
Humerus fracture after a bicycle accident on 28 September 1994. Emergency operation (with osteosynthesis). Wrist-drop with severe injury to the radial nerve and injury to the median nerve. Development of causalgia. On 6 December 1994, neurolysis of the radial nerve with subsequent deterioration in symptoms and edema formation. Three and a half months after the accident, the patient was referred to our outpatient pain department as therapy-resistant (calcitonin, antidepressants, physiotherapy) with a prognosis of "hopeless."

Findings on admission, 16 January 1995
In addition to the symptoms described above, there was the characteristic clinical picture of "frozen shoulder." Access to the axilla was therefore not possible in this patient (Fig. 7.42).

Therapy
At the patient's request, the calcitonin treatment and antidepressant administration were terminated. During the first three weeks, the patient received four blocks of the cervicothoracic (stellate) ganglion, followed by four blocks of the cervicobrachial plexus. There was no improvement in the original symptoms. However, the mobility of the shoulder improved sufficiently to allow partial abduction of the arm, making it possible to carry out axillary plexus blocks.

On 15 February 1995, a three-week series of six axillary blocks of the brachial plexus was started (each dosage 20 ml 0.25 % bupivacaine).

Following the blocks, this very cooperative patient received physiotherapy and carried out intensive exercise at home [32, 48]. On 6 March 1995 (Fig. 7.43), her condition had already clearly improved: the edema had resolved and the wrist was partly mobile.

Treatment was continued with a further 15 blocks (each dosage reduced to 10 ml 0.25 % bupivacaine). The constant neurological follow-up confirmed increasing improvement in the reinnervation of the hand.

Physiotherapy and home exercises were continued, the mobility of the hand continually increased and the pain declined (Fig. 7.44).

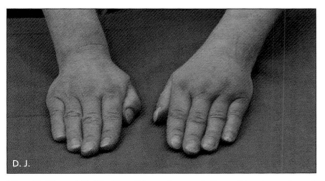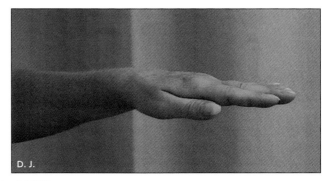

D. J.   D. J.

Figs. 7.45 and 7.46 Condition at completion of treatment on 25 April 1995

Final findings, 25 April 1995

Complete resolution of the edema and "frozen shoulder." Almost complete absence of pain, mobility of the hand restored to about 85 % (Figs. 7.45 and 7.46). The neurological follow-up showed 80 % recovery.

In March 1996, some of the osteosynthesis material was removed.

Interscalene, subclavian perivascular and axillary blocks of the brachial plexus: advantages and disadvantages

Interscalene block

Advantages

▨ Clear anatomical landmarks: interscalene groove, sternocleidomastoid muscle, transverse process (C6). Can therefore be carried out even with distorted anatomy, e. g. in obese patients.

▨ Cooperation by the patient is not absolutely necessary.

▨ No special positioning of the arm is required.

▨ Technically simple procedure.

▨ Due to proximal injection at the level of C6, most of the plexus is anesthetized and the block can be carried out even in cases of infection or malignant disease in the arm region. In addition, the caudal parts of the cervical plexus are included.

▨ Surgery and pain treatment are possible in the whole region of the shoulder and upper arm.

▨ Subsequent intraoperative injections are possible in extended interventions.

▨ The risk of pneumothorax is very low. The needle is advanced at an adequate distance from the pleural cupula.

Disadvantages

▨ It is necessary to produce paresthesias.

▨ The region of the ulnar nerve is not always adequately anesthetized.

▨ The potential complications – although these are extremely rare – include: Neural injury, epidural or subarachnoid injection, intravascular injection, CNS intoxication.

Subclavian perivascular block

Advantages

▨ Clear anatomical landmarks: caudal part of the interscalene groove, subclavian artery, midpoint of the clavicle.

▨ Injection of the local anesthetic is possible without repositioning the upper extremity.

▨ There is no risk of subarachnoid or epidural injection, nor of puncturing the vertebral artery.

▨ Infections in the arm region do not represent a contraindication to this technique.

Disadvantages

▨ Risk of pneumothorax.

▨ Puncture of the subclavian artery is possible.

▨ Very rarely, applying a tourniquet requires additional block of the intercostobrachial nerve (T2) and medial brachial cutaneous nerve.

▨ No application in pain therapy.

Axillary block

Advantages

- Clear anatomical landmarks: axillary artery.
- Easily carried out due to the superficial position of the neurovascular sheath. Can also be used in children and in patients with pulmonary problems or renal insufficiency (applying an arteriovenous shunt).
- Also applicable as a continuous block.
- A safe method of anesthesia for surgery and pain therapy measures, particularly in the forearm and hand.
- The following complications and side effects are excluded: pneumothorax, epidural or subarachnoid injection, concomitant anesthetization of the vagus, phrenic and recurrent laryngeal nerves or of the stellate ganglion.
- This is the method of choice for outpatients and emergency patients.

Disadvantages

- Abduction of the upper arm is required.
- The anesthesia is not sufficient for interventions in the shoulder or upper arm.
- The musculocutaneous nerve and/or axillary nerve are often not adequately anesthetized.
- Extremely rare, but possible complications are: neural injury, intravascular injection and CNS intoxication.

8 Suprascapular nerve

Anatomy

The suprascapular nerve receives fibers from the fifth and sixth cervical spinal nerves. It branches off from the superior trunk of the brachial plexus (Fig. 8.1) and courses through the supraclavicular fossa along the lateral edge of the plexus as far as the scapular notch. It enters the supraspinous fossa through the notch. Covered by the supraspinatus muscle, the suprascapular nerve passes to the neck of the scapula and under the transverse scapular ligament to the infraspinous fossa. It supplies the supraspinatus and infraspinatus muscles, and sends off fibers to the shoulder and acromioclavicular joint, as well as to the suprascapular vessels (Fig. 8.2).

Blocks of the suprascapular nerve

Indications
Diagnostic
- Painful conditions in the shoulder region and shoulder joint.

Therapeutic
- Rheumatic and degenerative diseases of the shoulder girdle.
- "Frozen shoulder", pseudoparetic shoulder, stiff shoulder (mobilization in shoulder ankylosis).
- Humeroscapular periarthritis after mechanical stress on the soft-tissue structures in the shoulder girdle, after immobilization of an arm, trauma, or surgery.
- Hemiplegia (shoulder-arm pain, increased load on the supraspinatus muscle or subluxation of the shoulder joint are reported in ca. 70 % of cases).
- Tumor pain in the area of the shoulder girdle (the catheter technique is preferable here, even when the treatment time is restricted). The block cannot replace oral medication, but is supportive.
- Post-herpetic neuralgia.

Specific contraindications
Anticoagulant treatment.

Procedure

Preparations
Check that the emergency equipment is complete and in working order. Sterile precautions, intravenous access, intubation kit, emergency medication.

Materials
5-ml syringe, 10-ml syringe, 22-G needle (5 cm or 7 cm), swabs, disinfectant (Fig. 8.3).

Skin prep
In all blocks.

Patient positioning
Sitting, with the neck tilted forward comfortably (so-called "pharaoh posture").

Landmarks
Acromion, spine of scapula (Fig. 8.4). A line is drawn along the course of the spine of the scapula between the acromion and the medial edge of the shoulder blade. A second line parallel to the line of the spinous processes of the vertebrae transects the connecting line. The injection site lies about 2.5–3 cm cranial to the intersection of the two straight lines (Fig. 8.5).

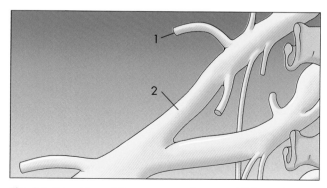

Fig. 8.1 Branching of the suprascapular nerve (1) from the superior trunk of the brachial plexus (2)

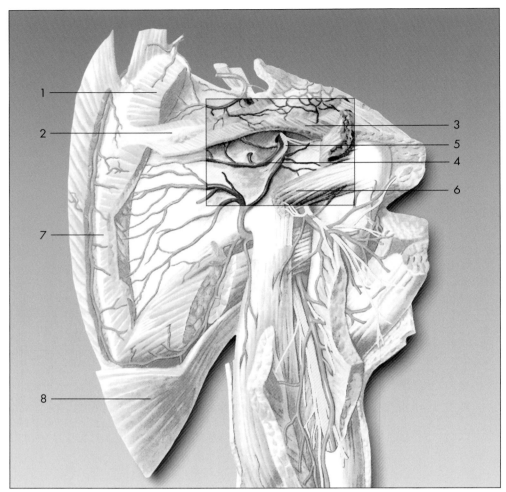

Fig. 8.2 Anatomy:
(1) supraspinatus muscle,
(2) spine of scapula,
(3) deltoid muscle,
(4) suprascapular artery,
(5) suprascapular nerve,
(6) teres minor muscle,
(7) infraspinatus muscle,
(8) latissimus dorsi muscle

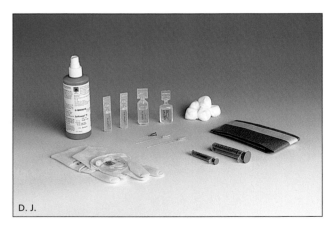

Fig. 8.3 Materials

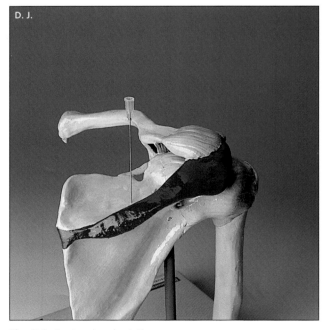

Fig. 8.4 Anatomic orientation

Injection technique

After skin prep, a needle 5 cm or 7 cm long, depending on the patient's anatomy, is slowly advanced perpendicular to the skin surface in the direction of the scapular notch (Fig. 8.6).

Depending on the anatomy, bone contact is made after 3.5–5 cm. The needle is then corrected medially and laterally, until the scapular notch is reached.

After careful aspiration, the local anesthetic is slowly injected; aspiration must be repeated during the injection.

> During the injection, the patient experiences an aching sensation in the upper arm and shoulder joint. Targeted elicitation of paresthesias is not necessary, but they may occur unintentionally.

Dosage

Diagnostic

5 ml local anesthetic, e. g. 1 % prilocaine or 1 % mepivacaine.

Therapeutic

5–10 ml local anesthetic, e. g. 0.75 % ropivacaine or 0.5 % bupivacaine.

In acute conditions, 2 mg dexamethasone can be added in each of the first and second blocks.

Combination with a block of the subscapular nerve is possible, and often desirable (see Chap. 9).

Block series

If there is a trend toward improvement after the first and second treatment, a series of six to eight blocks is useful in all indications.

Side effects

If the dosage is too high, transient weakness can occur in the supraspinatus and infraspinatus muscles, and outpatients in particular should be informed about this.

Complications

- Intravascular injection (suprascapular artery), extremely rare.
- Pneumothorax, extremely rare (Fig. 8.7).
  Prophylaxis: only advance the needle until bone contact is made.

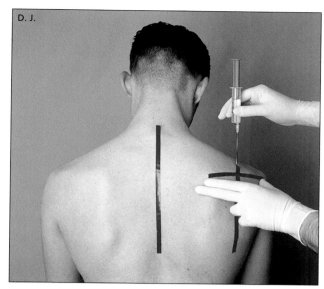

Fig. 8.5 Marking the injection site

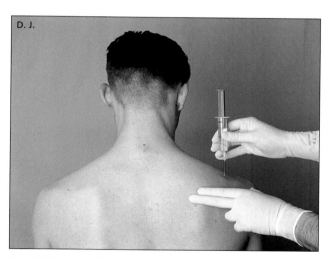

Fig. 8.6 Slow needle insertion in the direction of the scapular notch

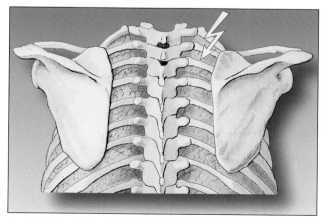

Fig. 8.7 To prevent pneumothorax, the needle should only be advanced until bone contact is made

9 Subscapular nerve blocks
Infiltration of subscapular muscle trigger points ("frozen shoulder")

Anatomy

The subscapular nerves consist of two or three nerves emerging from various parts of the brachial plexus for the subscapular, teres major, and latissimus dorsi muscles. The longest and most important of these is the thoracodorsal nerve, which runs along the axillary border of the scapula and supplies the latissimus dorsi muscle (Figs. 9.1 and 9.2).

The superior subscapular nerve emerges from C5 and C6 (C7), and enters the subscapular muscle. The medial subscapular nerve (C5–6) arises from the posterior secondary trunks and supplies the lateral lower part of the subscapular muscle and teres major muscle.

The inferior subscapular nerve (thoracodorsal nerve) is the largest in this group. It arises from the posterior secondary branches or from the axillary nerve, or more rarely from the radial nerve, and passes along the lateral edge of the scapula to the latissimus dorsi muscle.

Indications and contraindications

(See Chap. 8, p. 87)

Procedure

Preparations
Check that the emergency equipment is complete and in working order; sterile precautions, intravenous access.

Materials (Fig. 9.3)
Fine 2.5-cm long 26-G needle for local anesthesia, 7-cm long 20-G needle (with the needle shaft angled by about 20°), local anesthetic, disinfectant, swabs, 2 ml and 10 ml syringes.

Technique
Position
Sitting, with the neck comfortably tilted and the shoulders relaxed.

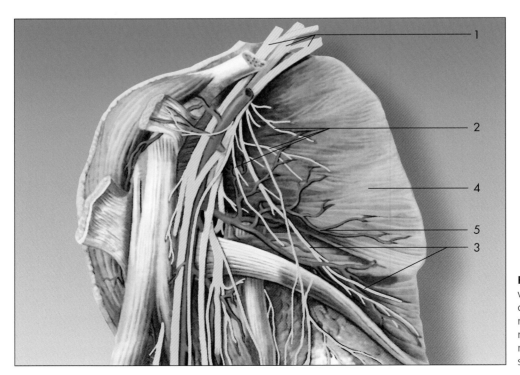

Fig. 9.1 Anatomy (anterior view): (1) cords of the brachial plexus, (2) subscapular nerve, (3) thoracodorsal nerve, (4) subscapular muscle, (5) circumflex scapular artery

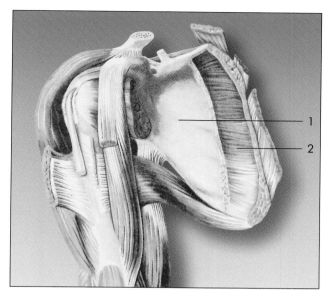

Fig. 9.2 Anatomy. (1) Subscapular fossa, (2) subscapular muscle

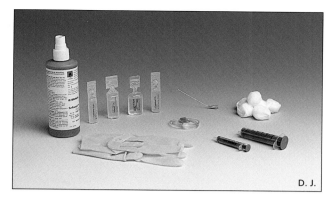

Fig. 9.3 Materials

Location (Fig. 9.4)
- The patient's ipsilateral arm is pulled back, so that the contours of the scapula are easily recognized.
- The center of the medial border of the scapula is marked as the injection point.
- Acromion.

Skin prep, local anesthesia, drawing up the local anesthetic, testing the injection needle for patency.

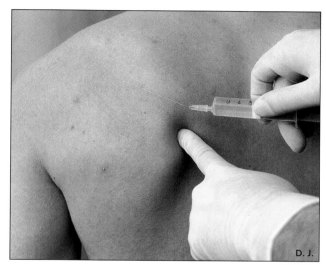

Fig. 9.4 Location. Marking the injection site (center of the medial border of the scapula)

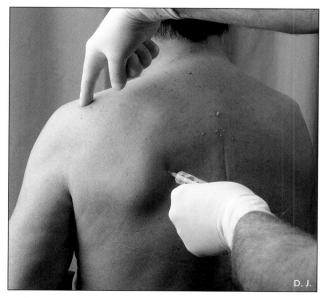

Fig. 9.5 Introducing the needle in the direction of the acromion

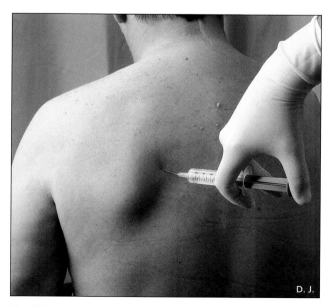

Fig. 9.6 Injection

91

Injection technique

- ▨ Introduce the 20° angled needle into the center of the medial border of the scapula, in the direction of the acromion (Fig. 9.5).
- ▨ The needle is introduced subscapularly parallel to the skin surface between the front surface of the scapula (costal surface) and the posterior thoracic wall (ribs), into the subscapular fossa (Fig. 9.2). If the needle meets the edge of the ribs, it is withdrawn as far as the subcutis and reintroduced.
- ▨ At a depth of 4 cm, then 5 cm and finally 6 cm – depending on the anatomy – a total of 10 ml local anesthetic is then injected after prior aspiration (Fig. 9.6).

The signs of a successful injection are: spread extending into the shoulder joint, upper arm, and often as far as the wrist, corresponding to the radiation pattern of the trigger points of the subscapular muscle [6].

Dosage

Diagnostic
5 ml local anesthetic, e. g. 1 % prilocaine or 1 % mepivacaine.

Therapeutic
10–15 ml local anesthetic, e. g. 0.5–0.75 % ropivacaine, 0.25–0.5 % bupivacaine. In acute pain, the addition of 4 mg dexamethasone has proved useful.

In our own experience, this block is superior to blocking the suprascapular nerve. A combination of the two techniques is possible, and often desirable.

Block series

In all indications, a series of six to eight blocks is useful, if an improvement trend is seen after the first and second treatments.

Side effects

If the dosage is too high, transient weakness may occur in the shoulder and upper arm region. Outpatients should be informed about this.

Complications

When the technique is carried out correctly: none.

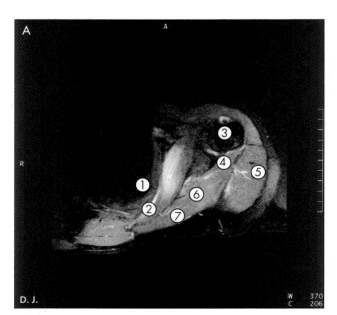 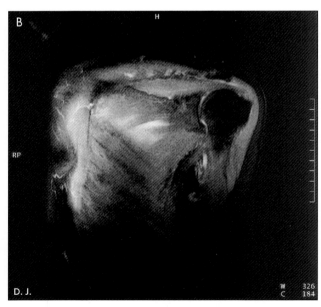

Fig. 9.7 A, B Magnetic resonance images 10 minutes after injection of 10 ml ropivacaine without radiographic contrast medium into the subscapular fossa. **A** Axial (cross-section), **B** paracoronal.
(1) Thorax wall, (2) subscapular muscle and subscapular fossa, (3) head of the humerus, (4) teres minor muscle, (5) deltoid muscle, (6) scapula, (7) infraspinatus muscle

10 Peripheral nerve blocks in the elbow region

Ulnar nerve

The ulnar nerve originates from the medial cord of the brachial plexus (C8–T1, C7). The nerve courses on the medial side of the lower third of the upper arm, in the groove of the ulnar nerve on the posterior side of the medial epicondyle of the humerus.

The nerve is easily palpated at this location. In the forearm, it runs between the humeral and ulnar head of the flexor carpi ulnaris muscle on the inner side of the forearm.

Median nerve

The median nerve originates from the medial and lateral cords of the brachial plexus (C5, C6–C8, T1). At the elbow, it lies medial to the brachial artery, courses along the medial surface of the brachial muscle downwards in the elbow, where it can be found behind the bicipital aponeurosis and in front of the insertion of the brachial muscle and elbow joint.

Radial nerve and lateral antebrachial cutaneous nerve (musculocutaneous nerve)

These two nerves innervate the radial half of the forearm and the back of the hand, and have a close anatomical relationship.

The **radial nerve** (C5–C8, T1) is the longest branch of the brachial plexus, and represents a direct continuation of the posterior cord. It courses in the middle of the upper arm in the groove of the radial nerve along the dorsal side of the humerus. Before the lateral epicondyle of the humerus and the elbow joint capsule, it then enters the fissure between the brachioradialis muscle and the biceps muscle. At the level of the head of the radius, it divides into the deep branch (anterior interosseous nerve, mainly motor) and the superficial branch (mainly sensory). The latter follows the course of the radial artery.

Lateral antebrachial cutaneous nerve

The musculocutaneous nerve (C4, C5–C7) arises from the lateral cord of the brachial plexus. At the level of the elbow joint, it passes between the biceps muscle and the brachioradialis muscle to the brachial fascia, which it penetrates, becoming the lateral antebrachial cutaneous nerve.

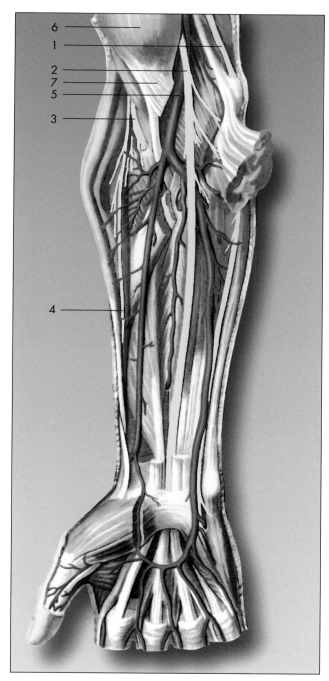

Fig. 10.1 Anatomy. (1) Ulnar nerve, (2) median nerve, (3) deep branch of the radial nerve (anterior interosseous nerve), (4) superficial branch of the radial nerve, (5) brachial artery, (6) biceps brachii muscle, (7) bicipital aponeurosis

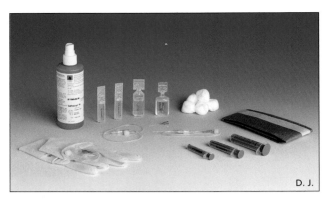

Fig. 10.2 Materials

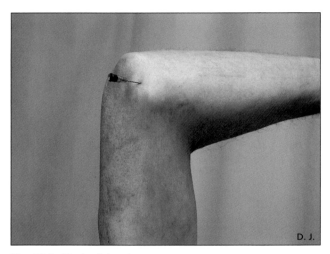

Fig. 10.3 Block of the ulnar nerve

Indications

Surgical
- Minor interventions in the innervated area.
- Supplementation of incomplete anesthesia of the brachial plexus.

> **Caution**
> Care must be taken to avoid neural injury, since paresthesias do not occur as a warning signal (see Chap. 7, p. 76).

Diagnostic
Differential diagnosis of painful conditions in the upper extremity.

Therapeutic
None.

Contraindications
Relative
- Local neuritis.
- Carpal tunnel syndrome (median nerve).

> **Caution**
> Distal blocks of the peripheral nerves of the arm are associated with a high incidence of neural injury (particularly the ulnar nerve). It is therefore advisable not to use these injections on a routine basis. During the injection, intraneural positioning of the needle must be excluded.

Procedure

Preparations
Check that the emergency equipment is complete and in working order; sterile precautions, intravenous access.

Materials (Fig. 10.2)
3.5–5 cm long atraumatic 25-G needle (15°), with injection lead ("immobile needle"), e. g. Stimuplex D (B. Braun Melsungen) or 24-G Plexufix needles, 2.5–5 cm long, local anesthetic, disinfectant, swabs, drape, syringes: 2, 5, and 10 ml.

Technique
Ulnar nerve (Fig. 10.3)
Positioning
Supine, with the arm rotated outward and the elbow bent to 90°.

Location
The medial epicondyle of the humerus and olecranon are palpated. The ulnar nerve runs in the groove of the ulnar nerve at a depth of 0.5–1 cm, and can usually be palpated.
Skin prep, local anesthesia, covering with a sterile drape, drawing up the local anesthetic, checking the patency of the needle and functioning of the nerve stimulator, attaching electrodes.

Injection
After definite localization of the groove of the ulnar nerve, the needle should be introduced using a skin spot ca. 1–2 cm above this point at an angle of 90° to the long axis of the humerus.
After paresthesias have been elicited and intraneural positioning of the needle has been excluded, withdraw the needle slightly and carry out a fan-shaped injection after aspiration.

Median nerve (Fig. 10.4)
Positioning
Supine, elbow joint extended.

Location
The intercondylar line is marked. Palpation of the brachial artery.

Injection technique
After palpation of the brachial artery, the needle is introduced through infiltrated skin, on the ulnar side of the artery. At a depth of 0.5–1 cm, paresthesias are elicited. After aspiration and exclusion of intraneural positioning of the needle, a fan-shaped injection is carried out.

Radial nerve and lateral antebrachial cutaneous nerve (musculocutaneous nerve) (Fig. 10.4)
These two nerves are closely related to one another anatomically, so that both can be blocked using this technique.

Positioning
Supine, elbow joint extended.

Location
Lateral humeral epicondyle, biceps tendon, brachioradial muscle.

Injection technique
At the level of the intercondylar line, the fissure between the brachioradial muscle and the biceps tendon is palpated. The needle is introduced through a spot about 2 cm lateral to the biceps tendon, in a proximal and lateral direction towards the lateral epicondyle.
After paresthesias are elicited, intraneural positioning has been excluded, and aspiration has been carried out, 5–8 ml of a local anesthetic are injected. After withdrawal of the needle, fan-shaped infiltration of 5 ml local anesthetic is carried out as far as the subcutaneous tissue.
If no paresthesias can be elicited, the needle is introduced as far as the lateral surface of the lateral humeral epicondyle, and after bone contact the first dose of 3–4 ml of the local anesthetic is injected. The needle is then withdrawn subcutaneously, and after altering the direction slightly medially the procedure is repeated two or three times. On each occasion, 2–3 ml of local anesthetic is injected. Finally, when withdrawing the needle, fan-shaped infiltration of 5 ml local anesthetic as far as the subcutaneous tissue is carried out.

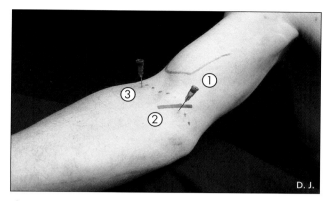

Fig. 10.4 Blocks of the median nerve and radial nerve.
(1) Median nerve, (2) brachial artery, (3) radial nerve

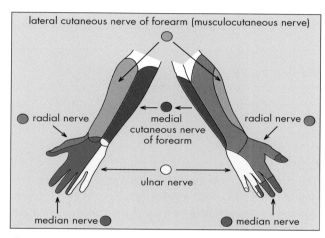

Fig. 10.5 Skin innervation

Dosage
Ulnar nerve: 2–5 ml local anesthetic.
Median nerve: 5 ml local anesthetic.
Radial nerve (and lateral antebrachial cutaneous nerve) 10–15 ml local anesthetic.

0.75 % ropivacaine
0.5 % bupivacaine
1 % prilocaine
1 % mepivacaine
1 % lidocaine

Skin innervation (Fig. 10.5)

Complications
Neuritis after nerve puncture (particularly in the ulnar nerve).

11 Peripheral nerve blocks in the wrist region

Ulnar nerve (Fig. 11.1)
In the medial distal third of the forearm, about 5 cm proximal to the wrist, the ulnar nerve divides into a sensory branch – the dorsal branch; and a mixed branch – the palmar branch. The latter runs along the tendon of the flexor carpi ulnaris muscle in a distal direction. The ulnar artery lies directly radially, alongside the nerve.

Median nerve (Fig. 11.1)
The median nerve lies between the tendons of the palmaris longus muscle and the flexor carpi radialis muscle. It courses in the direction of the long axis of the radius.

Radial nerve (Fig. 11.2)
The superficial branch of the radial nerve courses – together with the radial artery, initially – in the forearm along the medial side of the brachioradial muscle in the direction of the wrist. About 7–8 cm proximal to the wrist, it crosses under the tendon of the brachioradialis muscle and reaches the extensor side of the forearm. At the level of the wrist, the radial nerve divides into several peripheral branches.

Indications

Surgical
- Minor interventions in the innervated area.
- Supplementation in incomplete anesthetization of the brachial plexus.

Caution
Care must be taken to avoid neural injury, since paresthesias do not occur here as a warning signal (see Chap. 7, p. 76).

Diagnostic
Differential diagnosis of painful conditions in the hand.

Therapeutic
None.

Contraindications
Relative
Neuritis.

Procedure

Preparations
Check that the emergency equipment is complete and in working order; sterile precautions, intravenous access.

Materials (Fig. 11.3)
3.5–5 cm long atraumatic 25-G needle (15°), with injection lead, e. g. Stimuplex D (B. Braun Melsungen), exception: circular block of the radial nerve; fine 25-G needles, 2.5 cm long.
Local anesthetic, disinfectant, swabs, drape, syringes: 2, 5, and 10 ml.

Technique

Skin prep, local anesthesia, drawing up the local anesthetic, checking patency of the injection needle and functioning of the nerve stimulator, attaching electrodes.

Ulnar nerve (Fig. 11.4)
Positioning
Supine, with wrist slightly flexed.

Location
Styloid process of ulna, ulnar artery, flexor carpi ulnaris muscle.

Injection technique
Palmar branch: proximal to the styloid process of the ulna, the ulnar artery and tendon of the flexor carpi ulnaris muscle are palpated. The needle is introduced perpendicularly between the tendon and the artery, in the direction of the pisiform bone. After paresthesias have been elicited (1–2 cm), the needle is minimally withdrawn. After excluding intraneural positioning of the needle and aspiration, the needle is fixed and the local anesthetic is injected.
If no paresthesias can be elicited, the needle is advanced until bone contact is made, and 1 ml of local anesthetic is injected.
During withdrawal of the needle, fan-shaped infiltration is then carried out. A further 3–5 ml of the local anesthetic is used for this.
Dorsal branch: fan-shaped infiltration medial to the tendon of the flexor carpi ulnaris muscle, in the direction of the styloid process of the ulna.

Median nerve (Fig. 11.4)
Positioning
Supine, with the elbow stretched. The forearm musculature is tensed by making a fist, so that the muscular tendons become easily visible.

Location
Styloid process of the ulna, tendons of the palmaris longus and flexor carpi radialis muscles.

Injection technique
The needle is introduced perpendicularly at the level of the proximal bend of the wrist, through a skin spot between the tendons of the palmaris longus and flexor carpi radialis muscle. After paresthesias have been elicited (0.5–1 cm), the needle is minimally withdrawn, an intraneural location is excluded, and after aspiration the local anesthetic is injected.

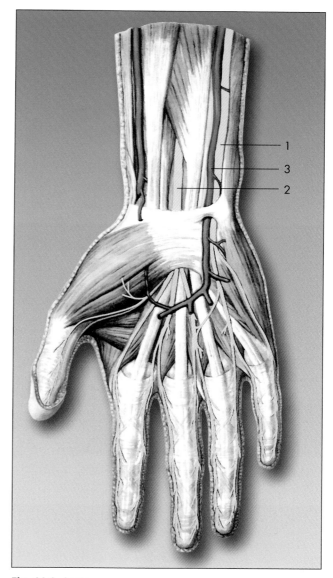

Fig. 11.1 Anatomy.
(1) Ulnar nerve, (2) median nerve, (3) ulnar artery

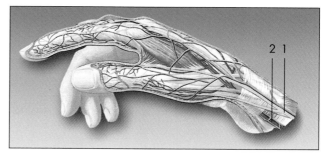

Fig. 11.2 Anatomy.
(1) Radial nerve (superficial branch), (2) radial artery

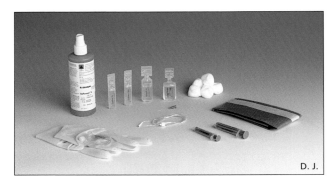

Fig. 11.3 Materials

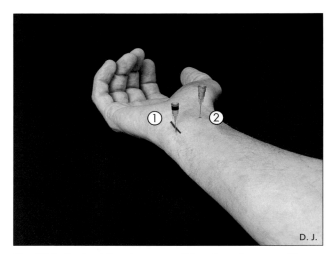

Fig. 11.4 Block of the ulnar nerve (1) and median nerve (2)

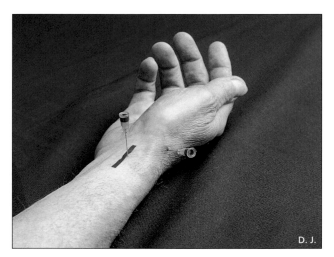

Fig. 11.5 Block of the radial nerve

Radial nerve (Fig. 11.5)
Positioning
Supine, with hand supinated.

Location
Level of the styloid process of the ulna, radial artery.

Injection technique
The needle is introduced through a skin spot perpendicular to the skin surface and lateral to the radial artery (0.5–1 cm). After paresthesias have been elicited, the needle is minimally withdrawn, an intraneural position is excluded, and after prior aspiration, the local anesthetic is injected. Supplementation of the block can be provided by subcutaneous infiltration of the peripheral branches between the extensor pollicis longus and brevis muscles on the dorsal side. It is helpful for the patient to extend the thumb.

Dosage
Ulnar nerve: 3–5 ml local anesthetic.
Median nerve: 3–5 ml local anesthetic.
Radial nerve: 5–8 ml local anesthetic.

0.75 % ropivacaine
0.5 % bupivacaine
1 % prilocaine
1 % mepivacaine
1 % lidocaine

Complications
Neuritis after puncture of a nerve.

12 Intravenous sympathetic block with guanethidine (Ismelin®)

Introduction

Guanethidine is an inhibitor substance that acts at the postganglionic sympathetic efferents. Its pharmacological effect is based on depleting norepinephrine stores, with consequent block of the reuptake of the transmitter for several days. The substance, also used as an antihypertensive drug, is much more effective for intravenous sympathetic block (microsympathectomy) than procaine, and is described as the "local anesthetic for the sympathetic nervous system" [2]. Other sympathetic blocking drugs have been used, such as reserpine or brotylium. There is controversy surrounding the need for guanethidine and whether it produces any useful effect.

Figures 12.1–12.3 show the most frequent areas of application for i.v. regional anesthesia.

Intravenous sympathetic block with guanethidine

Indications
Intravenous sympathetic block is a good alternative to stellate or plexus blocks when these are contraindicated or regional anesthesia cannot be used in patients receiving anticoagulant treatment.

Diagnostic
- Complex regional pain syndrome (CRPS).

Therapeutic
- Complex regional pain syndrome (CRPS) type I (sympathetic reflex dystrophy) and type II (causalgia).
- Perfusion disturbances in the extremities with burning pain, accompanied by hyperesthesia, hyperpathia, cold sensitivity.
- Postsympathectomy syndrome.
- Raynaud's disease.
- Ischemic ulcers.
- Diabetic angioneuropathy.
- Post-traumatic neuralgia [3].

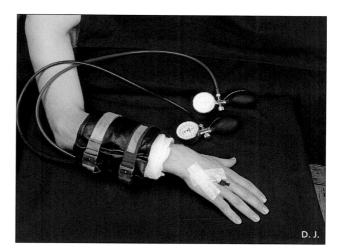

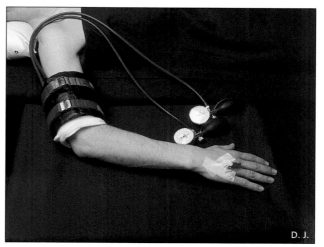

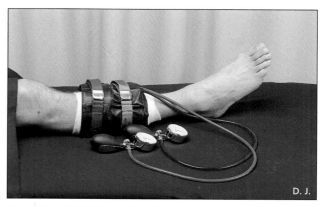

Figs. 12.1–12.3 Areas of application of i.v. regional anesthesia

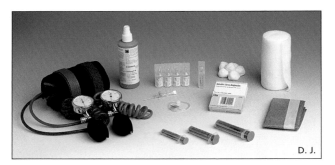

Fig. 12.4 Materials

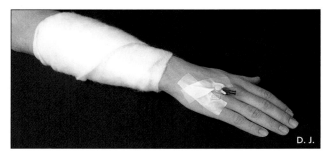

Fig. 12.5 The block area is wrapped

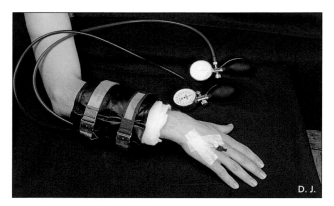

Fig. 12.6 Applying the cuff

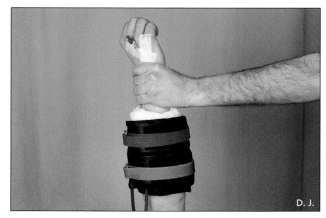

Fig. 12.7 Raising the extremity

Specific contraindications
Infected extremity.

Procedure

This block should only be carried out when full anesthesiological facilities are available.

Preparations
Check that the emergency equipment is complete and in working order. Sterile precautions. Two intravenous access points (healthy extremity and extremity being treated), BP and ECG monitoring, pulse oximetry, anesthetic machine.

Materials
5-ml syringe, 10-ml syringe, 20-ml syringe, 50-ml perfusion syringe, saline, cotton-wool cushioning, tourniquet (two-lumen with color-indicated proximal and distal parts), intubation kit, emergency drugs ready to hand, disinfectant (Fig. 12.4).

Skin prep
In all blocks.

Patient positioning
Supine, with the extremity free.

Technical procedure
  1. Place two plastic indwelling catheters, the first in a healthy extremity, and the second as distally as possible in the extremity being treated.
  2. Place the extremity being treated in a free position and bandage the block area for prophylaxis against neural injury (Fig. 12.5).
  3. Place the double-lumen cuff, with colored markers at the proximal and distal ends (Fig. 12.6).
  4. Raise the extremity for ca. 5 minutes and massage it (Fig. 12.7).
  5. Pump up the proximal cuff. The pressure must be ca. 100 mmHg higher than the patient's systolic blood pressure (Fig. 12.8). The change in the pulse wave amplitude is documented using a pulse oximeter.
  6. Place the extremity horizontally and inject 5 ml local anesthetic, e. g. 1 % mepivacaine, through the plastic indwelling catheter (Fig. 12.9). Administration of the local anesthetic serves to reduce both pressure pain and pain after guanethidine administration.

7. The distal cuff is then pumped up. Here again, the pressure must be ca. 100 mmHg higher than the patient's systolic blood pressure. The distal cuff now lies in the anesthetized area, and the cuff pressure is better tolerated. Release the proximal cuff. Inject the guanethidine, allow it ca. 20 minutes to bind (Figs. 12.10 and 12.11).

8. To improve the distribution of the sympatholytic substance, the extremity must be moved about during this period and constantly massaged (Fig. 12.12).

9. After ca. 20 minutes, pump up the proximal cuff once again (ca. 100 mmHg above the patient's systolic pressure, Fig. 12.13).

10. After a further 10 minutes, slowly release the distal and proximal cuffs alternately, step by step (Fig. 12.14). This reduces reperfusion of the still unbound guanethidine to a minimum, and prevents systemic sympatholysis with a fall in blood pressure and bradycardia. At the end of the block, the patient must be monitored for one hour.

> The tourniquet should be applied as far distally as possible. This allows an optimal dose-effect ratio. During the block, the pressure in the block cuff must be constantly checked.

> **Caution**
> Since accidental intravenous spread of the local anesthetic and/or the guanethidine can never be excluded, the patient must be carefully and constantly monitored.

Effects of the block

Two regularly occurring effects of the block are vasodilation (increased skin temperature and pulse wave) and inhibition of sweat gland function.

In particular, measurement of the skin temperature before and after the block and comparison with the contralateral side is a reliable criterion for a successful block. Usually, the extremity being treated feels warmest on the first day after the block. Measurable sympathetic blockade rarely lasts after this time.

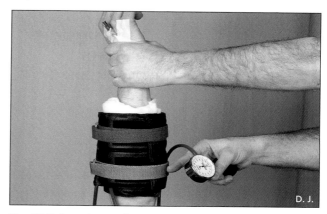

Fig. 12.8 Pumping up the proximal section

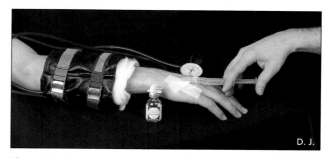

Fig. 12.9 Injecting 5 ml 1 % mepivacaine

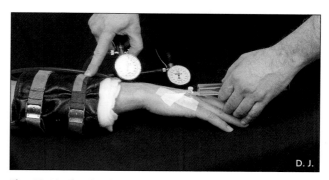

Fig. 12.10 The distal part of the cuff is pumped up, and the proximal part is released

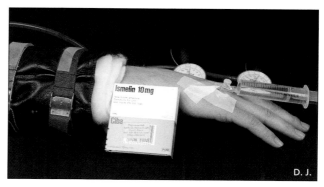

Fig. 12.11 The guanethidine is injected

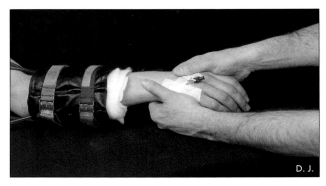

Fig. 12.12 The extremity must be constantly moved and massaged to ensure good distribution of the sympatholytic agent

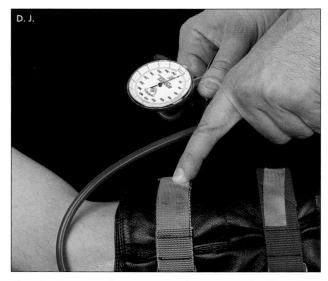

Fig. 12.13 Repeated pumping up of the proximal cuff section

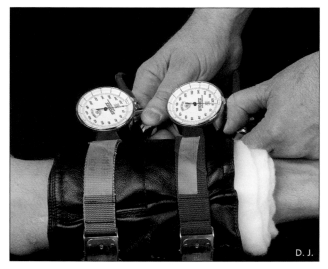

Fig. 12.14 The distal and proximal cuff sections are slowly and alternately released

During informed consent, the patient should be informed that fatigue, and rarely general weakness, may occur on the day of treatment or the following day. Complete elimination of the guanethidine takes up to three weeks.

Dosage
Diagnostic
5–10 mg guanethidine in 20 ml sodium chloride solution, distal to compression.

Caution
No prophylactic administration of local anesthetic.

Therapeutic
Prophylactic administration of 5 ml of a local anesthetic, e. g. 1 % mepivacaine.
Forearm: 10–15 mg guanethidine in 20 ml sodium chloride solution.
Upper arm: 15–20 mg guanethidine in 30 ml sodium chloride solution.
Lower leg: 20–25 mg guanethidine in 50 ml sodium chloride solution.

Block series
An initial series of two or three therapeutic blocks can be carried out at intervals of three to five days. Thereafter, and only if there is clear evidence of effectiveness, periodic repetition is possible.

Side effects
Injection pain, tourniquet pain (prophylactic administration of a local anesthetic in the therapeutic block, possibly with mild sedation), hypotension, diarrhea.

Complication
When the details of the technical procedure and dosage are precisely observed, no complications are expected.

Intravenous sympathetic block

Block no.   □ Right   □ Left

Record and checklist

Name: _____   Date: _____
Diagnosis: _____
Premedication: □ No   □ Yes _____

Purpose of block: □ Diagnosis   □ Treatment
i. v. access: □ No. 1   □ No. 2
Monitoring: □ ECG   □ Pulse oximetry
Ventilation facilities: □ Yes (equipment checked)
Emergency equipment (drugs): □ Checked
Patient: □ Informed   □ Consent

Position: □ Supine
Location of the tourniquet:
□ Forearm   □ Upper arm   □ Lower leg   □ Thigh
Local anesthetic: □ No   □ Yes _____ml _____% _____
Injection mixture: Guanethidine _____ mg
                                      NaCl 0.9% _____ ml
Ischemic time: On _____ Off _____ □ 20 min □ 25 min □ 30 min
Release of cuff over: □ 5 min □ 10 min fractionated

Patient's remarks during injection: □ None
□ Pain   □ Paresthesias   □ Warmth   □ Coldness
Objective block effect after 15 min:
                  □ Temperature measurement right _____°C left _____°C
□ Sensory   □ Motor
Monitoring after block: □ < 1 h   □ > 1 h
                  Time of discharge: _____

Complications and side effects:
□ Hypotension   □ Bradycardia   □ Fatigue
□ Cardiac rhythm disturbances   □ Other _____

Subjective effects of block: Duration: _____
□ None   □ Increased pain
□ Reduced pain   □ No pain

VISUAL ANALOG SCALE

|||||||||||||||||||||||||||||||||||||||||||||||||||||||||||||||||||||||||||||||||||||||||||||||||||||
0   10   20   30   40   50   60   70   80   90   100

Special notes:
_____
_____
_____
_____
_____
_____

	1. h			2. h		
	15	30	45	15	30	45
220						
200						
180						
160						
140						
120						
100						
80						
60						
40						
20						

mm Hg

O₂

Thorax, abdomen and lumbar spinal region

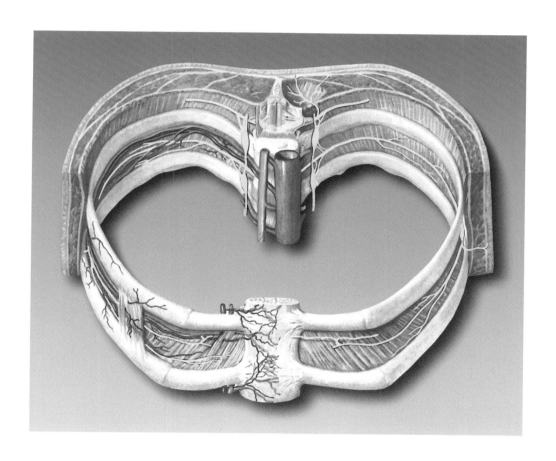

Thorax

13 Thoracic spinal nerve blocks

Anatomy

The thoracic spinal nerves form 12 pairs, which with the exception of the first two are narrow compared with the lower half of the cervical nerves. These spinal nerves emerge from the spinal cord with two roots – the receptor sensory dorsal root (posterior) and the effector motor ventral root (anterior) (Fig. 13.1).
After leaving the dural sac, the two roots are surrounded by a dural sheath. The sensory root expands by taking up numerous nerve cells to form the **spinal ganglion**. Beyond the ganglion, the roots form a common mixed spinal nerve trunk, which divides into four branches after exiting through the intervertebral foramen:

 The **dorsal primary rami,**
 the **ventral primary rami,**
 the **meningeal branches**
 (which supply the spinal canal and the meninges), and

 The **white and gray communicating branches,** which anastomose with each neighboring ganglion of the sympathetic trunk and thus extend to the viscera and vessels, mediating and involving the sympathetic nervous system.

The **dorsal rami** of the thoracic nerves pass between the two transverse processes to their area of distribution, and divide into the two typical branches, the medial and lateral branches; they give off muscular branches (back muscles) and cutaneous branches (spinous processes, posterior wall of the thorax, and lumbar region).
The **ventral rami** of the thoracic nerves are also termed **intercostal nerves**, and they course segmentally (Fig. 13.2).
The 11 upper nerves are (relative to the thoracic ribs) genuinely intercostal, while the twelfth lies caudal to the twelfth rib and is known as the **subcostal nerve.** The six upper intercostal nerves course entirely in the intercostal spaces, as far as the edge of the sternum; the six lower ones reach the area of the linea alba. All of the

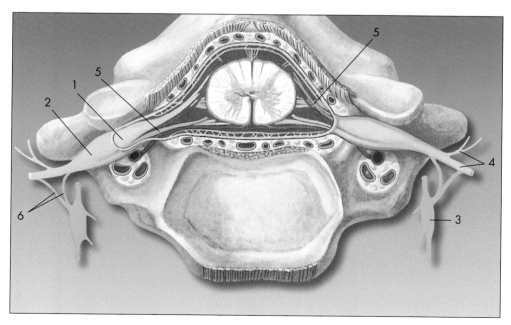

Fig. 13.1 Anatomy of the thoracic spinal nerves.
(1) Spinal ganglion,
(2) spinal nerve, (3) ganglion of the sympathetic trunk,
(4) dorsal and ventral branch, (5) dorsal and ventral root, (6) white and gray communicating branches

intercostal nerves, with the exception of the twelfth, course in the relevant intercostal space in front of the superior costotransverse ligament and on the inner surface of the **external intercostal muscles.**

The **internal intercostal muscles** are absent from the spine far as the costal angle. Over this area, the intercostal nerves are only covered by the **endothoracic fascia** and **costal pleura.**

At the start of the internal intercostal muscles, the nerves lie between these muscles and the external intercostal muscles, and they are accompanied by the **intercostal vessels (the intercostal artery and vein).** They lie caudal to the vessels.

Special care needs to be taken during procedures, as due to the proximity of blood vessels to the nerves, toxic concentrations can easily be reached.

Branches of the intercostal nerves
Muscular branches

It is advisable to distinguish between the six upper intercostal nerve pairs (which supply the subcostal muscle, serratus posterior superior muscle, and transversus thoracis muscle) and the lower five (which supply the subcostal muscle, serratus posterior inferior muscle, and transversus, obliquus, and rectus abdominis muscles).

Lateral cutaneous branches

for the skin and lateral sides of the thorax and abdomen. A small part of the first intercostal nerve (inferior trunk of the brachial plexus) supplies the skin of the axilla.

Anterior cutaneous branches

supply the anterior side of the thorax.

Pleural and peritoneal branches

supply the pleura and thoracic wall and the peritoneum of the lateral and anterior abdominal wall, as well as the pleural and peritoneal covering at the origin of the diaphragm.

Thoracic paravertebral somatic nerve block

Definition
A dorsal somatic block of the thoracic intercostal nerve below the transverse process, in its area of origin just after it exits from the intervertebral foramen and courses through the paravertebral space.

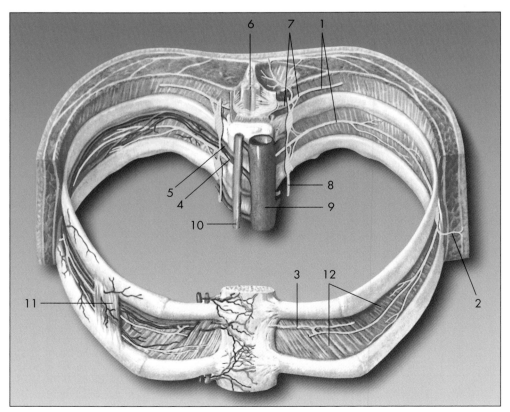

Fig. 13.2 Intercostal nerves. (1) Ventral branches (intercostal nerves), (2) lateral cutaneous branch, (3) anterior cutaneous branch, (4) posterior intercostal artery, (5) posterior intercostal vein, (6) spinal cord, (7) spinal nerve, (8) sympathetic trunk, (9) thoracic aorta, (10) azygos vein, (11) external intercostal muscles, (12) internal intercostal muscles

Indications

Diagnostic
- Differential diagnosis of somatic and autonomic pain.
- Differentiation and localization of intercostal neuralgia, causalgia, cardiac pain, etc.

Therapeutic
- A series of blocks in the appropriate dermatome is particularly useful in the acute phase of herpes zoster.
- Pain in the intercostal area (neuralgia, causalgia).
- Painful conditions after fractured ribs or contusions of the thoracic wall.
- Postoperative pain after upper abdominal or thoracic interventions (providing relief for expectoration and deep breathing).

In most of the indications mentioned, an indwelling epidural catheter is preferred (see Chaps. 33 and 34).

Block series
A series of six to eight blocks is recommended. When there is evidence of improvement in the symptoms, additional blocks can also be carried out.

Surgical
- Inguinal herniectomies (in combination with a lumbar paravertebral somatic block, T10–L2) [9, 14]. High doses of local anesthetic will be required.

Contraindications

Specific
- Anticoagulant treatment.
- Infections and skin diseases in the injection area.

Relative
- Asthenic patients.
- Chronic obstructive lung diseases.

Procedure

This block should only be carried out by experienced anesthetists, or under their supervision. A specific indication is required.

Preparations
Check that the emergency equipment is complete and in working order; sterile precautions, intravenous access, ECG monitoring, pulse oximetry, intubation kit, ventilation facilities, emergency medication.

Materials (Fig. 13.3)
Fine 26-G needle, 2.5 cm long, for local anesthesia.
Atraumatic 24-G needle, 0.7 × 80 mm (15°) with injection lead (e.g. Stimuplex D, B. Braun Melsungen) or 24-G spinal needle, 0.6 × 80 mm.
Syringes: 2, 5, and 10 ml.
Local anesthetic, disinfectant, swabs, sterile gloves and drape; flat, firm pillow.

Patient positioning
- **Prone position:** cushioned with a pillow under the lower thorax and upper abdomen. The patient's arms hang to the sides (Fig. 13.4).
  For blocks of the upper four thoracic nerves, it is recommended that the patient's head is positioned projecting over the end of the table, supported by an assistant (see Fig. 13.10, p. 114).
- **Sitting:** with the trunk leaning forward (see Fig. 13.13 B, p. 115).

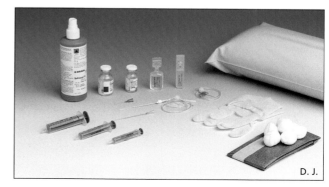

Fig. 13.3 Materials

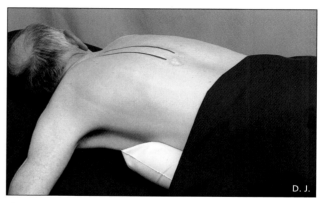

Fig. 13.4 Prone position

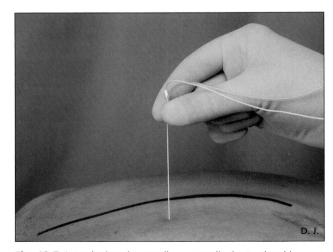

Fig. 13.5 Introducing the needle perpendicular to the skin surface

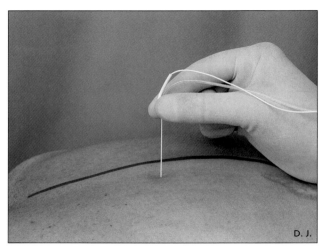

Fig. 13.6 A Bone contact (transverse process)

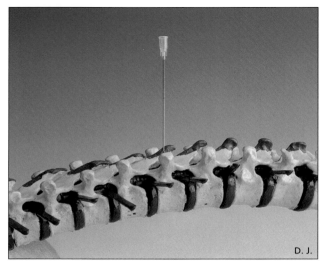

Fig. 13.6 B In the skeleton

Location
- Vertebra prominens (nuchal tubercle) (count down caudally).
- Iliac crest line of L4 (count up cranially).
- Upper edge of the transverse process selected;
  A horizontal line is drawn on the segment above the level being blocked. The injection point is located ca. 3.5–4 cm (two fingerbreadths) paramedian to this.

Skin prep, local anesthesia, covering with a sterile drape, drawing up the local anesthetic, testing the patency of the injection needle.

> **Caution**
> During the injection, the following points must be observed without fail:
> - The person carrying out the injection must stand on the side being blocked.
> - The injection point must not be located more than 4 cm lateral to the midline (rib contact, risk of pneumothorax!)
> - There is a risk of perforating the dural cuff if the injection is made too far medially (epidural or subarachnoid injection).
> - The transverse process is ca. 0.6–0.7 cm thick.
> - If there is no bone contact after 2.5–5 cm (depending on the anatomy), the direction of the needle must be corrected (the transverse process has been missed; risk of pleural puncture).
> - If the patient coughs, it indicates pleural irritation. The procedure should be halted.
> - Eliciting paresthesias is not obligatory.
> - The injection should be carried out on an incremental basis, with frequent aspiration (blood, CSF?).

Injection technique
- The injection needle is introduced perpendicular to the skin surface (Fig. 13.5) until bone contact is made (transverse process) (Fig. 13.6 A, B).
  Depending on the anatomy, bone contact is made at a depth of 2.5–5 cm. The depth of the needle is marked visually.

The needle is withdrawn to lie subcutaneously, and introduced at an angle of 15–20° in a caudal or cranial direction, past the transverse process, up to 2 cm deeper (Fig. 13.7 A, B).
Eliciting paresthesias is helpful, and confirms the correct position of the needle, but it is not obligatory, since optimal effectiveness of the block can be achieved with the diffusion of the local anesthetic.

After aspiration at various levels (blood, CSF?), incremental injection of local anesthetic is carried out.

Caution

After a successful somatic paravertebral block of the thoracic nerves, the injected local anesthetic diffuses via the plethora of communicating branches that are present, towards the neighboring sympathetic chain, which is almost always blocked as well.

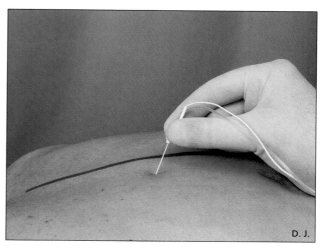

Fig. 13.7 A The needle is withdrawn subcutaneously and then introduced 2 cm deeper past the transverse process

Dosage

Diagnostic
5 ml local anesthetic per segment, e. g. 0.5 % prilocaine, 0.5 % mepivacaine, 0.5 % lidocaine.

Therapeutic
5–10 ml local anesthetic per segment, e. g. 0.375 % ropivacaine, 0.25–0.375 % bupivacaine. In acute conditions (e. g. herpes zoster in the innervated area), 2 to 4 mg dexamethasone can be added.

Surgical
5 ml local anesthetic per segment (T10–L2), e. g. 0.5 % bupivacaine with the addition of epinephrine 1 : 400 000 [9] or 1 % ropivacaine.

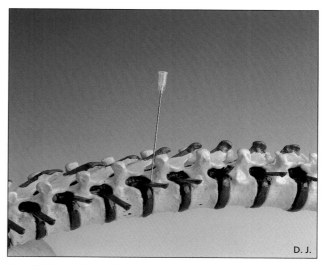

Fig. 13.7 B In the skeleton

Complications

Pneumothorax (Fig. 13.8):
This is a rare complication if the technique is carried out correctly. It is usually a small pneumothorax with spontaneous resorption. If there is any suspicion, however, a thoracic radiograph is required after four to six hours.

Epidural or subarachnoid injection (avoid injecting too medially!) (see Chapt. 28, p. 200 and Chap. 33, p. 231).

Intravascular injection with toxic reactions (see Chap. 4, pp. 42, 43).

Hypotension due to accompanying sympathetic block (e. g. with larger volumes of the local anesthetic).

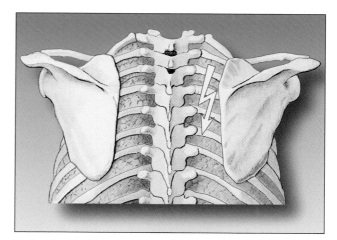

Fig. 13.8 Complications: risk of pneumothorax

Record and checklist

Thoracic paravertebral nerve block

Block no.   □ Right   □ Left

Name: _____   Date: _____

Diagnosis: _____

Premedication: □ No   □ Yes

Neurological abnormalities: □ No   □ Yes _____

Purpose of block: □ Diagnosis   □ Treatment   □ Surgery

Needle: G _____ Length _____ cm

i. v. access: □ Yes

Monitoring: □ ECG   □ Pulse oximetry

Ventilation facilities: □ Yes (equipment checked)

Emergency equipment (drugs):   □ Checked

Patient: □ Informed   □ Consent

Position: □ Prone   □ Sitting

Injection level: □ T _____ _____ _____

Injection:

Local anesthetic: _____ ml _____ %
(incremental)

Addition to LA: □ Yes _____ µg/mg   □ No

Patient's remarks during injection:

□ None   □ Paresthesias   □ Warmth   □ Pain

Neural area: _____

Objective block effect after 15 min:

□ Cold test   □ Temperature measurement right _____°C   left _____°C

Segments affected: T _____

Monitoring after block: □ < 1 h   □ > 1 h

                           Time of discharge: _____

Complications:

□ None   □ Intravascular   □ Subarachnoid/epidural

□ Pneumothorax   □ Other

Subjective effects of block: Duration: _____

□ None   □ Increased pain

□ Reduced pain   □ No pain

VISUAL ANALOG SCALE

|￼|￼|￼|￼|￼|￼|￼|￼|￼|￼|￼
0   10   20   30   40   50   60   70   80   90   100

Special notes:

_____

_____

_____

_____

_____

	1. h			2. h		
	15	30	45	15	30	45

220
200
180
160   mm Hg
140
120
100
80
60   O₂
40
20

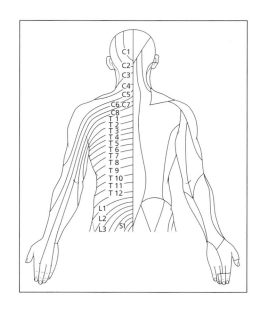

Blocks of the intercostal nerves

Definition

Block of one or more intercostal nerves at various points in their course, most often paravertebrally in the area of the costal angle, or dorsomedially in the area of the posterior axillary line; more rarely in the area of the anterior axillary line, or parasternally.

Indications

Diagnostic
▨ Differential diagnosis of somatic and autonomic pain conditions.

Therapeutic
▨ Pain in the intercostal area (neuralgia and causalgia).
▨ Painful conditions after rib fractures or contusions of the thoracic wall, pleuritic pain.
▨ Acute phase of herpes zoster (in combination with a somatic paravertebral block).
▨ Postoperative pain therapy after upper abdominal and thoracic interventions, to relieve muscular spasms and wound pain (relief of expectoration and deep breathing).

In most of the indications mentioned, an epidural catheter procedure is preferred (see Chaps. 33 and 34).

Surgical
▨ Superficial interventions in the innervation area.
▨ Placement of a thoracic drain.

Contraindications

Specific
▨ Anticoagulant treatment.
▨ Infections and skin diseases in the injection area.

Relative
▨ Asthenic patients.
▨ Chronic obstructive lung diseases.

Procedure

Preparations
Check that the emergency equipment is complete and in working order; sterile precautions, intravenous access, ECG monitoring, pulse oximetry, endotracheal anesthesia set, ventilation facilities, emergency medication.

Materials (Fig. 13.9)
Fine 26-G needle, 2.5 cm long, for local anesthesia.
Atraumatic 25-G needle, 0.5 × 35 mm (15°) with injection lead (e. g. Stimuplex D, B. Braun Melsungen) or 24-G Plexufix needle, 0.55 × 25 mm.
Syringes: 2, 5, and 10 ml.
Local anesthetic, disinfectant, swabs, sterile gloves and drape; flat, firm pillow (prone position).

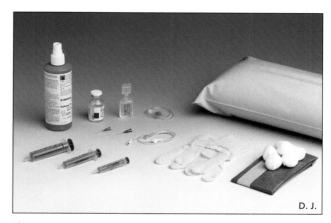

Fig. 13.9 Materials

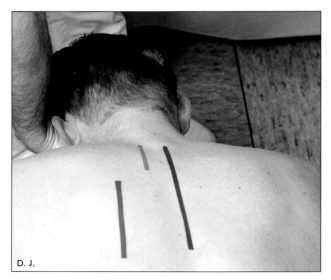

Fig. 13.10 Block of the first four intercostal nerves is carried out paravertebrally (green line)

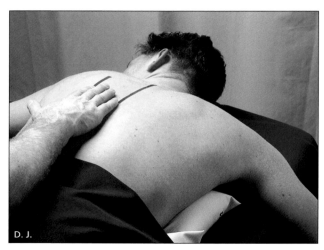

Fig. 13.11 Prone position

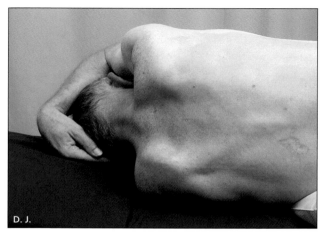

Fig. 13.12 Lateral recumbent position

> **Caution**
> The first four intercostal nerves are blocked para-vertebrally, ca. 3.5–4 cm (ca. two fingerbreadths) lateral to the spinous processes (Fig. 13.10).

Intercostal block in the area of the costal angle

Patient positioning
- **Prone position:** with a pillow under the mid-abdomen, between the arch of the ribs and the iliac crest line, with the patient's arms hanging (Fig. 13.11). This position is particularly preferred with bilateral blocks.
- **Lateral recumbent:** more rarely, and with unilateral blocks (Fig. 13.12).
- **Supine:** (Fig. 13.13 A).
- **Sitting:** e. g., in rib fractures (Fig. 13.13 B).

Location
- Twelfth rib (count cranially).
- Costal angle (ca. 7–8 cm – four fingerbreadths – lateral to the midline and lateral to the musculature of the erector muscle of the spine) (Fig. 13.11).
- Caudal boundary of the rib being blocked (Fig. 13.14).

Skin prep, local anesthesia, covering with a sterile drape, drawing up the local anesthetic, checking the patency of the injection needle.

> **Caution**
> During the injection, the following points must be observed without fail:
> ■ The person carrying out the injection must stand on the side being blocked.
> ■ The intercostal nerve courses dorsocaudal to the vessels in the inferior costal groove.
> ■ The rib is ca. 0.6–0.7 cm thick.
> ■ Start with the lowest rib.
> ■ The injection must only be carried out after definite localization of the rib being blocked.
> ■ Targeted paresthesias are not elicited.
> ■ If the patient coughs, it indicates pleural irritation. The procedure should be interrupted.
> ■ Injection should be carried out on an incremental basis, with frequent aspiration.

Injection technique

▨ The index and middle fingers of the left hand palpate the rib being blocked, and press the skin around the contours of the ribs.
The index finger locates the lower edge of the rib.
▨ Through a skin puncture, directed by the right hand, a 3.5-cm long needle is advanced at an angle of 80° to the skin surface, until bone contact (costal periosteum) is made (Fig. 13.15).
▨ The needle is withdrawn slightly, and the skin and needle are then simultaneously pushed caudally until the needle slides under the lower edge of the rib (Fig. 13.16 A).
▨ After loss of bone contact, the needle must only be introduced 2–3 mm deeper (Fig. 13.16 B).
▨ The cone of the needle is fixed between the thumb and index finger as this is done; the middle finger fixes the shaft and directs the needle.
The side of the left hand (left hypothenar) rests on the patient's back; initially it serves as a brake, and then during the injection it serves for fixation (Fig. 13.17).
▨ After aspiration at various levels, the local anesthetic is injected on an incremental basis.

> **Caution**
> Due to overlap, at least three nerves have to be blocked in order to achieve a complete segmental block.

Effects of the block

Block of the skin, lateral and anterior thoracic wall, motor block of the intercostal muscles, as well as of the pleura and thoracic wall.
The six lower intercostal nerves reach the area of the linea alba, leading to motor block of the abdominal musculature and sensory block of the skin and abdomen, as well as of the peritoneum and lateral and anterior thoracic wall.

Dosage

3–5 ml local anesthetic per segment, e. g. 0.5–0.75 % ropivacaine, 0.25–0.5% bupivacaine.

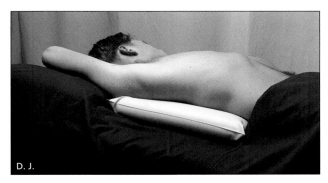

Fig. 13.13 A Supine position

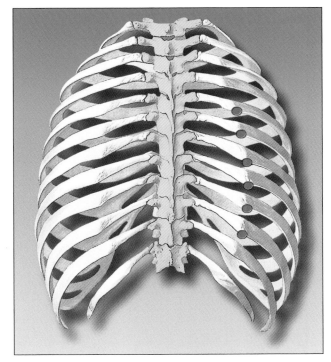

Fig. 13.13 B Sitting

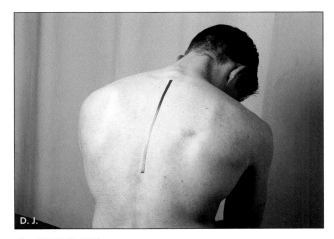

Fig. 13.14 Thoracic skeleton, showing the costal angles

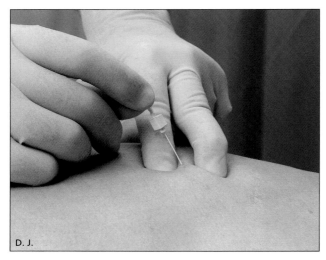

Fig. 13.15 The needle is advanced as far as the costal periosteum

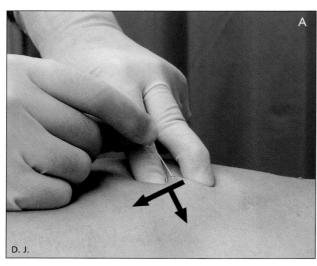

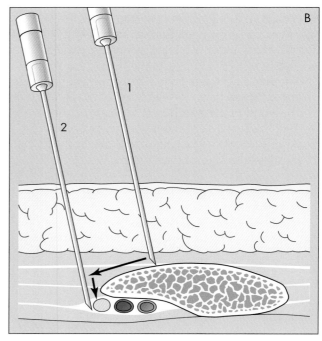

Fig. 13.16 A, B The skin and the needle are simultaneously pushed caudally, and the needle is then introduced a further 2–3 mm

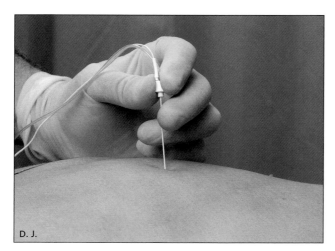

Fig. 13.17 Guiding the needle

Caution

As intercostal block is the procedure in which the highest blood levels of local anesthetic per milligram are administered (due to very fast resorption), there is a risk of overdosage here.
The individual maximum dose must be carefully calculated, and must never be exceeded.

Dorsolateral intercostal block in the area of the posterior axillary line

This block is carried out ca. 2 cm dorsomedial to the posterior axillary line, with the patient in a supine position. Cushioning with a flat pillow under the back allows the relevant side of the chest to be raised at a slight angle. The patient's ipsilateral arm lies under the neck (Fig. 13.18).
This technique is suitable for blocking the lateral cutaneous branch of the intercostal nerve.
The materials and preparation, injection technique, dosage and complications are the same as those for the block of the costal angle described above.
More rarely, blocks of the intercostal nerves are carried out in the area of the anterior axillary line (distal third of the ribs and sternum), or parasternally (e. g. in sternum fractures).

Complications
░ Pneumothorax (see Chap. 13, p. 111).
░ Toxic reactions due to overdosage (see Chap. 4, p. 43).
░ Intravascular injection (see Chap. 4, p. 42).

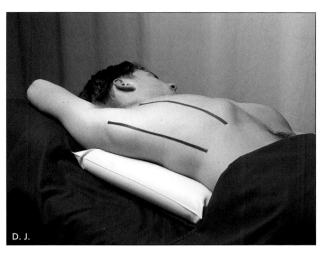

D. J.

Fig. 13.18 Posterior axillary line (red), anterior axillary line (blue)

Record and checklist

Block of the intercostal nerves

Block no.
☐ Right   ☐ Left

Name: _____   Date: _____

Diagnosis: _____

Neurological abnormalities: ☐ No   ☐ Yes _____

Purpose of block: ☐ *Diagnosis*   ☐ *Treatment*   ☐ *Surgery*

Needle: *G* _____ *Length* _____ *cm*

i. v. access: ☐ *Yes*   ☐ *No*

Monitoring: ☐ *ECG*   ☐ *Pulse oximetry*

Ventilation facilities: ☐ *Yes (equipment checked)*

Emergency equipment *(drugs):*   ☐ *Checked*

Patient: ☐ *Informed*   ☐ *Consent*

Position: ☐ *Prone*   ☐ *Lateral recumbent*   ☐ *Sitting*   ☐ *Supine*

Approach: ☐ *Costal angle* ☐ *Posterior axillary line* ☐ *Anterior axillary line* ☐ *Parasternal*

No. of nerves blocked: T _____ _____ _____ _____

Injection:

Local anesthetic: _____ *ml* _____ %

Addition to LA: ☐ *Yes* _____ *μg/mg*   ☐ *No*

Patient's remarks during injection:

☐ *None*   ☐ *Paresthesias*   ☐ *Warmth*   ☐ *Pain*

Neural area: _____

Objective block effect after 15 min:

☐ *Cold test*   ☐ *Temperature measurement right* _____ °C *left* _____ °C

Monitoring after block: ☐ *< 1 h*   ☐ *> 1 h*

 Time of discharge: _____

Complications:

☐ *None*   ☐ *Intravascular injection*   ☐ *Pneumothorax*   ☐ *Toxic reaction*

Subjective effects of block: *Duration:* _____

☐ *None*   ☐ *Increased pain*

☐ *Reduced pain*   ☐ *No pain*

VISUAL ANALOG SCALE

| 0 | 10 | 20 | 30 | 40 | 50 | 60 | 70 | 80 | 90 | 100 |

Special notes:

_____

_____

_____

_____

_____

_____

_____

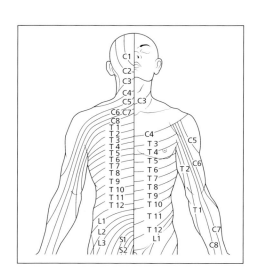

	1. h			2. h		
	15	30	45	15	30	45
220						
200						
180						
160						
140						
120						
100						
80						
60						
40						
20						

mm Hg

O₂

Posterior branches of the thoracic spinal nerves

Anatomy

The posterior branches of the spinal nerve supply the skin of the back and the back musculature. Their area of distribution in the thoracic section stretches over the area between the spinous processes of the vertebrae and the costal angles (Fig. 13.19).

The posterior branches of the thoracic nerves each run between two transverse processes to their area of distribution, and divide shortly thereafter into a medial branch and a lateral branch. Together, these both supply the deep muscles of the back, but only one of each pair penetrates the subcutaneous tissue to become a cutaneous nerve.

Normally, the posterior branches of the eight upper thoracic nerves send off thick medial cutaneous branches, while the four lower ones send off thick lateral cutaneous branches.

The medial cutaneous branches pass through the trapezius muscle alongside the spinous processes of the vertebrae. The point of exit of the lateral cutaneous branches lies in the area of the musculotendinous line of the latissimus dorsi muscle.

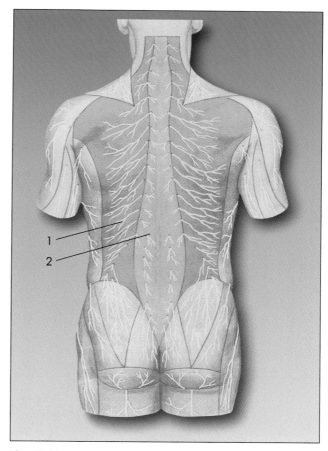

Fig. 13.19 Anatomy. Posterior branches of the thoracic nerves: (1) lateral cutaneous branches, (2) medial cutaneous branches

Indications

Therapeutic
- Muscular tension in the area of the trapezius muscle, serratus anterior and posterior muscles, rhomboideus muscle, levator scapulae muscle, splenius capitis muscle, and splenius cervicis muscle.
- Spasm of the deep paraspinal musculature.
- Shoulder pain, supplementing a block of the suprascapular and subscapular nerves (see Chaps. 8 and 9).

Specific contraindications

None.

Procedure

Preparations
Check that the emergency equipment is complete and in working order. Sterile precautions.

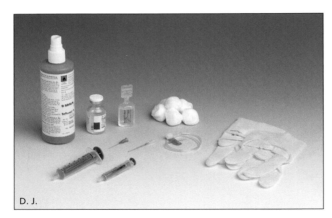

Fig. 13.20 Materials

Materials (Fig. 13.20)
2-ml syringe, 5-ml syringe, fine 23-G needle (4 cm long), disinfectant.
Skin prep in all blocks.

Patient positioning
Sitting, with the head tilted forward slightly and the back muscles relaxed ("pharaoh posture").

Location
Spinous processes of the vertebral column in the C7–T1 and T2–T7 areas.

Injection technique
The intervertebral space between two neighboring spinous processes is palpated, and the needle is introduced at an angle of ca. 45° laterally, up to a depth of ca. 3–4 cm (Fig. 13.21).
After aspiration at various levels, the local anesthetic is injected slowly. When indicated, the neighboring segments can be anesthetized, starting at C7–T1 up to T7 and further along the spine (Fig. 13.22).

Effects of the block
Relaxation and pain relief in the area of the nape musculature and paraspinal musculature of the spine.
C7–T1: After the injection, a pleasant sensation of warmth develops, which radiates laterally to the shoulder and often also cranially as far as the suboccipital area.
T2–T7: The lateral thoracic spread, with a sensation of warmth and slight itching, is about 20 cm.

Dosage
1–1.5 ml local anesthetic per segment, e. g. 0.5–0.75 % ropivacaine, 0.25–0.5 % bupivacaine.
Up to 10–15 ml local anesthetic in total.

Side effects
No side effects are expected.

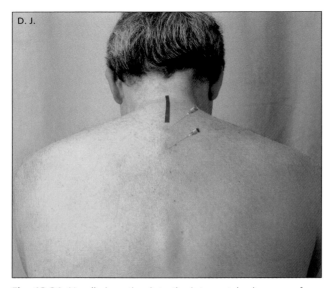

Fig. 13.21 Needle insertion into the intervertebral spaces of neighboring spinous processes

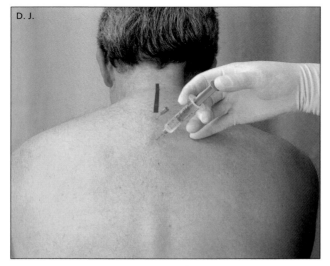

Fig. 13.22 Slow injection after careful aspiration

Spinal nerves (posterior branches)

Block no.   ☐ Right   ☐ Left   ☐ Bilateral

Name: _____   Date: _____
Diagnosis: _____

Purpose of block:		☐ *Diagnosis*	☐ *Treatment*
Needle:	☐ *23 G*	☐ *30 mm*	☐ *40 mm*
i. v. access:		☐ *Yes*	☐ *No*
Monitoring:		☐ *ECG*	☐ *Pulse oximetry*

Position: ☐ *Sitting*
Access route: ☐ *Median, angle ca. 45°, segment(s)* _____
Local anesthetic: _____ *ml* _____ *% per segment*
Addition to LA: ☐ *No*   ☐ *Yes* _____

Patient's remarks during injection:
☐ *None*   ☐ *Pain*   ☐ *Paresthesias*   ☐ *Warmth*

Objective block effect after 15 min:
☐ Cold test   ☐ *Temperature measurement right* _____ °C *left* _____ °C
Segments affected: _____ *(numbness, warmth)*

Monitoring after block: ☐ *< 30 min*   ☐ *> 30 min*
                            Time of discharge: _____

Complications:
☐ *None*   ☐ *Yes (which?)* _____

Subjective effects of block: Duration: _____
☐ *None*   ☐ *Increased pain*
☐ *Reduced pain*   ☐ *No pain*

VISUAL ANALOG SCALE

```
|||||||||||||||||||||||||||||||||||||||||||||||||||||||||||||||||||||||||
0    10    20    30    40    50    60    70    80    90    100
```

Special notes:

_____
_____
_____
_____
_____
_____
_____
_____
_____
_____
_____
_____

Record and checklist

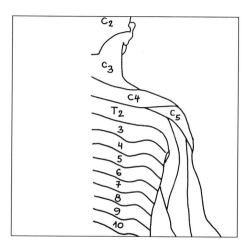

Lumbar spinal region

14 Lumbar paravertebral somatic nerve block

Definition
Dorsal somatic block of a lumbar nerve below the transverse process in its area of origin, just after it exits from the intervertebral foramen and runs through the paravertebral space.

Anatomy

Shortly after they exit from the intervertebral foramina, the spinal nerves divide into ventral branches (anterior) and dorsal branches (posterior). The smaller posterior branches turn dorsally and supply the skin and musculature of the back.

Together with the twelfth thoracic nerve, the longer ventral branches of the first four lumbar nerves form the lumbar plexus. The shorter muscular branches supply the psoas muscle and quadratus lumborum muscle (pp. 148, 149).

The lumbar plexus is connected with the lumbar part of the sympathetic chain via the 2–3 cm long communicating branches.

Indications
Diagnostic
- Differentiation and localization of painful conditions in the lower abdominal quadrants, back, and lower extremities.

Therapeutic
- Pain in the lumbar, inguinal, and thigh region.
- Acute phase of herpes zoster in the appropriate dermatome.

Block series
A series of six to eight blocks is recommended. When there is evidence of improvement, additional blocks can be carried out.

Surgical
- Inguinal herniectomies (in combination with a lumbar paravertebral somatic block, T10–L2) [9, 14]. High doses of local anesthetic are usually required.

Contraindications
Specific
- Anticoagulant treatment.
- Infections and skin diseases in the injection area.

Procedure

This block should only be carried out by experienced anesthetists, or under their supervision.

Preparations
Check that the emergency equipment is complete and in working order; sterile precautions, intravenous access, ECG monitoring, pulse oximetry, intubation kit, ventilation facilities, emergency medication.

Materials (Fig. 14.1)
Fine 26-G needle, 2.5 cm long, for local anesthesia.
Atraumatic 24-G needle, 0.7 × 80 mm (0.7 × 120 mm) (15°) with injection lead (e. g. Stimuplex D, B. Braun Melsungen) or 24-G spinal needle, 0.6 × 80 mm, or 21-G spinal needle, 0.8 × 120 mm.
Syringes: 2, 5, and 10 ml.
Local anesthetics, disinfectant, swabs, sterile gloves, drape, flat, firm pillow.

Patient positioning
■ Prone position: cushioned with a pillow in the mid-abdomen, to eliminate lumbar lordosis. The patient's arms are hanging.
It is also possible to carry out the injection with the patient in a sitting or lateral position.

Location
■ Iliac crest line L4 (count cranially).
■ Upper edge of the selected spinous process.

> **Caution**
> Each of the lumbar somatic nerves leaves the intervertebral foramina slightly caudal and ventral to the transverse process.
> The upper edge of each spinous process in the lumbar region lies more or less on the same horizontal line as its own transverse process. After palpation of the upper edge of the spinous process, a horizontal line is drawn laterally. The injection point is located ca. 2.5–4 cm paramedian.

Skin prep, local anesthesia, covering with a sterile drape, drawing up the local anesthetic, checking the patency of the injection needle.

> **Caution**
> During the injection, the following points must be observed without fail:
> ■ The person carrying out the injection must stand on the side being blocked.
> ■ There is a risk of perforating the dural cuff if the injection is made too far medially (epidural or subarachnoid injection).
> ■ The transverse process is ca. 0.6–0.7 cm thick.
> ■ If there is no bone contact after 3.5–5 cm (depending on the anatomy), the direction of the needle must be corrected (the needle is located between two transverse processes).
> ■ Producing paresthesias is not obligatory.
> ■ The injection should be carried out incrementally, with frequent aspiration (blood, CSF?).
> ■ Motor weakness in the leg must always be expected. Patients should be informed about this.

Injection technique
■ The injection needle is introduced perpendicular to the skin surface (Fig. 14.2) until bone contact is made (transverse process).
Depending on the anatomy, bone contact is made at a depth of ca. 3–5 cm. The depth of the needle is marked visually (Fig. 14.3 A, B).

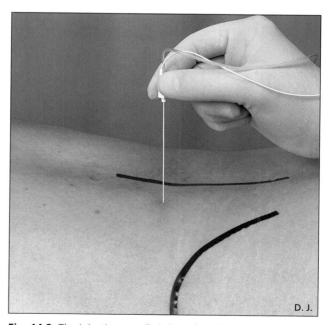

Fig. 14.2 The injection needle is introduced perpendicular to the skin surface

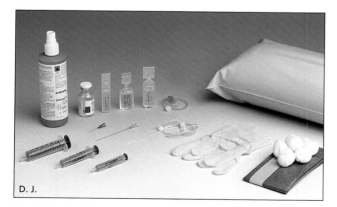

Fig. 14.1 Materials

The needle is then withdrawn subcutaneously, and introduced at an angle of ca. 15–20° caudally (or cranially), past the transverse process, for a further 2–2.5 cm deeper (Fig. 14.4 A, B).
Eliciting paresthesias is helpful, and confirms the correct positioning of the needle, but it is not obligatory, since the optimal effect of the block can be achieved by diffusion of local anesthetic.

After aspiration at various levels (blood, CSF?), the local anesthetic is injected on an incremental basis.

Caution
After a successful somatic paravertebral block in the lumbar region, the injected local anesthetic diffuses through the plethora of communicating branches that are present (particularly in the first and second lumbar nerves, but more rarely in the third) towards the neighboring sympathetic chain, which is almost always blocked as well.

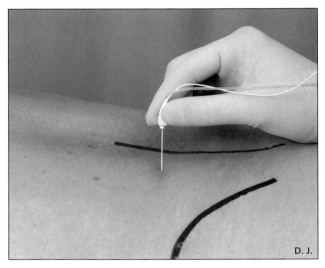

Fig. 14.3 A Bone contact with the transverse process. Visual marking of the depth

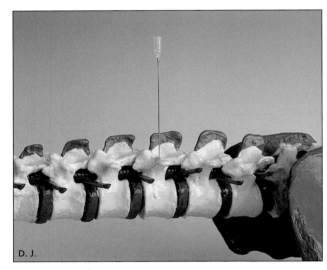

Fig. 14.3 B In the skeleton

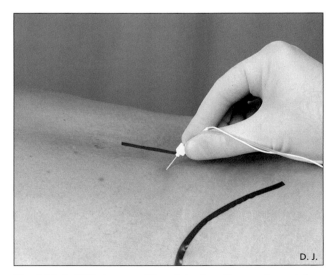

Fig. 14.4 A Withdraw, and then introduce the needle past the transverse process

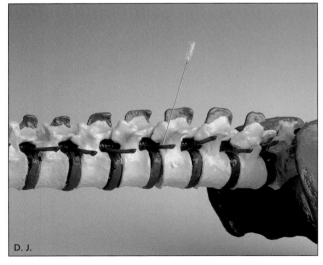

Fig. 14.4 B In the skeleton

Dosage

Diagnostic

5 ml local anesthetic per segment, e. g. 0.5 % prilocaine, 0.5 % mepivacaine, 0.5 % lidocaine.

Therapeutic

5–10 ml local anesthetic per segment, e. g. 0.5 % ropivacaine, 0.25–0.375 % bupivacaine.

In acute conditions (e. g. herpes zoster), 2–4 mg dexamethasone can be added.

Surgical

5 ml local anesthetic per segment (T10–L2), e. g. 0.5 % bupivacaine with 1 : 400 000 epinephrine [9] or 1 % ropivacaine.

Important notes for outpatients

(See Chap. 18, p. 155)

Complications

- Epidural or subarachnoid injection (avoid injecting too medially! See Chap. 28, p. 200, and Chap. 33, p. 231).
- Intravascular injection with toxic reactions (see Chap. 4, pp. 42, 43).
- Intra-abdominal and retroperitoneal injection, or injection into the peritoneum (severe complications are not expected).
- Hypotension due to accompanying sympathetic block (e. g. with larger volumes of local anesthetic or too deep an injection).

Record and checklist

Lumbar paravertebral nerve block

Block no.　　　　　　　　　☐ Right　　☐ Left

Name: _____　Date: _____

Diagnosis: _____

Premedication:　　　　　　☐ No　　☐ Yes

Neurological abnormalities:　☐ No　　☐ Yes _____

Purpose of block:　☐ *Diagnosis*　☐ *Treatment*　☐ *Surgery*

Needle:　G _____　Length _____ *cm*

i. v. access:　　　　☐ *Yes*

Monitoring:　　　　☐ *ECG*　　☐ *Pulse oximetry*

Ventilation facilities:　　　　☐ *Yes (equipment checked)*

Emergency equipment *(drugs)*:　☐ *Checked*

Patient:　　　　☐ *Informed*　☐ *Consent*

Position:　　　☐ *Prone*

Injection level:　☐ *L* _____ _____ _____

Injection:

Local anesthetic: _____ *ml* _____ %
(incremental)

Addition to LA:　☐ *Yes* _____ *µg/mg* _____ ☐ *No*

Patient's remarks during injection:

☐ *None*　☐ *Paresthesias*　☐ *Warmth*　☐ *Pain*

Neural area: _____

Objective block effect after 15 min:

☐ *Cold test*　☐ *Temperature measurement right* _____ *°C left* _____ *°C*

Segments affected: *L* _____

Monitoring after block:　☐ *< 1 h*　☐ *> 1 h*

Time of discharge: _____ *Motor/sensory function tested*

Complications:

☐ *None*　☐ *Intravascular injection*　☐ *Subarachnoid/epidural*　☐ *Other*

Subjective effects of block:　　　　　*Duration:* _____

☐ *None*　　　　　　☐ *Increased pain*
☐ *Reduced pain*　　　☐ *No pain*

VISUAL ANALOG SCALE

| 0 | 10 | 20 | 30 | 40 | 50 | 60 | 70 | 80 | 90 | 100 |

Special notes:

_____
_____
_____
_____

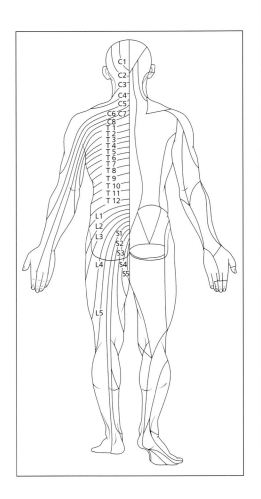

	1. h			2. h		
	15	30	45	15	30	45
220						
200						
180						
160						
140						
120						
100						
80						
60						
40						
20						

mm Hg

O₂

15 Lumbar sympathetic block

Definition

Injection of a local anesthetic or neurolytic in the sympathetic ganglia of the lumbar sympathetic trunk.

Anatomy (Figs. 15.1, 15.2 A, B)

From the T12 ganglion, the stem of the sympathetic trunk continues into the abdominal cavity. The abdominal part of the trunk reaches the anterolateral surface of the lumbar vertebrae, lying directly medial to the origin of the psoas here, to the right behind the inferior vena cava and cisterna chyli and to the left beside the aorta.

The lumbar part of the sympathetic trunk usually contains only four lumbar ganglia (due to fusion of the twelfth thoracic and first lumbar ganglion), with a spindle shape or oval shape. The final ganglion is usually the largest.

The average length of the ganglia is ca. 3–5 mm (more rarely, up to 10–15 mm). The psoas muscle and its fascia separate the sympathetic nerve trunk from the lumbar somatic spinal nerves.

The sympathetic trunks send off and receive communicating and visceral branches, as well as vascular, muscular, osseous and articular branches.

White communicating branches only reach the lumbar sympathetic ganglia from the two cranial spinal nerves, as well as from the three lumbar spinal nerves. They carry preganglionic fibers and visceral afferents. Gray communicating branches are sent off from the corresponding ganglia to all the lumbar spinal nerves. They contain vasomotor, sudomotor and pilomotor fibers, which are distributed with the lumbar spinal nerves.

From the lumbar part of the sympathetic chain, some branches run to the renal plexus, but most pass to the abdominal aortic plexus and the hypogastric plexus. Most of the sympathetic nerve fibers responsible for the lower extremity pass through the L2 (dominant) and L3 ganglia.

Indications

Diagnostic and prognostic

- Differentiation between various forms of vasospastic disease in the area of the lower extremities.
- Prognostic block to establish an indication for surgical sympathectomy or a neurolytic block.
- Checking (confirmation) of a surgical sympathectomy.

Therapeutic

- Pain caused by perfusion disturbances in vasospastic diseases in the region of the lower extremities, in the form of arterial or venous dysfunction or a combination of the two.
- Intermittent claudication.
- Embolism and thrombosis.
- Thrombophlebitis and post-phlebitic edema.
- Post-reconstructive vascular procedures.
- Post frostbite or trauma.
- Complex regional pain syndrome (CRPS) types I and II.
- Phantom stump pain.
- Erythromelalgia.
- Acrocyanosis.
- Phlegmasia alba dolens (milk leg).
- Persistent infection of the leg.
- Poorly healing ulcers.
- Neuropathy after radiotherapy.
- Hyperhidrosis of the lower body.
- Acute phase of herpes zoster.
- Visceral pain (e. g. renal colic).

Block series

A series of six to eight blocks is recommended. When there is evidence of improvement in the symptoms, additional blocks can also be carried out.

Contraindications

▨ Anticoagulant treatment.
▨ Infections and skin diseases in the injection area.
▨ Addition of vasopressors in patients with peripheral circulatory disturbances.

Procedure

This block should only be carried out by experienced anesthetists, or under their supervision.

Preparations
Check that the emergency equipment is complete and in working order; sterile precautions, intravenous access, ECG monitoring, pulse oximetry, intubation kit, ventilation facilities, emergency medication.

Materials (Fig. 15.3)
Fine 26-G needle, 2.5 cm long, for local anesthesia.
Atraumatic 22-G needle, 0.7 × 120 mm (15°) with injection lead (e.g. Stimuplex D, B. Braun Melsungen) or spinal needle, 0.7 (0.9) × 120 mm (150 mm), 20–22 G (e. g. Spinocan, B. Braun Melsungen).
Syringes: 2, 5 and 10 ml.
Disinfectant, swabs, compresses, sterile gloves and drape, flat, firm pillow.

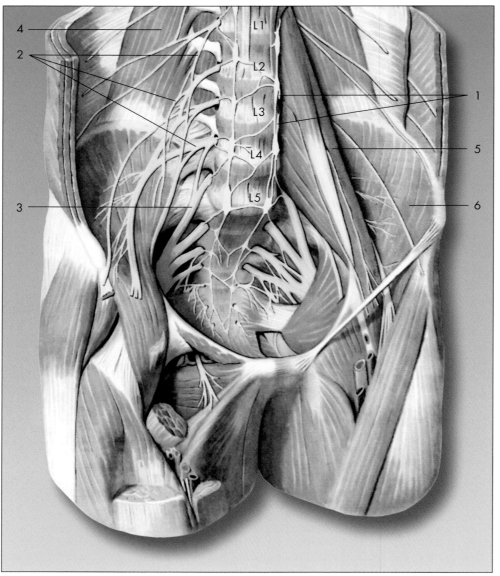

Fig. 15.1 Anatomy (anterior view):
(1) sympathetic trunk with communicating branches,
(2) lumbar plexus,
(3) lumbosacral trunk,
(4) quadratus lumborum muscle,
(5) psoas major muscle,
(6) iliac muscle

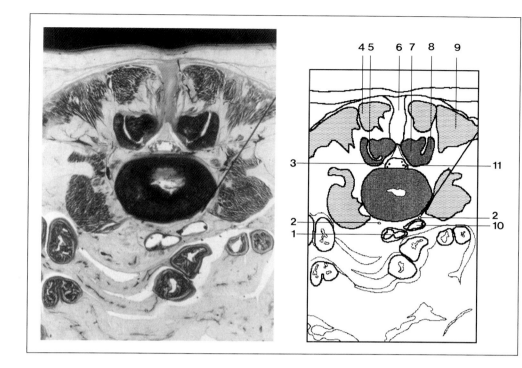

Fig. 15.2 A Lumbar sympathetic block (anatomy and diagram). (1) Aorta, (2) sympathic ganglion, (3) epidural space, (4) medial tract of back muscles, (5) intervertebral joint, (6) interspinal ligament, (7) superior articular process of L3, (8) inferior articular process of L4, (9) lateral tract of back muscles, (10) vena cava, (11) filum terminale

[From Grönemeyer and Seibel, Interventionelle Computertomographie. Lehrbuch und Atlas zur interventionellen Operationstechnik und Schmerztherapie, Vienna/Berlin: Ueberreutter Wissenschaft, 1989.]

Patient positioning

▨ Prone position: support with a pillow in the mid-abdomen (to eliminate lumbar lordosis). The patient's arms hang down.

The patient should breathe with the mouth open, to reduce tension in the back muscles.

This position is preferable, particularly when the block is carried out under X-ray control using an image intensifier.

▨ Lateral decubitus: the flank is supported with a pillow. The side being blocked should be uppermost.

Landmarks (Fig. 15.4 A, B)

▨ L4 iliac crest line.

▨ L2: a parallel line is drawn ca. 4 fingerbreadths (7 cm) from the midline. The intersection point between this line and the twelfth rib is at the level of L2.

▨ Midpoint of each spinous process of the relevant lumbar vertebra.

Disinfection, generous local anesthetic infiltration of the injection channel, covering with a sterile drape, drawing up the local anesthetic, testing the patency of the injection needle.

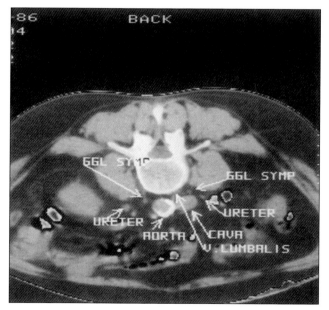

Fig. 15.2 B CT section in the center of the L4 vertebra. The sympathetic ganglia are well delineated in the fatty tissue on each side. Neighboring structures, such as the vessels and ureters, can also be precisely differentiated

[From Grönemeyer and Seibel, Interventionelle Computertomographie. Lehrbuch und Atlas zur interventionellen Operationstechnik und Schmerztherapie, Vienna/Berlin: Ueberreutter Wissenschaft, 1989.]

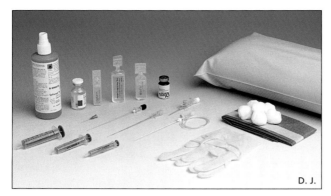

Fig. 15.3 Materials

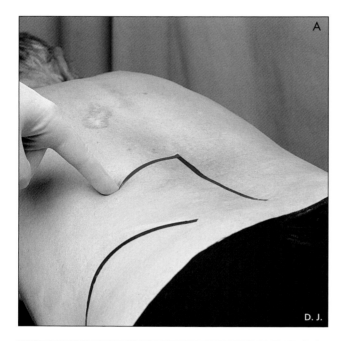

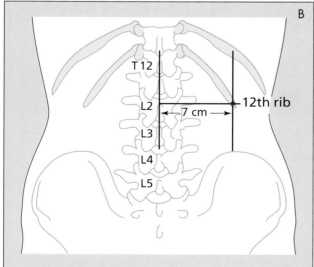

Fig. 15.4 A, B Localization

Caution
During the injection, the following points must be observed:
- A sympathetic block is at the L2 segment; block of segment L4 follows.
- The person carrying out the injection must stand on the side being blocked.
- Usually, the injection point should not be located more than 8 cm lateral to the midline (risk of renal puncture) and no more than 5 cm medial from it (lateral side of the vertebra is more difficult to reach).
- Paresthesias occur relatively frequently during introduction of the needle and indicate irritation of the lumbar somatic nerves.
- Inadvertent block of the lumbar somatic nerves can lead to motor weakness of the contralateral leg. The patient should be informed of this risk.
- There is a risk of perforating the dural cuff if the injection is made too far medially (epidural or subarachnoid injection).
- Aspirate frequently and inject incrementally.
- No neurolytics should be administered without precise confirmation of the needle position using X-ray control with an image intensifier.

Injection technique
- The injection needle is introduced in the direction of the intended vertebra, ca. four fingerbreadths (7 cm) lateral to the midline and at an angle of ca. 30–40° to the skin surface and slightly cranially (Fig. 15.5).
- Locating the transverse process at a depth of ca. 3–5 cm is helpful. The depth of the transverse process is marked visually (Fig. 15.6 A, B).
- The needle is withdrawn subcutaneously.
- The needle is then reintroduced slightly more steeply, with stepwise correction of the direction cranially or caudally (to avoid the transverse process) and medially (to obtain contact with the vertebral periosteum).

After contact with the periosteum, the needle is rotated 180°, so that the opening of the needle tip is directed toward the vertebra and can slide off the bony edge. After sliding off, the needle is further advanced by 1–2 cm (Fig. 15.8 A–C).

Caution

The lumbar sympathetic trunk lies about twice as deep as the distance between the skin and the transverse process (Fig. 15.7).

The distance from the transverse process and the ganglia of the lumbar sympathetic trunk is ca. 3.8–5 cm and is relatively constant.

The distance from the skin to the transverse process depends on the anatomy and is rather more variable.

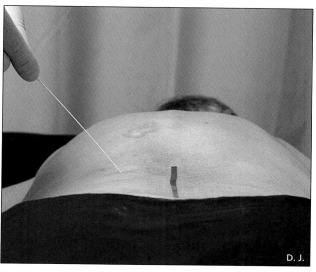

Fig. 15.5 Introducing the injection needle

Confirming the correct needle position

- X-ray control.
- Loss-of-resistance technique with 0.9 % NaCl or air. Perforation of the psoas fascia is similar to that experienced when carrying out an epidural.

  A false loss of resistance can occur when the needle is positioned superficially between the psoas muscle and the quadratus lumborum muscle, leading to inadvertent block of the lumbar somatic nerves, with consequent numbness of the lower extremity during the period of effect of the local anesthetic.

  Injection of a neurolytic into this area without prior X-ray control of the position can have fatal consequences.
- After careful aspiration testing at all levels, resistance-free incremental injection of the local anesthetic is carried out.

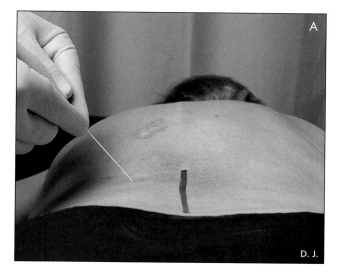

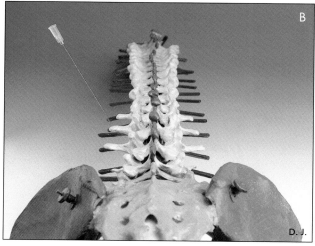

Fig. 15.6 A, B Bone contact with the transverse process. **A** On a patient, **B** On a skeleton

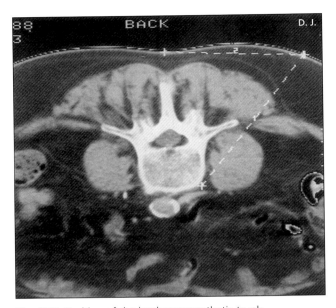

Fig. 15.7 Position of the lumbar sympathetic trunk

[From Grönemeyer and Seibel, Interventionelle Computertomographie. Lehrbuch und Atlas zur interventionellen Operationstechnik und Schmerztherapie, Vienna/Berlin: Ueberreutter Wissenschaft, 1989.]

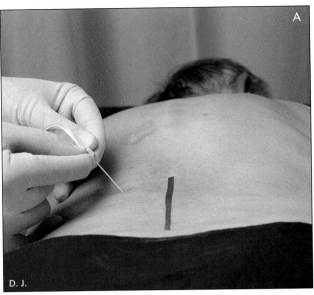

Fig. 15.8 A After the needle has been withdrawn subcutaneously, it is reintroduced at a steeper angle, followed by contact with the vertebral periosteum and rotation of the needle by 180°. The needle is then advanced 1–2 cm

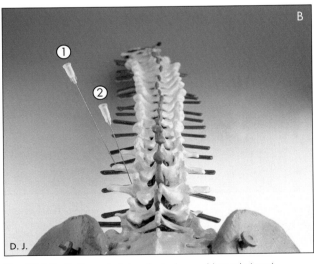

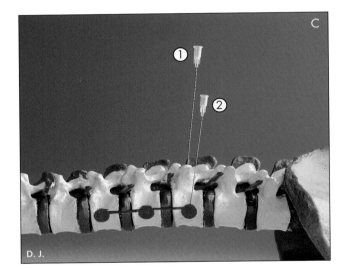

Fig. 15.8 B, C On a skeleton (anterior and lateral views)

Neurolytic block

Injection of neurolytics – 45–95 % ethanol, 7 % phenol in water or 7–10 % phenol in Conray (iothalamate meglumine) – at the lumbar sympathetic ganglia.
Prerequisite:
The procedure must be carried out under radiographic guidance.
Usually, three needles are introduced at the level of L2, L3 and L4 and the neurolytic is only injected after definite confirmation of the correct needle position. After this, 1 ml of air is injected per needle, to clear any residual neurolytic from the needle.

Effects of the block
Signs of vascular dilation in the area of the ipsilateral leg are:

- Increase in skin temperature.
- Hyperthermia and anhidrosis.
- Loss of the sympathogalvanic reflex.
- Reduced pain or absence of pain.
- No signs of sensory or motor block (assuming that the lumbar somatic nerves have not been concomitantly anesthetized).

Dosage

Diagnostic
5 ml local anesthetic with contrast medium, e. g. 0.5 % prilocaine, 0.5 % mepivacaine, 0.5 % lidocaine.

Therapeutic
20 ml local anesthetic (single-needle technique).
10 ml local anesthetic per needle (in the two-needle or three-needle technique), e. g. 0.2–0.375 % ropivacaine, 0.25 % bupivacaine.

Neurolytics
3 ml per segment.

Side effects

- Transient motor weakness due to anesthetization of the lumbar somatic nerves. Paresthesias during the injection are a warning signal. This undesired effect is always liable to occur and is caused by superficial injection in the area of the lumbar somatic nerves or by resorption after the administration of large volumes of a local anesthetic. It is therefore necessary to monitor the patient for at least one hour after the block (see Chap. 18, section on Important Notes for Outpatients, p. 155).
- Fall in blood pressure due to sympathetic block.

Complications

Severe
- Intravascular injection (aorta, vena cava) with toxic reactions (see Chap. 4, pp. 42, 43).
- Epidural or subarachnoid injection (see Chap. 28, p. 200 and Chap. 33, p. 231).

Potential
- Retroperitoneal hemorrhage.
- Hemorrhage in the psoas area (with subsequent pain in the thigh and transient weakness in the quadriceps muscle).
- Renal injury accompanied by hematuria.
- Back pain.
- Perforation of an intervertebral disk.
- Ejaculation disturbances (in younger patients with bilateral block).

Complications of neurolytic block
- Injury to the lumbar somatic nerves (neuritis, 1 %).
- Neuralgia in the genitofemoral nerve (5–10 %).
- Ureteral stricture.
- Impotence.
- Neurological deficit.

Record and checklist

Lumbar sympathetic block

Block no. _____   ☐ Right   ☐ Left

	1. h			2. h		
	15	30	45	15	30	45

220
200
180
160
140
120
100
80
60
40
20

mm Hg

O₂

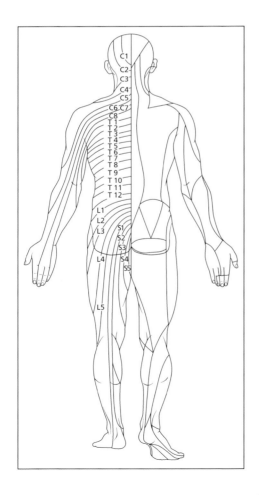

Name: _____   Date: _____
Diagnosis: _____
Premedication: ☐ No   ☐ Yes
Neurological abnormalities: ☐ No   ☐ Yes _____

Purpose of block: ☐ *Diagnosis*   ☐ *Treatment*
Needle: G _____ Length _____ cm
i. v. access and infusion: ☐ *Yes*
Monitoring: ☐ *ECG*   ☐ *Pulse oximetry*
Ventilation facilities: ☐ *Yes (equipment checked)*
Emergency equipment *(drugs):*   ☐ *Checked*
Patient: ☐ *Informed*   ☐ *Consent*

Position: ☐ *Prone*   ☐ *Lateral decubitus*
Injection level: ☐ *L* _____ _____ _____
Injection technique: ☐ *X-ray image converter* ☐ *Loss of resistanc* ☐ *CT-guided*
Injection:
Local anesthetic: _____ *ml* _____ %
(incremental)
Addition to LA: ☐ *Yes* _____ *µg/mg* ☐ *No*
Neurolytic: _____ *ml* _____ %
Addition: ☐ *Yes*   ☐ *No*

Patient's remarks during injection:
☐ *Non*   ☐ *Paresthesias*   ☐ *Warmth*   ☐ *Pain*
Neural area: _____
Objective block effect after 15 min:
☐ *Cold test*   ☐ *Temperature measurement right* _____ °C *left* _____ °C
Segments affected: *L* _____
Monitoring after block: ☐ *< 1 h*   ☐ *> 1 h*
Time of discharge: _____ ☐ *Motor / sensory function tested*

Complications:
☐ *None*   ☐ *Intravascular injection*   ☐ *Subarachnoid / epidural*
☐ *BP reduction*   ☐ *Other*

Subjective effects of block: *Duration:* _____
☐ *None*   ☐ *Increased pain*
☐ *Reduced pain*   ☐ *No pain*
VISUAL ANALOG SCALE

|||||||||||||||||||||||||||||||||||||||||||||||||||||||||||||||||||||||||||||||||||||||||||||||||
0   10   20   30   40   50   60   70   80   90   100

Special notes:
_____
_____

16 Iliolumbosacral ligaments

Definition

Injection of a local anesthetic or a sclerosant solution along the ligamentous insertion points in the lumbosacral area.

Anatomy (Fig. 16.1)

(See Chap. 27)

The ligaments of the sacral and coccygeal region are very important, since they transfer the entire weight of the trunk via the hip bones to the lower extremities. This occurs through firm anchoring of the vertebrae, hip bones and sacrum.

The pelvic girdle only has one ligamentous connection of its own, the obturator membrane of the hip bone. **Ventrally**, the connection between the two hip bones is created by the pubic symphysis. **Dorsally**, there are connections with the trunk or spinal column – with the sacrum and coccyx, as well as the lumbar spine, via the sacroiliac joint and a number of ligaments.

The sacroiliac joint

The articular bones are the sacrum, hip bone and iliac bone. The joint capsule is under firm tension and posteriorly its place is taken by the interosseous sacroiliac joint. The joint cavity is narrow and fissure-like. A number of ligaments are present as special features.

The **direct strengthening ligaments** are the anterior sacroiliac ligament **ventrally**, the posterior sacroiliac ligament **dorsally** and the interosseous sacroiliac ligament.

The iliolumbar ligament, sacrospinal ligament and sacrotuberous ligament serve as **indirect strengthening ligaments**.

The **anterior sacroiliac ligaments** are usually not particularly thick and lie on the pelvic side of the joint capsule. They run from the pelvic fascia of the sacrum to the iliac bone.

The **posterior sacroiliac ligaments**, 1 cm thick, are anchored with their long fibers on the posterior superior iliac spine and the lateral parts of the third and fourth segments of the sacrum.

The **interosseous sacroiliac ligament** fills the deep cavity between the iliac tuberosity and the sacral tuberosity. The strongest ligament in this region, it is one of the body's thickest ligaments.

The **iliolumbar ligament** originates, with its strong bands, from the transverse processes of the fourth and fifth lumbar vertebrae, radiating over the iliac crest and the neighboring parts of the anterior and posterior surfaces of the iliac bone.

The **sacrotuberous ligament** is attached to the interior surface of the ischial tuberosity and originates from the lateral margin of the sacrum and coccyx. It extends up as far as the posterior and superior inferior iliac spine.

The **sacrospinous ligament** is shorter and thinner than the previous one and is connected to it. Its base is also attached to the lateral margin of the sacrum and coccyx, but its tip attaches to the ischial spine.

The sacrotuberous ligament and sacrospinous ligament represent an essential part of the pelvic diaphragm.

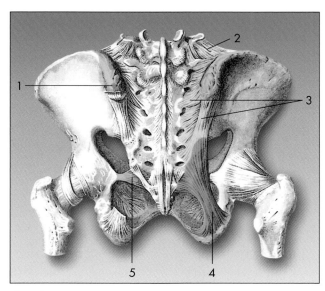

Fig. 16.1 Anatomy.
(1) Posterior superior iliac spine, (2) iliolumbar ligament,
(3) dorsal sacroiliac ligament, (4) sacrotuberous ligament,
(5) sacrospinal ligament

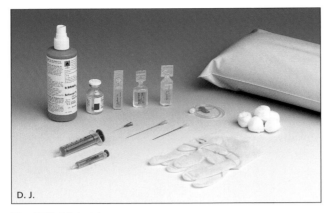

Fig. 16.2 Materials

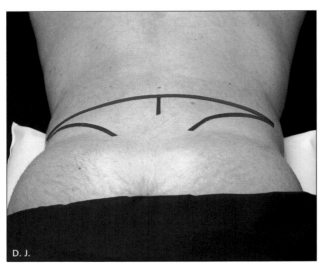

Fig. 16.3 The spinous process of L5 is located about two fingerbreadths below the iliac crest line

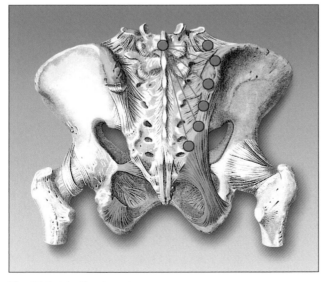

Fig. 16.4 Injection targets

Indications

Diagnostic
- Differential diagnosis of various pain syndromes in the lumbosacral region.

Therapeutic
- Pain in iliolumbosacral ligamentous insufficiency.

Block series
A series of six to eight blocks is recommended. When there is evidence of improvement in the symptoms, additional blocks can also be carried out.

Contraindications

- Anticoagulant treatment.
- Infections and skin diseases in the injection area.

Procedure

Preparations
Check that the emergency equipment is complete and in working order; sterile precautions, intravenous access.

Materials (Fig. 16.2)
Fine 26-G needle, 2.5 cm long, for local anesthesia.
20–22-G needle, 7–8 cm long.
Syringes: 2 ml and 10 ml.
Local anesthetic, disinfectant, swabs, sterile gloves and flat, firm pillow.

Patient positioning
- Prone position: pillow under the mid-abdomen (to eliminate lumbar lordosis). The patient's arms are hanging.

Landmarks (Fig. 16.3)
- Iliac crest line of L4.
- The spinous process of the fifth lumbar vertebra is located about two fingerbreadths below the iliac crest line. The injection point is above the spinous process.

Injection targets (Fig. 16.4)
- Transverse process of the fifth lumbar vertebra.
- Dorsal cranial iliac spine.
- Lateral edge of the caudal part of the sacral bone.

Skin prep, local anesthesia, drawing up the local anesthetic, testing the patency of the injection needle.

Injection technique

Iliolumbar ligament

- The needle is introduced through a skin puncture in the direction of the lateral part of the transverse process of the fifth lumbar vertebra, at an angle of 45° to the surface of the skin (Fig. 16.5).
- Bone contact is made after about 4–5 cm; the needle is then withdrawn by 1 mm and after aspiration, 1–2 ml of local anesthetic is administered.
- The needle is then withdrawn subcutaneously.
- The needle is then reintroduced at an angle of ca. 30° in the direction of the iliac crest, which is marked on the outside by the operator's index finger (Fig. 16.6).
  After bone contact, the needle is withdrawn by 1 mm and after aspiration, 1 ml of local anesthetic is injected.

Sacroiliac, sacrotuberous and sacrospinal ligament

- The needle is withdrawn subcutaneously.
- The needle is reintroduced at an angle of 30° in the direction of the dorsal cranial iliac spine, which is marked on the outside by the operator's index finger. After aspiration, 1 ml of local anesthetic is injected at two further points along the iliac spine.

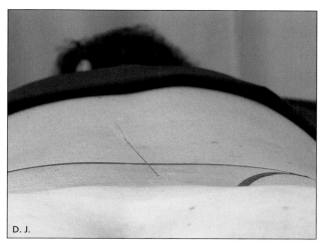

Fig. 16.5 Introducing the injection needle in the direction of the transverse process of L5 (45°)

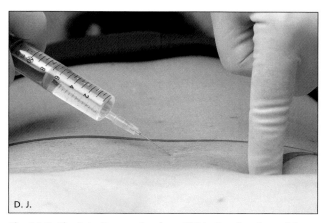

Fig. 16.6 The injection angle of ca. 30° in the direction of the iliac crest

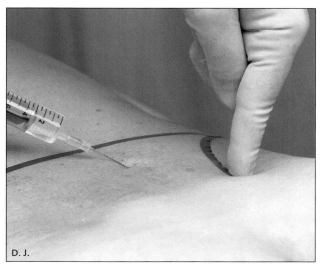

Fig. 16.7 Injection in the direction of the dorsal cranial iliac spine and then along the lower half of the sacrum

The needle is withdrawn subcutaneously once more and then reintroduced two or three times at an angle of 20° along the lower half of the sacrum. The lateral edge is infiltrated with 1 ml local anesthetic at each level (Fig. 16.7).

> **Caution**
> Pain may increase during the injection.

Dosage

Diagnostic
10–15 ml local anesthetic, e. g. 0.5–1 % prilocaine, 0.5–1 % mepivacaine.

Therapeutic
- Unilateral block: 10 ml local anesthetic, e. g. 0.75 % ropivacaine, 0.5 % bupivacaine.
- Bilateral block: 15 ml local anesthetic, e. g. 0.5–0.75 % ropivacaine, 0.25–0.5 % bupivacaine, distributed on both sides.

In acute cases 4 mg dexamethasone can be added with benefit.

Sclerosant solution [4]
- 6 ml 40 % glucose + 4 ml 15 mepivacaine (1 ml per injection site)
- Barbour solution with local anesthetic:
  Phenol crist. 2.0 vol %
  Glucose monohydrate 27.5 vol %
  Anhydrous glycerine 30.0 vol %
  Methylene blue 1.0 vol %
  Distilled water 39.5 vol %
  6 ml Barbour solution + 4 ml 0.5 % bupivacaine = 10 ml (1 ml per injection site)

Repeated injection of sclerosant solution shows no benefit compared with a block series with a local anesthetic.

Complications
Block of a lumbar somatic nerve, with accompanying motor weakness (prophylaxis: no injection without bone contact).
Monitoring is obligatory after the block. The patient should be supported by a nurse when he first stands up. Complications are extremely rare and occur mainly from poor technique.

Abdomen

17 Celiac plexus block

Definition
Injection of a local anesthetic or neurolytic in the region of the celiac plexus.

Anatomy (Fig. 17.1)

The celiac plexus is the largest of the three large sympathetic plexuses (cardiac plexus – thorax; celiac plexus – abdomen; hypogastric plexus – pelvis).
It receives its primary innervation from the preganglionic splanchnic nerves (greater splanchnic nerve T5–10, lesser splanchnic nerve T10–11 and lowest splanchnic nerve T11–12), the postganglionic fibers of which, after synapsing in the celiac ganglion, radiate to the associated plexus and innervate most of the abdominal organs. This large network, with a diameter of about 50 mm, surrounds the origins of the celiac artery and superior mesenteric artery, extends laterally as far as the adrenal glands, upward as far as the aortic hiatus and downward as far as the root of the renal artery. It lies on the initial part of the abdominal aorta, at the level of the first lumbar vertebra, anterior to the medial crus of the diaphragm.
The most important roots of the celiac plexus are the splanchnic nerves, the abdominal branches of the vagus nerves and several branches of the last thoracic ganglion and two highest lumbar ganglia. Cranially, the celiac plexus is connected to the thoracic aortic plexus and caudally it continues into the abdominal aortic plexus. A paired celiac ganglion forms the basis for the celiac plexus. The left ganglion lies closer to the midline and partly on the aorta, while the right one (ventrolateral to the vena cava) lies slightly more to the side in the area of the fissure between the medial and lateral crura of the diaphragm. The two ganglia are connected to one another. With closer approximation and fusion, the double ganglion takes on a ring shape, which is also known as the solar ganglion (solar plexus). The smaller superior mesenteric ganglion and aorticorenal ganglion are associated with the celiac ganglion.

The lesser splanchnic nerve usually enters the latter ganglion, while the greater splanchnic nerve passes to the posterior surface of the lateral part of the celiac ganglion. The phrenic ganglion is a third, unpaired, ganglion. The following, sometimes paired and sometimes unpaired, secondary (associated) plexuses emerge from the celiac plexus:
- Paired (phrenic plexus, suprarenal plexus, renal plexus and spermatic plexus).
- Unpaired (superior gastric plexus, hepatic plexus, splenic plexus and superior mesenteric plexus).

Indications

Diagnostic
- Differential diagnosis of pain in the abdominal region (visceral, epigastric or cardiac pain).

Prognostic
- In upper abdominal carcinoma pain, before a neurolytic block.

Therapeutic
- Relief of upper abdominal pain (pancreas, stomach).
- Treatment of dumping syndrome.
- Injection of neurolytics as a palliative measure in malignant intra-abdominal processes (pancreas, stomach).

Contraindications

■ Anticoagulant treatment.
■ Infections and skin diseases in the injection area.
■ Hypovolemia.
■ General debility.

■ Injection of a neurolytic without precise identification of the needle position (with guidance by CT or image intensifier).

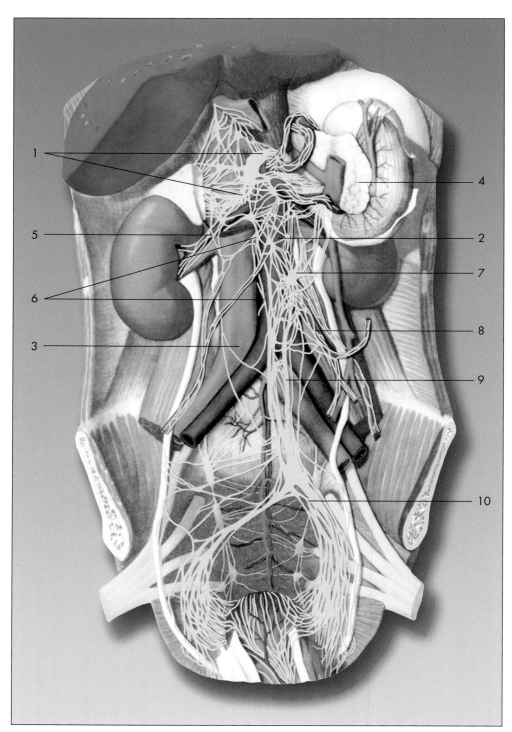

Fig. 17.1 Anatomy.
(1) Celiac plexus, (2) aorta,
(3) inferior vena cava,
(4) pancreas, (5) renal plexus, (6) abdominal aortic plexus, (7) inferior mesenteric ganglion, (8) inferior mesenteric plexus, (9) superior hypogastric plexus,
(10) inferior hypogastric plexus

Procedure

This block should be carried out by very experienced anesthetists.

Preparations
Check that the emergency equipment is complete and in working order; sterile precautions, intravenous access, ECG monitoring, pulse oximetry, intubation kit, ventilation facilities, emergency medication.

Materials (Fig. 17.2)
Fine 26-G needle for local anesthesia.
20–22-G spinal needle, 0.7 (0.9) × 120 mm (150 mm) (e. g. Spinocan, B. Braun Melsungen).
Syringes: 2, 10 and 10 ml.
Disinfectant, swabs, compresses, sterile gloves and drape, flat, firm pillow.

Patient positioning
- Prone position: supported with a pillow in the mid-abdomen (to relieve lumbar lordosis). The patient's arms are hanging, with head lying to the side. The patient breathes with the mouth open, to reduce tension in the back muscles.
This position is preferable.
- Lateral decubitus position, with support under the flank. The side being blocked lies upward.

Location
- L4 iliac crest line (count the spinous processes cranially).
- L2: a parallel line is drawn about 7–8 cm lateral to the midline. The intersection between this line and the lower edge of the twelfth rib determines the level of the upper edge of L2 (see Chap. 15, Fig. 15.4 B).
- T12–L1 is located in the midline and joined with dots to the lower edge of the twelfth rib. This produces a triangle, the equal sides of which provide basic guidance for the needle direction (Fig. 17.3).

Skin prep, generous local anesthetic infiltration of the injection channel, covering with a sterile drape, drawing up the local anesthetic, checking the patency of the injection needle.

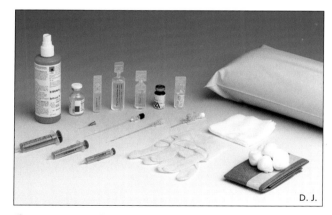
Fig. 17.2 Materials

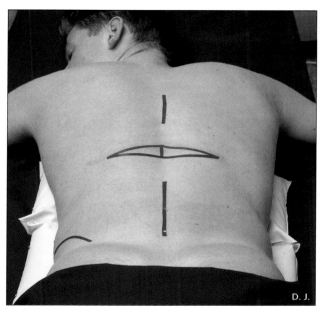
Fig. 17.3 Location

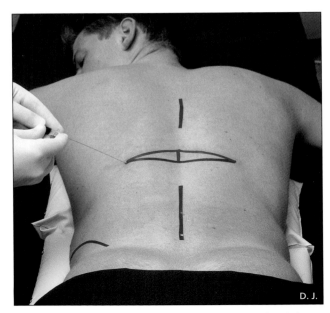

Fig. 17.4 Introducing the injection needle at an angle of about 45° to the skin surface

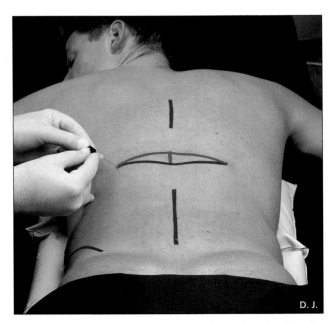

Fig. 17.5 Bone contact with the L1 vertebra. After visual marking of the depth, the needle is withdrawn back to the subcutis

Caution
During the injection, the following points must be observed without fail:

■ In bilateral injections, it is advantageous to inject the left side first.
■ For a diagnostic block a bilateral injection is unnecessary.
■ The operator performing the injection must stand on the side being blocked.
■ In most patients, the distance between the skin and the celiac plexus is about 9–11 cm.
■ Superficial bone contact (after 3–5 cm) indicates contact with the transverse process and requires correction.
■ Paresthesias during the introduction of the needle arise due to stimulation of the lumbar somatic nerves.
■ There is a risk of perforating the dural cuff (epidural or subarachnoid injection).
■ If the patient coughs, it indicates pleural irritation or injury. The procedure should be interrupted.
■ Aspirate frequently and inject on an incremental basis.
■ The method of choice when administering neurolytics is CT-guided injection.

Injection technique (dorsal, retrocrural)

■ About 7–8 cm lateral to the midline (lower edge of the twelfth rib), at an angle of 45° to the skin surface and directed slightly cranially, the injection needle is advanced toward the L1 vertebra (Fig. 17.4). Bone contact is usually made at a depth of about 7–9 cm (Figs. 17.5, 17.7).
■ The depth of the needle is marked visually.
■ The needle is withdrawn subcutaneously.
■ The needle is then redirected at a steeper angle of 60° to the skin surface, so that it can just slide past the lateral edge of the L1 vertebra (Figs. 17.6, 17.7).
■ The needle introduced on the left (the aorta side) can then be carefully advanced a further 1.5–2 cm deeper. After the needle is positioned in the periaortal space, pulsations are transmitted via the needle shaft to the fingertips. The needle introduced on the right side can be advanced in a similar fashion or slightly deeper (2–3 cm) (Figs. 17.7, 17.8).

- The end of the needle must be observed for spontaneous backflow of liquid (blood, CSF, urine?).
- Aspiration test at all four levels.
- Test dose of the local anesthetic.
- Resistance-free, incremental injection of a local anesthetic.

Caution
It is essential to carry out this injection under image intensifier or CT guidance (X-ray control).

Neurolytic block
Unilateral or bilateral injection of neurolytics (50 % ethanol) in the region of the celiac plexus.

Caution
It is essential that, the block should be carried out under X-ray control, in order to reduce potential complications to a minimum and increase accuracy. Several access routes are possible (Figs. 17.8, 17.9).

A diagnostic block with local anesthetics can be helpful.
This measure can only achieve the desired result if the disease is not too far advanced and is not producing additional neuropathic pain (e. g. extension to the epigastric nerves, intercostal nerves or lumbar plexus) [5].

Effects of the block
- Hyperthermia in the upper abdominal region (vascular dilatation in the splanchnic region).
- Increased intestinal motility.
- Pain reduction.

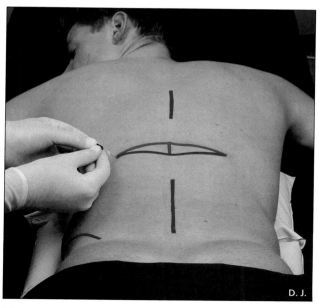

Fig. 17.6 Redirection of the needle at an angle of 60° to the skin surface

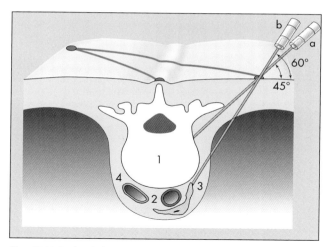

Fig. 17.7 Path of the needle to the celiac plexus. Diagram: (a) contact with the L1 vertebra, (b) introduction of the needle at a steeper angle of 60° to the skin surface. (1) L1 vertebra, (2) aorta, (3) celiac plexus, (4) inferior vena cava

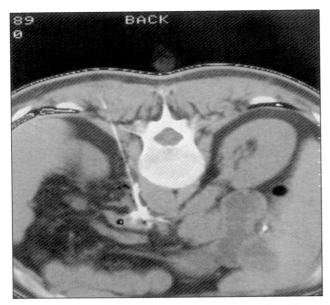

Fig. 17.8 Dorsal CT-guided celiac plexus injection. After injection of contrast medium, a good spread in the area of the celiac plexus can be seen

[From Grönemeyer and Seibel, Interventionelle Computertomographie. Lehrbuch und Atlas zur interventionellen Operationstechnik und Schmerztherapie. Vienna/Berlin: Uebberreuter Wissenschaft, 1989]

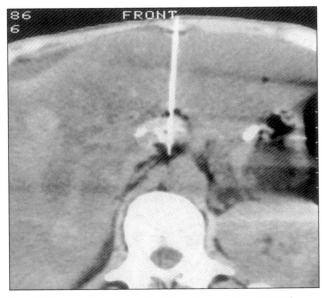

Fig. 17.9 Ventral transhepatic CT-guided injection. Several access routes are possible in celiac plexus injection. In this case, the injection was carried out using a ventral transhepatic approach. The tip of the needle lies directly alongside the celiac trunk. The alcohol spreads precisely within the celiac plexus

[From Grönemeyer and Seibel, Interventionelle Computertomographie. Lehrbuch und Atlas zur interventionellen Operationstechnik und Schmerztherapie. Vienna/Berlin: Uebberreuter Wissenschaft, 1989]

Dosage
Diagnostic
20–30 ml local anesthetic, e. g. 0.5–1 % prilocaine, 0.5–1 % mepivacaine, 0.5–1 % lidocaine.

Therapeutic
- Local anesthetics
  20–30 ml local anesthetic, e. g. 0.375–0.5 % ropivacaine, 0.25–0.375 % bupivacaine.
  A mixture with methylprednisolone is recommended in acute conditions.
- Neurolytics
  25–50 ml 50 % ethanol in combination with 0.2 % ropivacaine or 0.125 % bupivacaine.
  Some authors recommended prior administration of 5 ml 2 % lidocaine to relieve the pain of the ethanol injection.

Side effects
Hypotension due to sympathetic block (caution in older patients).

Complications
Severe
- Intravascular injections (aorta, vena cava, celiac artery, renal artery) with toxic reactions (see Chap. 4, pp. 42, 43).
- Epidural or subarachnoid injection (see Chap. 28, p. 200 and Chap. 33, p. 231).
- Pneumothorax.

Potential
- Vascular injury (hemorrhage, retroperitoneal hematoma formation).
- Injection into kidneys and other intra-abdominal organs.
- Aortal pseudoaneurysm.
- Abscess or cyst formation.
- Intraosseous or psoas injection.

Complications of neurolytic block
- Paraplegia [3, 15].
- Monoparesis, with loss of sphincter function in the rectum and bladder.
- Sexual dysfunction.
- Diarrhea.
- Retroperitoneal fibrosis.
- Renal necrosis.
- Chemical peritonitis [2].
- Chemical pericarditis [12].

Celiac plexus block

Block no.   ☐ Right   ☐ Left

Record and checklist

Name: _____   Date: _____

Diagnosis: _____

Premedication: ☐ No   ☐ Yes

Neurological abnormalities: ☐ No   ☐ Yes _____

Purpose of block: ☐ *Diagnosis*   ☐ *Treatment*

Needle: *G* _____ *Length* _____ *cm*

i. v. access and infusion: ☐ *Yes*

Monitoring: ☐ *ECG*   ☐ *Pulse oximetry*

Ventilation facilities: ☐ *Yes (equipment checked)*

Emergency equipment *(drugs):*   ☐ *Checked*

Patient: ☐ *Informed*   ☐ *Consent*

Contraindications excluded: ☐

Position: ☐ *Prone*   ☐ *Lateral decubitus*

Injection level: ☐ *L1*

Injection technique: ☐ *Dorsal* ☐ *Ventral* ☐ *X-ray image intensifier guidance*
                       ☐ *CT-guided*

Injection:

Local anesthetic: _____ *ml* _____ %
(incremental)

Addition to LA: ☐ *Yes* _____ ☐ *No* _____

Neurolytic: _____ *ml* _____ %

Addition: ☐ *Yes*   ☐ *No*

Patient's remarks during injection:

☐ *None*   ☐ *Paresthesias*   ☐ *Warmth*   ☐ *Pain*

Neural area: _____

Objective block effect after 15 min:

☐ *Cold test* ☐ *Temperature measurement before* _____ °C *after* _____ °C

Monitoring after block: ☐ *< 1 h*   ☐ *> 1 h*

                    Time of discharge: _____

Complications:

☐ *None*   ☐ *Intravascular injection*   ☐ *Subarachnoid / epidural*
☐ *Pneumothorax* ☐ *BP reduction*   ☐ *Neurological injury*   ☐ *Other*

Subjective effects of block: Duration: _____

☐ *None*   ☐ *Increased pain*
☐ *Reduced pain*   ☐ *No pain*

VISUAL ANALOG SCALE

|︱︱︱︱|︱︱︱︱|︱︱︱︱|︱︱︱︱|︱︱︱︱|︱︱︱︱|︱︱︱︱|︱︱︱︱|︱︱︱︱|︱︱︱︱|
0   10   20   30   40   50   60   70   80   90   100

Special notes:

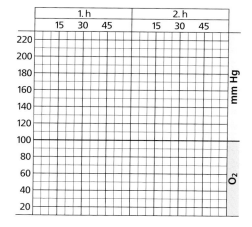

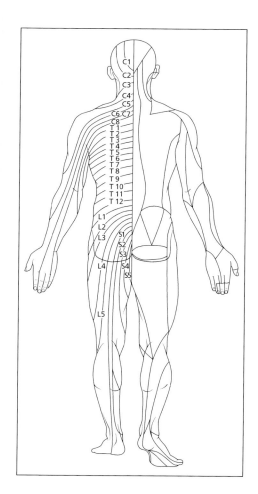

Lower extremities

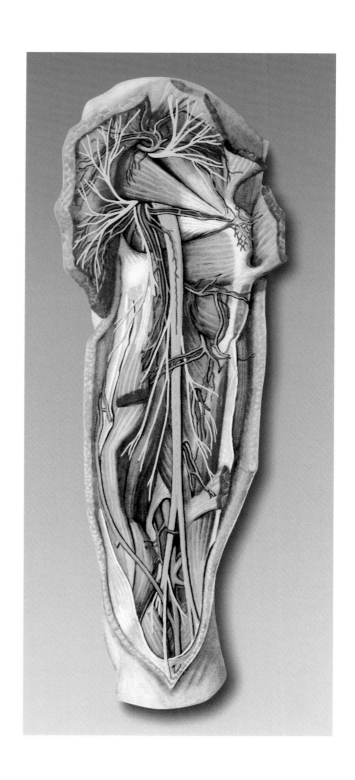

Lumbar plexus, sacral plexus and coccygeal plexus

Anatomy

These plexuses, closely related to one another, are formed by the lumbar, sacral and coccygeal spinal nerves.

The **lumbar plexus** lies in front of the transverse processes of the lumbar vertebrae. It mainly arises from the ventral branches, the first three lumbar nerves, most of the fourth lumbar nerve and the twelfth thoracic nerve (subcostal nerve).

The most important branches of the plexus are located in **a fascial compartment** that is enclosed ("sandwiched") by the quadratus lumborum, psoas major and iliacus muscles.

The first lumbar nerve, which contains a branch from the twelfth thoracic nerve, divides into an upper branch (iliohypogastric nerve and ilioinguinal nerve) and a lower branch (genitofemoral nerve).

Most of the second, third and parts of the fourth lumbar nerves form ventral and dorsal branches, from which the femoral nerve and obturator nerve branch off. The lateral femoral cutaneous nerve is formed from fibers of the dorsal branches of L2/L3.

The caudal parts of the ventral branches of L4 and L5 combine to form the **lumbosacral trunk.** Together with the ventral branches of the first three sacral nerves and the upper part of the ventral branch of the fourth sacral nerve, the lumbosacral trunk forms the sacral plexus, the largest branch of which is the sciatic nerve. The lumbar plexus is also connected with the lumbar part of the sympathetic nervous system via two or three long communicating branches.

The thickness of the ventral branches of the lumbar nerves increases markedly from the first to the fifth nerve (L1 has a diameter of ca. 2.5 mm, L2 is already ca. 4 mm, L3 and L4 are ca. 6 mm and L5 is as large as 7 mm).

The **coccygeal plexus** arises from the lower part of the ventral branches of the fourth and fifth sacral nerves, as well as the coccygeal nerves.

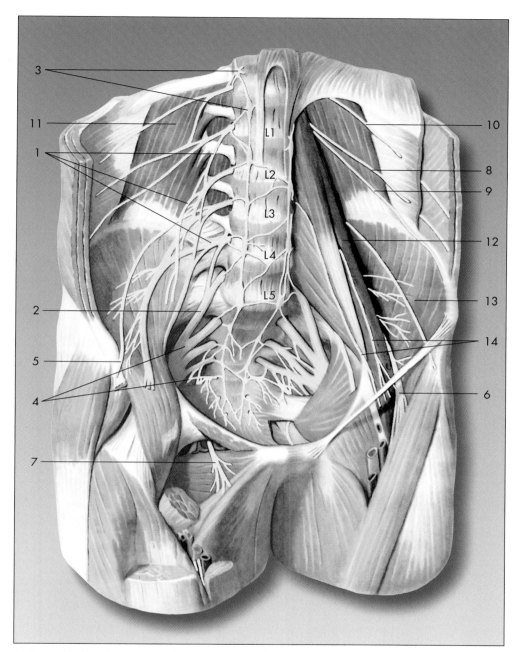

Anatomy: lumbar plexus, sacral plexus and coccygeal plexus.
(1) Lumbar plexus, (2) lumbosacral trunk, (3) sympathetic trunk, (4) sacral plexus, (5) lateral femoral cutaneous nerve, (6) femoral nerve, (7) obturator nerve, (8) iliohypogastric nerve, (9) ilioinguinal nerve, (10) subcostal nerve, (11) quadratus lumborum muscle, (12) psoas major muscle, (13) iliacus muscle, (14) genitofemoral nerve

Lumbar plexus blocks

Introduction

The concept underlying blocks of the lumbar plexus is that the course of the neural network from the transverse processes to the inguinal ligament lies within a perivascular and perineural space. Like the epidural space, this space limits the spread of the local anesthetic and conducts it to the various nerves.

Within the connective tissue and neural sheath, the concentration and volume of the local anesthetic determine the extent of the block's spread.

Two techniques are described that belong to the standard methods for blocking the lumbar plexus:

- The caudal (ventral) psoas compartment block ("three-in-one" inguinal femoral paravascular block).
- The cranial (dorsal) psoas compartment block.

18 Inguinal femoral paravascular block ("three-in-one" block)

Definition

The "three-in-one" block is an infero-antero approach to the femoral nerve, lateral femoral cutaneous nerve and obturator nerve. These three nerves (Fig. 18.1) are blocked with a single injection into the common connective tissue and neural sheath (Fig. 18.2) immediately below the inguinal ligament.

A volume of at least 30–40 ml of local anesthetic is necessary to block all three nerves.

The success of the block depends directly on the amount of local anesthetic injected. To produce complete anesthesia of the leg, it should be combined with a sciatic nerve block (Figs. 18.7, 18.8).

Advantages
- Suitable for postoperative or post-traumatic analgesia and for therapeutic blocks.
- Suitable for patients in whom a unilateral block is desired – particularly in outpatient procedures.

Disadvantages
- Success is unpredictable.
- Larger amounts of local anesthetic are necessary (particularly if the sciatic nerve is also being anesthetized).
- The likelihood of systemic toxicity is increased.
- Longer times to onset of effect must be expected (surgical indications).
- Not all nerves in the plexus are blocked (e. g. the lateral femoral cutaneous nerve).
- For surgical procedures with ischemia or tourniquet, neuraxial anesthesia is preferable.

Indications

Surgical
- Superficial surgical interventions in the innervated area:
  wound care, skin transplantation, muscle biopsies.
- Blocking of the obturator reflex in transurethral prostate resection.
- Analgesia for positioning for neuraxial block anesthesia in femoral neck fractures.
- Performing surgical interventions in the area of the lower extremity in ischemia or tourniqet, in combination with block of the sciatic nerve.
  Larger volumes of local anesthetic must be used here (toxicity!).
- Outpatient procedures.

Therapeutic
- Postoperative pain therapy (e. g. after femoral neck, femoral shaft, tibial and patellar fractures, knee joint operations).
- Post-traumatic pain.
- Post-surgical neurolysis or nerve reimplantations for better innervation.
- Early mobilization after hip or knee joint operations.
- Arterial occlusive disease and poor perfusion in the lower extremities.
- Complex regional pain syndrome (CRPS) types I and II.
- Postamputation pain.
- Edema in the leg after radiotherapy.
- Diabetic polyneuropathy.
- Knee joint arthrosis.
- Elimination of adductor spasm in paraplegic patients.

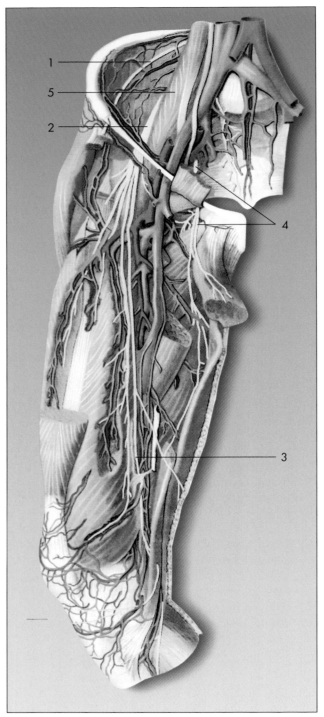

Fig. 18.1 Anatomy: femoral nerve, lateral femoral cutaneous nerve and obturator nerve.
(1) Lateral femoral cutaneous nerve, (2) femoral nerve,
(3) saphenous nerve, (4) obturator nerve, (5) psoas major muscle

Block series
A series of six to eight blocks is recommended. When there is evidence of improvement in the symptoms, additional blocks can also be carried out.

Prophylactic
- Postoperative analgesia.
- Prophylaxis against postamputation pain.
- Prophylaxis against Sudeck's atrophy (CRPS).

Contraindications

Specific
- Infections (e. g. osteomyelitis, pyoderma) or malignant diseases in the inguinal region.
- Local hematoma.
- Anticoagulant treatment.
- Distorted anatomy (due to prior surgical interventions or trauma to the inguinal and thigh region).

Relative
The decision should be taken after carefully weighing up the risks and benefits:
- Hemorrhagic diathesis.
- Stable central nervous system disorders.
- Local neural injury (caution when there is unclear responsibility between surgery and anesthesia).
- Contralateral neural paresis.
- Patients with a femoral bypass.

Procedure

This block should be carried out by experience anesthetists, or under their supervision.

Preparations
Check that the emergency equipment is complete and in working order. Sterile precautions, intravenous access, ECG monitoring, pulse oximetry, intubation kit, ventilation facilities, emergency medication.

Materials (Fig. 18.3)
Fine 26-G needle, 2.5 cm long, for local anesthesia.
80 mm long atraumatic 22-G needle (15°) with injection lead ("immobile needle," e. g. Stimuplex D, B. Braun Melsungen). Nerve stimulator (e. g. Stimuplex HNS 11, B. Braun Melsungen).
In continuous techniques: catheter set, e. g. Contiplex (Contiplex catheter 0.45 × 0.85 × 400 mm, with 18-G indwelling needle (15–30°), B. Braun Melsungen).
Syringes: 2 and 20 ml.
Local anesthetics, disinfectant, swabs, compresses, sterile gloves and drape.

Patient positioning
Supine, with the thigh slightly abducted. The patient's ipsilateral hand lies under the head. The person carrying out the injection must stand on the side being blocked.

Landmarks
The femoral artery is palpated 1–2 cm distal to the inguinal ligament. It is held between the spread index and middle finger. The injection point lies about 1–1.5 cm laterally.
Skin prep, subcutaneous local anesthesia, sterile drapes, draw up local anesthetic into 20-ml syringes, check patency of injection needles and functioning of nerve stimulator, attach electrodes.

Preliminary puncture with a large-lumen needle or hemostylet.

> **Caution**
> The **quadriceps femoris muscle** and the **patella** must be observed throughout the procedure.

Injection technique

Single injection technique
　The injection is carried out in a cranial direction at an angle of about 30–40° to the skin surface, almost parallel to the course of the femoral artery.
Stimulant current of 1–2 mA and 2 Hz is selected for a stimulation period of 0.1 ms (Fig. 18.4).

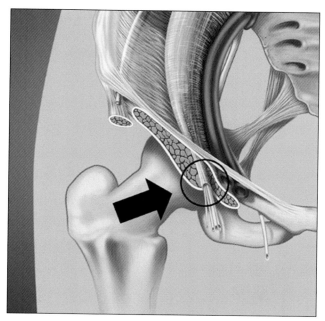

Fig. 18.2 Common connective tissue and neural sheath

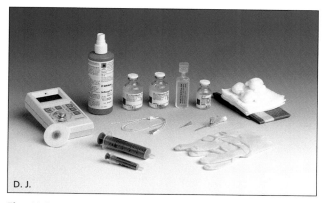

Fig. 18.3 Materials

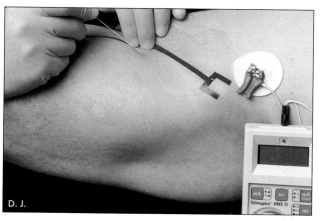

Fig. 18.4 Injection. Cranial direction, at an angle of about 30–40° to the skin surface

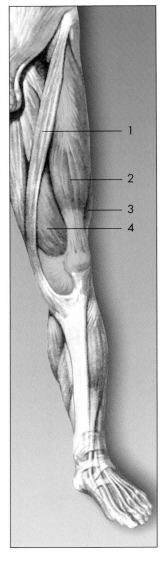

Fig. 18.5 Note the contractions of the quadriceps femoris muscle and patellar movements! (1) Sartorius muscle, (2) rectus femoris muscle, (3) vastus lateralis muscle, (4) vastus medialis muscle

▨ The needle is advanced until contractions of the **quadriceps femoris muscle** and **patellar** movements become visible ("dancing patella"). Contractions of the sartorius muscle alone suggest incorrect positioning and are inadequate (Fig. 18.5).

▨ Do **not** advance the needle further!
The stimulant current is reduced to 0.3 mA. Slight twitching suggests that the stimulation needle is in the immediate vicinity of the nerve.

▨ Aspiration test.

▨ Test dose of 3 ml local anesthetic (e. g. 1 % prilocaine). During the injection, the twitching slowly disappears.

▨ Incremental injection of a local anesthetic (injection-aspiration after each 3–4 ml).

▨ After the injection, **compression massage** of the injection area is carried out and then **flexing of the thigh** for about 1 minute (Fig. 18.6).

▨ Cardiovascular monitoring.

Caution
During the injection, distal compression should be applied with the finger to encourage proximal spread of the local anesthetic.

The distribution of the anesthetic is indicated in Figure 18.7.

Continuous technique
The site is located in the same way as described for the unilateral technique. Puncture is carried out about 2–2.5 cm below the inguinal ligament and 1–1.5 cm lateral to the femoral artery and in a cranial direction at an angle of about 30–40°.

Using the Seldinger technique, the catheter is advanced at least 10 cm deep into the fascial compartment.

An aspiration test, administration of a test dose, fixation of the catheter and placement of a bacterial filter then follow. After aspirating again, a local anesthetic is administered on an incremental basis.

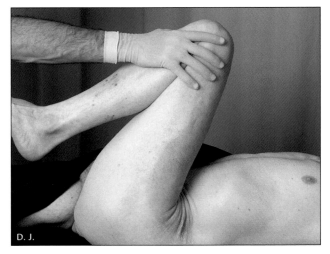

D. J.

Fig. 18.6 After the injection – flexing the thigh for about 1 minute

Dosage

Surgical
30–40 ml local anesthetic, e. g. 0.75 % ropivacaine, 0.5 % bupivacaine, 1 % prilocaine, 1 % mepivacaine.
A combination of local anesthetics with longer-term and medium-term effect has proved valuable for surgical indications – e. g. 1 % prilocaine (20 ml) + 0.5–0.75 % ropivacaine (20 ml) or 1 % prilocaine (20 ml) + 0.25–0.5 % bupivacaine (20 ml).

Therapeutic
20 ml local anesthetic, e. g. 0.2–0.375 % ropivacaine, 0.125–0.25 % bupivacaine.

Important notes for outpatients
Long standing block can occur (even after administration of low-dose local anesthetics, e. g. 0.125 % bupivacaine or 0.2 % ropivacaine).
The blocked leg can give way, even 10–18 hours after the injection.
The patient must therefore use walking aids during this period. The same rules apply to the treatment of post-amputation pain. During the period of effect of the local anesthetic the patient should not wear a prosthesis.

> **Caution**
> A record must be kept of patient information and consent.

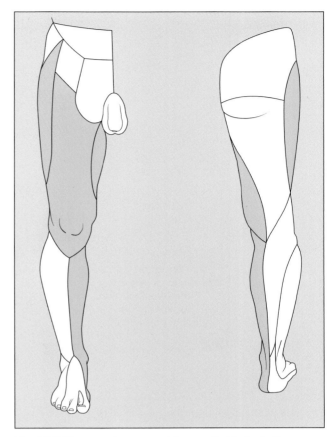

Fig. 18.7 The neural areas most frequently blocked after administering a "three-in-one" block

Continuous technique
Test dose: 3–5 ml 1 % prilocaine (1 % mepivacaine).
Bolus administration: 30 ml 0.5–0.75 % ropivacaine or 0.25–0.5 % bupivacaine.
Maintenance dose:
Intermittent administration: 15–20 ml of local anesthetic every 4–6 hours (0.5–0.75 % ropivacaine or 0.25–0.5 % bupivacaine) after a prior test dose.
Reduction of the dose and/or adjustment of the interval, depending on the clinical picture.
Continuous infusion: infusion of the local anesthetic via the catheter should be started 30–60 minutes after the bolus dose. A test dose is obligatory.

Ropivacaine: 0.2–0.375 %	**6–14 ml/h**
Bupivacaine: 0.125 %	**10–14 ml/h**
Bupivacaine: 0.25 %	**8–10 ml/h**

If necessary, the infusion can be supplemented with bolus doses of 5–10 ml 0.5–0.75 % ropivacaine (0.25–0.5 % bupivacaine).

> **Caution**
> Individual adjustment of the dosage and period of treatment is essential.

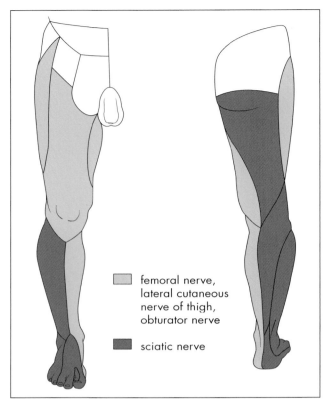

Fig. 18.8 Comparison of the innervation areas of the femoral nerve, lateral femoral cutaneous nerve and obturator nerve with the innervation area of the sciatic nerve

femoral nerve, lateral cutaneous nerve of thigh, obturator nerve

sciatic nerve

Complications

- Nerve injury

  Traumatic nerve injury is a rare complication with this technique. It can occur as a result of the use of sharp needles (due to nerve puncture), intraneural or microvascular injury (hematoma and its sequelae), prolonged ischemia, as well as toxic effects of intraneurally injected local anesthetic (see Chap. 7, p. 76). Probable effects of intraneural injection include a transient neurological deficit (unexpectedly long period of effect of the block, lasting up to 10 days) [5, 9].

  A suspicion of intraneural positioning arises if there is strong twitching even at low levels of stimulant current (e. g. 0.2 mA) and if there is no interruption of the twitching after administration of the test dose. The local anesthetic may also be difficult to inject. Correction of the needle position is essential. (On prophylaxis, see Chap. 7, p. 76).

- Intravascular injection (see Chap. 4, p. 42).
- CNS intoxication (see Chap. 4, p. 43).
- Infection in the injection area (continuous techniques).
- Hematoma formation (note the obligatory prophylactic compression).

19 Psoas compartment block

Definition

The psoas compartment block represents a **superoposterior access route** to the lumbar plexus.

The concept is to block the closely juxtaposed branches of the lumbar plexus and parts of the sacral plexus by injecting local anesthetic through an accessible access route to the plexus (L4–5).

When the quality of the block is good, the area of distribution is comparable with that of the "three-in-one" block (see Chap. 18, Fig. 18.7).

The following nerves are affected: lateral femoral cutaneous nerve, femoral nerve, genitofemoral nerve, obturator nerve, and parts of the sciatic and posterior femoral cutaneous nerve.

To achieve complete numbness of the lower extremity, a combination of this block with block of the sciatic nerve is necessary (see Chap. 18, Figs. 18.7, 18.8).

Advantages
- Better block quality in comparison with the "three-in-one" block.
- Suitable for patients in whom a unilateral block is desired, particularly in outpatient procedures.
- The method is suitable for postoperative and post-traumatic analgesia and for therapeutic blocks.

Disadvantages
- Success of the block is unpredictable.
- Larger quantities of local anesthetic are needed (particularly if the sciatic nerve is also being anesthetized).
- There is an increased likelihood of systemic toxicity.
- There is a potential risk of intrathecal or epidural injection.
- Longer periods to onset of effect must be expected (surgical indications).
- For surgical procedures with ischemia or tourniquet, neuraxial anesthesia is preferable.

Indications

Surgical
- As a continuous or single technique block for all surgical procedures in the region of the lower extremity in ischemia/tourniquet, but in combination with a block of the sciatic nerve. A need for larger volumes of local anesthetics must be expected (toxicity!) (see Chap. 18, pp. 151, 156).
- Outpatient procedures.

Therapeutic
- Postoperative and post-traumatic pain therapy.
- Early mobilization after hip and knee joint operations.
- Arterial occlusive disease and poor perfusion of the lower extremities.
- Complex regional pain syndrome (CRPS), types I and II.
- Post-surgical neurolysis or nerve reimplantations for better innervation.
- Edema after radiotherapy.
- Postamputation pain.
- Diabetic polyneuropathy.
- Tumors and metastases in the hip joint and lesser pelvis.

Block series
A series of six to eight blocks is recommended. When there is evidence of improvement in the symptoms, additional blocks can also be carried out.

Prophylactic
- Postoperative analgesia.
- Prophylaxis against postamputation pain.
- Prophylaxis against Sudeck's atrophy (CRPS).

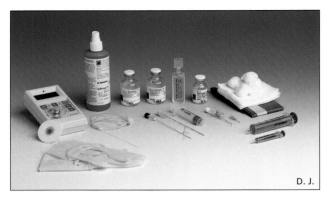

Fig. 19.1 Materials

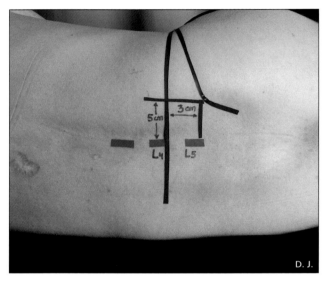

Fig. 19.2 Location

Contraindications

Specific
- Infection or hematoma in the injection area.
- Anticoagulant treatment.
- Lesion in the nerves to be stimulated distal to the injection site.

Relative
The decision should be taken after carefully weighing up the risks and benefits:
- Hemorrhagic diathesis.
- Stable systemic neural diseases.
- Local nerve injury (caution when there is unclear responsibility between surgery and anesthesia).
- Contralateral nerve paresis.

Procedure

This block should be carried out by experienced anesthetists, or under their supervision.

Preparations
Check that the emergency equipment is complete and in working order. Sterile precautions, intravenous access, ECG monitoring, pulse oximetry, intubation kit, ventilation facilities, emergency medication.

Materials (Fig. 19.1)
Fine 26-G needle, 2.5 cm long, for local anesthesia.
- Electrostimulation technique:
  Nerve stimulator (e. g. Stimuplex HNS 11, B. Braun Melsungen).
  120 mm long atraumatic 22-G needle (15°) with injection lead ("immobile needle", e. g. Stimuplex D, B. Braun Melsungen).
- Loss-of-resistance technique:
  120 mm (150 mm) long spinal needle, 20–22 G (e. g. Spinocan 0.7–0.9 × 120 mm (150 mm), B. Braun Melsungen) and a smoothly moving 10-ml plastic or glass syringe.
- Continuous technique:
  18-G Crawford or 18-G (15°) Contiplex D cannula (1.3 × 110 mm with plexus catheter, B. Braun Melsungen).

Syringes: 2 and 20 ml.
Local anesthetics, disinfectant, swabs, compresses, sterile gloves and drape.

Patient positioning
Lateral decubitus or sitting, depending on the position of the neuraxial anesthesia, legs drawn up, with the leg being blocked positioned higher.

Location
The iliac crest and the midline of the spinous process are located. From the intersection between these (L4 spinous process), a line is drawn 3 cm caudally, and from the end of it another line is drawn 5 cm laterally as far as the medial edge of the iliac crest, and marked as the injection point (Fig. 19.2).

Skin prep, local anesthesia, sterile draping, drawing up the local anesthetic into 20-ml syringes, checking the patency of the injection needle and functioning of the nerve stimulator, attaching the electrodes.

Preliminary puncture with a large-lumen needle or hemostylet.

> **Caution**
> The quadriceps femoris muscle must be watched throughout the procedure (see Chap. 18, Fig. 18.5, p. 154).

Injection technique

Electrostimulation technique

▨ Introduce an electrostimulation needle perpendicular to the skin surface until bone contact is made with the transverse process of L5 (Figs. 19.3, 19.5). It is then withdrawn slightly and advanced further cranially, past the transverse process (Figs. 19.4, 19.5). Stimulant current of 1 mA and 2 Hz is selected for a stimulation period of 0.1 ms.

▨ Advance the needle further until contractions of the **quadriceps femoris muscle** become visible.

▨ Reduce the stimulant current to 0.3 mA. If contractions of the muscle are still visible at this level of current, the needle is in the correct position.

▨ Aspiration test.

▨ Test dose of 3–5 ml of a local anesthetic.

▨ Incremental injection of a local anesthetic (injection-aspiration after each 3–4 ml).

▨ Precise cardiovascular monitoring.

Loss-of-resistance technique

▨ A 120 mm (150 mm) long 20–22-G spinal needle is introduced perpendicularly until bone contact is made with the transverse process of L5.
After bone contact, the needle is withdrawn slightly, as in the paravertebral block, and then advanced in a cranial direction past the transverse process as far as the quadratus lumborum muscle.

▨ Removal of the stylet and aspiration.

▨ A syringe filled with air or 0.9 % NaCl is attached.

▨ The needle is slowly advanced with constant pressure on the plunger.

▨ After initial resistance from the surrounding muscle mass, perforation of the muscle fascia occurs and there is penetration into the fascial compartment between the quadratus lumborum muscle and the psoas major muscle, characterized by "loss of resistance". Experience shows that this occurs at a depth of about 12 ± 2 cm. Paresthesias are often, but not always, produced.

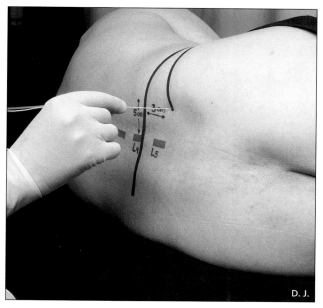

Fig. 19.3 The injection needle is introduced perpendicular to the skin surface until bone contact is made with the transverse process of L5

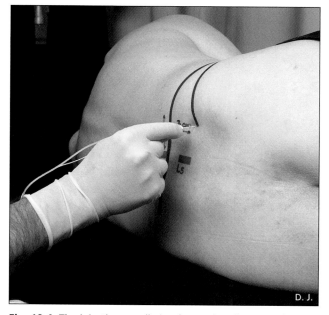

Fig. 19.4 The injection needle is advanced until contractions of the quadriceps femoris muscle become visible

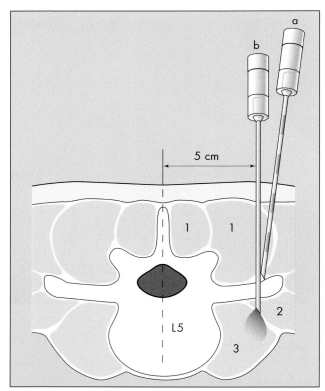

Fig. 19.5 Diagram: (a) contact with the transverse process of L5; (b) the needle is advanced past the transverse process until contractions of the quadriceps femoris muscle become visible. (1) Erector spinae muscle, (2) quadratus lumborum muscle, (3) Psoas muscle

- Once the psoas compartment has been reached, 10–20 ml of air is injected in order to dilate the space.
- Aspiration test.
- Test dose of 3–5 ml of a local anesthetic.
- Incremental injection of local anesthetic (injection-aspiration after each 3–4 ml).
- The patient must remain in the same position for about 5 minutes.
- Precise cardiovascular monitoring.

Continuous technique
The plexus catheter is advanced through the previously placed 18-G Crawford cannula about 5 cm deep into the fascial compartment. An alternative that has become available more recently involves use of the electrostimulation technique with a 100 mm Contiplex D cannula. However, this technique is associated with a higher rate of failures.

Dosage
Surgical
40–50 ml local anesthetic, e. g. 1 % prilocaine (20–30 ml) + 0.5–0.75 % ropivacaine (20 ml); 1 % prilocaine (20–30 ml) + 0.25–0.5 % bupivacaine (20 ml).

Therapeutic
30 ml local anesthetic, e. g. 0.2–0.375 % ropivacaine, 0.125–0.25 % bupivacaine.

Important notes for outpatients
(See Chap. 18, p. 155)

Continuous
(See Chap. 18, p. 155)

Complications
- Nerve injury (extremely rare; see Chap. 18, p. 156).
- Intravascular injection (see Chap. 4, p. 42).
- CNS intoxication (see Chap. 4, p. 43).
- Subarachnoid or epidural injection (see Chap. 28, p. 200, and Chap. 33, p. 231).
- Hematoma formation.
- Intra-abdominal injuries.
- Postinjection pain due to spasm in the lumbar paravertebral musculature.

20 Sciatic nerve block

Definition

Block of the largest of the four nerves supplying the leg at the lower end of the lumbosacral plexus, after it exits from the greater sciatic foramen or infrapiriform foramen.

Anatomy (Fig. 20.1)

The **sciatic nerve** arises from the ventral branches of the spinal nerves from L4 to S3. Exiting from the pelvic cavity at the lower edge of the piriformis muscle (in about 2 % of individuals, the nerve pierces the piriformis), its 16–20 mm thick trunk courses between the ischial tuberosity and the greater trochanter, turns downward over the gemeli, the obturator internus tendon and the quadratus femoris, which separate it from the hip joint, and leaves the buttock to enter the thigh beneath the lower border of the gluteus maximus. Distal to this, the nerve lies on the posterior surface of the adductor magnus muscle, where it is covered by the flexor muscle originating from the ischial tuberosity and thus extends as far as the popliteal fossa. Here it lies slightly laterally and above the popliteal vein and artery, with thick popliteal fascia overlying it. In the proximal angle of the popliteal fossa, the nerve usually divides into the thicker **tibial nerve,** which continues the trunk and the smaller **common peroneal (fibular) nerve.**

The **sensory** branches of the nerve innervate the dorsal thigh, the dorsolateral lower leg and lateral half of the foot, the hip and knee joint, as well as the femur. Its **muscular branches** are responsible for supplying the biceps femoris, semimembranosus, semitendinosus and adductor magnus muscles.

Indications

Surgical
- Superficial procedures in the innervated area.
- Carrying out surgical procedures in the region of the lower extremity under ischemia/tourniquet, but in combination with a block of the lumbar plexus ("three-in-one" block or dorsal psoas compartment block). A need for larger volumes of local anesthetics must be expected (toxicity!) (see Chap. 18, Fig. 18.8).

Therapeutic
An isolated block of the sciatic nerve is rarely indicated. A combination with block of the lumbar plexus or femoral nerve is recommended (see Chaps. 18, 19 and 21).

Block series
A series of six to eight blocks is recommended. When there is evidence of improvement in the symptoms, additional blocks can also be carried out.

Contraindications

Specific
- Infection or hematoma in the injection area.
- Anticoagulant treatment.
- Lesion in the nerves to be blocked distal to the injection site.

Relative
The decision should be taken after carefully weighing up the risks and benefits:
- Hemorrhagic diathesis.
- Stable central nervous system diseases.
- Local nerve injury.

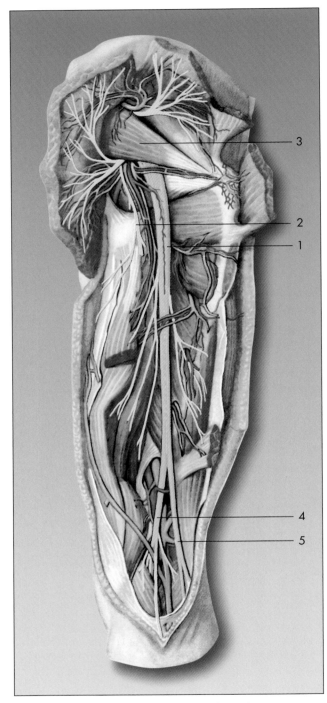

Fig. 20.1 Anatomy of the sciatic nerve. (1) Sciatic nerve, (2) posterior femoral cutaneous nerve, (3) piriformis muscle, (4) tibial nerve, (5) common peroneal (fibular) nerve

Procedure

This block should be carried out by experienced anesthetists, or under their supervision.

Preparations
Check that the emergency equipment is complete and in working order. Sterile precautions, intravenous access, ECG monitoring, pulse oximetry, intubation kit, ventilation facilities, emergency medication.

Materials (Fig. 20.2)
Nerve stimulator (e. g. Stimuplex HNS 11, B. Braun Melsungen).
80 mm long (120–150 mm in ventral access), atraumatic 22-G needle (15°) with injection lead ("immobile needle"), e. g. Stimuplex D, B. Braun Melsungen).
Syringes: 2, 10 and 20 ml.
Local anesthetics, disinfectant, swabs, compresses, sterile gloves and drape.

Classic dorsal transgluteal technique

Patient positioning (Fig. 20.3)
Lateral decubitus, with the leg being blocked lying upwards (Sims' position).
The upper leg is bent at the hip and knee joints and the upper knee lies on the table. The lower leg is outstretched.

Landmarks (Fig. 20.4)
The important orientation points are: the greater trochanter and posterior superior iliac spine (and/or sacral hiatus). The greater trochanter and posterior superior iliac spine are located. From the mid-point of the connecting line, a line is drawn medially and the injection point is marked after 5 cm (Labat line). To check this, another line connecting the greater trochanter and the sacral hiatus is bisected (Winnie line). The two points coincide.
Skin prep, local anesthesia, sterile draping, drawing up local anesthetic into a 20-ml syringe, checking patency of the injection needle and correct functioning of the nerve stimulator, attaching the electrodes.

Preliminary puncture with a large-lumen needle or hemostylet.

During the procedure, the **biceps femoris, semimembranosus** and **semitendinosus muscles** and the **foot** must be observed.

Injection technique

Electrostimulation

▨ The injection needle is introduced perpendicular to the skin surface (Fig. 20.5). Stimulation current of 1 mA and 2 Hz is selected for a stimulation period of 0.1 ms.

▨ After about 1–4 cm, there should be direct stimulation of the **gluteus maximus muscle.**

▨ At a depth of about 5 cm, contractions of the **biceps femoris, semimembranosus** and **semitendinosus muscles** are produced (Fig. 20.6).

▨ After the needle is advanced further, at a depth of about 6–8 cm there is **plantar** and **dorsal flexion** of the foot as a response to the stimulus from the tibial or peroneal part of the sciatic nerve (Fig. 20.6).

▨ Do **not** advance the needle any further.

▨ The stimulation current is reduced to 0.3 mA. Slight twitching suggests that the needle is positioned in the immediate vicinity of the nerve.

▨ Aspiration test.

▨ Test dose of 3 ml local anesthetic (e. g. 1 % prilocaine). During the injection, the twitching should slowly disappear.

▨ Incremental injection of a local anesthetic (injection–aspiration after each 3–4 ml).

▨ Precise cardiovascular monitoring.

The complete spread of the anesthesia is shown in Figure 20.9.

Producing paresthesias

An atraumatic injection needle 80 mm long (rarely longer) is advanced using the technique described above until paresthesias are elicited that extend to the sole of the foot, or until bone contact is made, with subsequent correction of the needle direction. This technique is associated with a higher failure rate.

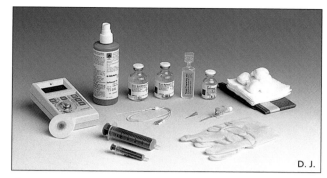

Fig. 20.2 Materials

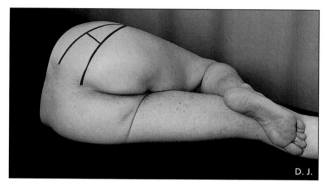

Fig. 20.3 Classic dorsal transgluteal technique (positioning)

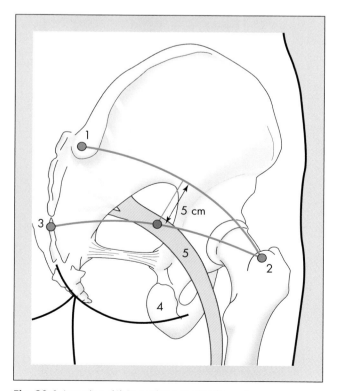

Fig. 20.4 Location. (1) Posterior superior iliac spine, (2) greater trochanter, (3) sacral hiatus, (4) ischial tuberosity, (5) sciatic nerve

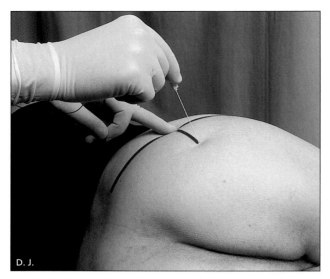

Fig. 20.5 The injection needle is introduced perpendicular to the skin surface

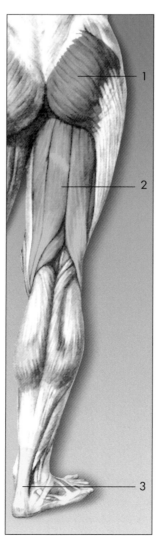

Fig. 20.6 Sequence of muscle contractions. (1) Gluteus maximus muscle, (2) semitendinosus muscle, semimembranosus muscle, biceps femoris muscle (3) plantar/dorsal flexion of the foot

Problem situations

▨ Bone contact at a depth of 8 cm without visible twitching. The injection needle should be withdrawn and the direction should be altered laterally.
▨ Intraneural positioning
The following signs suggest intraneural positioning of the injection needle:
– Strong twitching (even at a stimulant current of 0.2 mA).
– No disappearance of the twitching during injection of a test dose.
– Resistance and severe pain during the injection.

The injection must be interrupted immediately and the needle must be withdrawn.

Ventral approach

Patient positioning
A supine position that is comfortable for the patient, with slight outward rotation of the leg being blocked.

Landmarks
Important orientation points are: anterior superior iliac spine, pubic tubercle and greater trochanter.
Two lines are drawn for orientation:
– A line connecting the anterior superior iliac spine with the pubic tubercle, which is marked into thirds.
– A second line parallel to the first, from the greater trochanter across the thigh.

A perpendicular line is drawn from the intersection of the medial and central third of the upper inguinal ligament line to the parallel line and marked as the injection point (Figs. 20.7, 20.8).

Injection technique
A 22-G (15°) atraumatic injection needle 120–150 mm long, with an injection lead, is advanced perpendicular to the skin until bone contact is made with the femur. The needle is then withdrawn slightly and introduced about 5 cm deeper, past the femur. The correct needle position is confirmed when paresthesias or twitches are produced during electrostimulation. After aspiration and administration of a test dose, incremental injection of a local anesthetic is carried out.

Dosage

Surgical

20–30 ml local anesthetic, e. g. 0.75 % ropivacaine, 0.5 % bupivacaine, 1 % prilocaine, 1 % mepivacaine. A combination of long-lasting and medium-term local anesthetics has proved particularly useful for surgical indications.

Therapeutic

10–20 ml local anesthetic, e. g. 0.2–0.375 % ropivacaine, 0.125–0.25 % bupivacaine.

Important notes for outpatients

(See Chap. 18, p. 155)

Complications

Complications are rare, but possible:

- Nerve injury (see Chap. 7, p. 76 and Chap. 18, p. 156).
- Intravascular injection (see Chap. 4, p. 42).
- CNS intoxication (see Chap. 4, p. 43).
- Infection in the area of the injection.
- Hematoma formation.

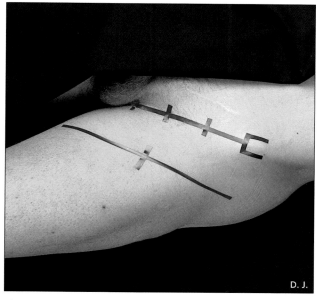

D. J.

Fig. 20.7 Location (in patient)

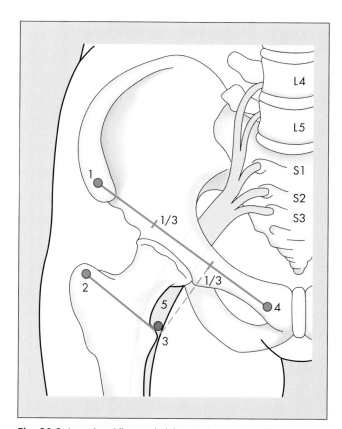

Fig. 20.8 Location (diagram). (1) Anterior superior iliac spine, (2) greater trochanter, (3) injection site, (4) pubic tubercle, (5) sciatic nerve

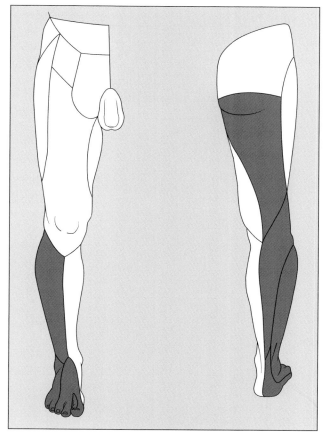

Fig. 20.9 Cutaneous innervated area of the sciatic nerve

Record and checklist

Lumbosacral plexus and individual nerves in the plexus

Block no.   ☐ Right   ☐ Left

Name: _____   Date: _____

Diagnosis: _____

Premedication: ☐ No   ☐ Yes

Neurological abnormalities: ☐ No   ☐ Yes _____

Purpose of block: ☐ Diagnosis   ☐ Treatment   ☐ Surgery

Needle: G _____ Length _____ cm   ☐ 15°   ☐ 30°   ☐ Other

i. v. access: ☐ Yes

Monitoring: ☐ ECG   ☐ Pulse oximetry

Ventilation facilities: ☐ Yes (equipment checked)

Emergency equipment (drugs):   ☐ Checked

Patient: ☐ Informed (post-block activity)   ☐ Consent

Position: ☐ Supine   ☐ Lateral decubitus   ☐ Sims' position   ☐ Sitting

Approach: ☐ Inguinal "3-in-1" block   ☐ Dorsal psoas compartment block
☐ Sciatic nerve   ☐ Femoral nerve   ☐ Lateral femoral cutaneous nerve
☐ Obturator nerve   ☐ Ilioinguinal/hypogastric nerves

Location technique: ☐ Electrostimulation   ☐ Paresthesias   ☐ Other

Plexus (nerve):   ☐ Located   ☐ Aspiration test   ☐ Test dose

Injection:

Local anesthetic: _____ ml _____ %
(incremental)

☐ Inguinal "3-in-1" block _____ ml   ☐ Dors. psoas compartment _____ ml
☐ Sciatic nerve _____ ml ☐ Femoral nerve _____ ml ☐ Lat. fem. cut. nerve ____ ml
☐ Obturator nerve _____ ml   ☐ Ilioinguinal/hypogastric nerves _____ ml
☐ Addition to LA: _____ µg/mg

Patient's remarks during injection:

☐ None   ☐ Paresthesias   ☐ Warmth   ☐ Pain (intraneural position?)

Neural area: _____

Objective block effect after 15 min:

☐ Cold test   ☐ Temperature measurement before _____ °C   after _____ °C
☐ Sensory   ☐ Motor

Monitoring after block: ☐ < 1 h   ☐ > 1 h

Time of discharge: _____ ☐ Motor / sensory function tested

Complications:

☐ None   ☐ Intravascular injection   ☐ Toxic signs
☐ Hematoma   ☐ Neurological complications   ☐ Other

Subjective effects of block: Duration: _____

☐ None   ☐ Increased pain   ☐ Reduced pain   ☐ No pain

VISUAL ANALOG SCALE

|꜒꜒꜒|
0   10   20   30   40   50   60   70   80   90   100

Special notes:

	1. h			2. h		
	15	30	45	15	30	45
220						
200						
180						
160						
140						
120						
100						
80						
60						
40						
20						

mm Hg

O₂

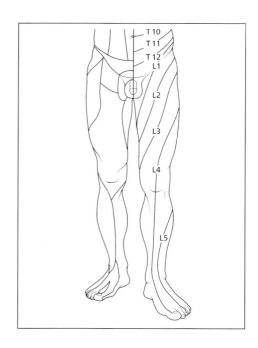

T 10
T 11
T 12
L1
L2
L3
L4
L5

Blocking individual nerves in the lumbar plexus

21 Femoral nerve

Definition
Block of the largest nerve emerging from the lumbar plexus below the inguinal ligament.

Anatomy (Fig. 21.1)

The nerve, which is about 12 mm wide, arises from the ventral branches of the spinal nerves from **L2–L4,** runs through the psoas major muscle and the iliacus muscle and reaches the thigh behind the inguinal ligament. Above the inguinal ligament, the femoral nerve is located in a fascial compartment, which is surrounded by the iliac fascia laterally, the psoas fascia medially and the transversalis fascia ventrally. After passing the inguinal ligament, the nerve continues dorsolateral to the iliopsoas fascia, ventral to the inguinal ligament and fascia lata and medial to the iliopectineal fascia. Four to five centimeters below the inguinal ligament, the nerve divides into an anterior, mainly sensory, branch and a posterior, mainly motor one.

Its largest sensory branch is the saphenous nerve, which separates from it in the femoral triangle. The femoral nerve provides the sensory supply to the upper thigh and shares in the innervation of the hip and knee joints as well as of the femur. Its sensory end branch, the saphenous nerve, innervates the medioventral lower leg and the medial half of the foot. Its muscular branches supply the pectineus, sartorius and quadriceps femoris muscles (see Chap. 18, Fig. 18.1).

Indications (see Chap. 18, p. 151)

Surgical
- Superficial surgical procedures in the area of innervation, usually in combination with block of the neighboring lumbar plexus nerves or the sciatic nerve.

Therapeutic
Excellent results can be achieved with combined block of the femoral nerve and sciatic nerve (block series), particularly in:
- Postamputation pain.
- Complex regional pain syndrome (CRPS), types I and 2 (see case report, p. 169).

In addition: in perfusion problems of the lower extremity, arterial occlusive disease (caution in patients with a femoral bypass), polyneuropathies, arthrosis of the knee joint, etc.

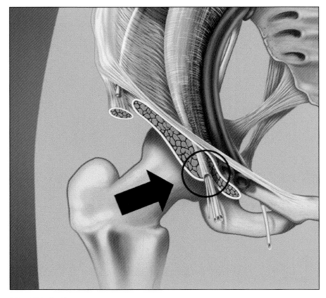

Fig. 21.1 Anatomy

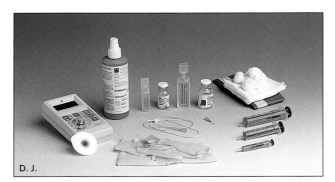

Fig. 21.2 Materials

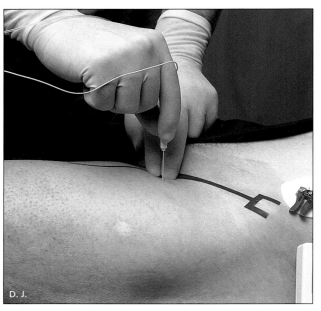

Fig. 21.3 Injection

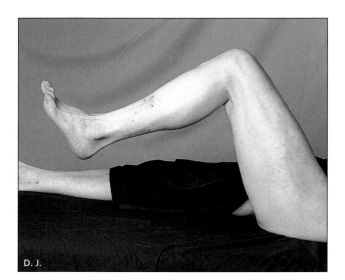

Fig. 21.4 The leg is maintained in the flexed position for several minutes after the injection

Procedure

Preparations (see Chap. 18, p. 152)

Materials (Fig. 21.2)
40 mm long, atraumatic 23–25-G needle (15°) with injection lead ("immobile needle," e. g. Stimuplex D, B. Braun Melsungen).
Syringes: 2, 10 and 20 ml.
Local anesthetics, disinfectant, swabs, compresses, sterile gloves and drape.

Patient positioning
Supine, with the thigh slightly abducted, with the ipsilateral hand under the head.

Landmarks
The femoral artery is palpated 1–2 cm distal to the inguinal ligament. It is held between the spread index finger and middle finger. The injection site is located about 1–1.5 cm lateral to this. The person performing the injection stands on the side being injected.
Skin prep, subcutaneous local anesthesia, covering with a sterile drape, drawing up the local anesthetic into a 10-ml or 20-ml syringe, checking the patency of the injection needle and correct functioning of the nerve stimulator, attaching the electrodes.

Injection technique
After a **preliminary puncture,** the injection needle is introduced perpendicular to the skin surface, with the femoral artery being pushed in a medial direction by the palpating finger (Fig. 21.3). The femoral nerve is located at a depth of ca. 2–3 cm. Producing paresthesias is helpful, but not obligatory.
After aspiration and administration of a test dose, incremental injection of a local anesthetic is carried out. If no paresthesias are produced, some of the local anesthetic is injected lateral to the artery in a fan-shaped fashion. The onset of effect is slow. A successful block is indicated if the patient is unable to extend the leg (Fig. 21.4).
It is helpful to use a nerve stimulator, as this allows a more targeted location of the nerve.
The distribution of anesthesia is shown in Figure 21.5.

Dosage

Surgical
30 ml local anesthetic, e. g. 0.75 % ropivacaine, 0.5 % bupivacaine, 1 % prilocaine, 1 % mepivacaine.

Therapeutic
Single block of the femoral nerve:
10–15 ml local anesthetic, e. g. 0.2 % ropivacaine, 0.125–0.25 % bupivacaine.
In combination with a sciatic nerve block:
Femoral nerve: 5–8 ml local anesthetic.
Sciatic nerve: 8–10 ml local anesthetic, e. g. 0.2–0.375 % ropivacaine, 0.125–0.25 % bupivacaine.

Important notes for outpatients
(See Chap. 18, p. 155)

Complications
(See Chap. 18, p. 156)

Example case
Patient W. W., aged 54, with a four-month history.
The following symptoms developed after an Achilles tendon strain:
Livid soft-tissue swelling in the area of the left foot and ankle joint, with sensitivity to touch and severe pain, resistant to treatment.
Radiography showed osteoporosis, with thinning of cortical bone.
Investigations indicated a diagnosis of Sudeck's atrophy (CRPS).
Prior treatment with calcitonin, cortisone, NSAIDs and opioids had not led to any relief of the symptoms.

Start of treatment, 4 August 1994 (Fig. 21.6)
A series of blocks [18] of the femoral nerve and sciatic nerve with 0.5 % bupivacaine, 25 ml (femoral nerve 15 ml, sciatic nerve 10 ml).

End of treatment, 24 October 1994 (Fig. 21.7)
Complete resolution of the symptoms.

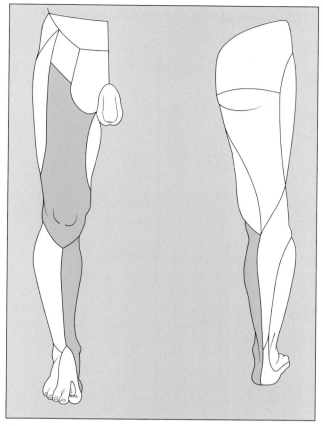

Fig. 21.5 Cutaneous innervation area of the femoral nerve

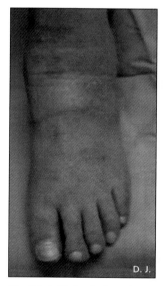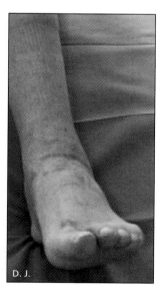

Fig. 21.6 Status before the start of treatment

Fig. 21.7 Status at the completion of treatment

22 Lateral femoral cutaneous nerve

Definition
Block of this sensory nerve, as it emerges from the lumbar plexus below the lateral inguinal ligament.

Anatomy (Fig. 22.1)

The lateral cutaneous femoral nerve arises from the ventral branches of the L2 and L3 spinal nerves, passing lateral to the psoas muscle and then to the iliacus muscle. Covered by the iliac fascia, it then runs to the region of the anterior superior iliac spine. It passes under the inguinal ligament and under the deep circumflex iliac artery, enters the thigh, where it lies under the superficial sheet of the fascia and divides into a thicker descending branch and a smaller posterior branch, which penetrate the fascia separately. The posterior branch runs posteriorly over the tensor fascia lata muscle and reaches the gluteal region. The anterior branch runs 3–5 cm below the inguinal ligament, then downwards along the anterior surface of the vastus lateralis muscle as far as the lateral knee area, where it sends off lateral branches (see Chap. 18, Fig. 18.1).

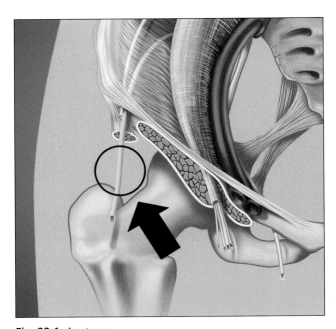

Fig. 22.1 Anatomy

Indications

Surgical
- Mainly for relief of tourniquet pain in combination with block of the neighboring nerves from the lumbar plexus and of the sciatic nerve.

Diagnostic
- Differentiation of various neuralgias in the thigh region.

Therapeutic (block series)
- Meralgia paraesthetica.

Contraindications

Infection at the injection site.

Procedure

Preparations
(See Chap. 18, p. 152)

Materials (Fig. 22.2)
40 mm long, atraumatic 25-G needle (15°/30°) with injection lead ("immobile needle", e. g. Stimuplex D, B. Braun Melsungen).

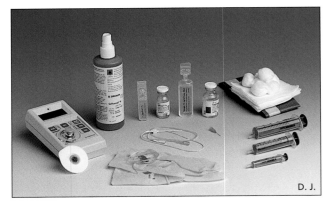

Fig. 22.2 Materials

Syringes: 2, 5, and 10 ml.
Local anesthetic, disinfectant, swabs, sterile gloves, drape.

Patient positioning
Supine, with the ipsilateral hand under the head.

Landmarks
The anterior superior iliac spine is palpated. The injection point lies about 2.5 cm medial and 2.5 cm caudal to it. The person carrying out the injection stands on the side being injected.
Skin prep, subcutaneous local anesthesia, drawing up the local anesthetic, checking the patency of the injection needle and correct functioning of the nerve stimulator if used, attaching the electrodes.

Injection technique (Fig. 22.3)
The injection needle is introduced slowly and perpendicularly in the direction of the fascia lata, penetration of which is recognized by loss of resistance or "fascial clicks".
Paresthesias are not elicited. Fan-shaped injection of the local anesthetic is carried out medially and laterally, subfascially as far as the ilium and also subcutaneously when withdrawing the needle.
When the *electrostimulation technique* is used, stimulation of the sensory nerve fibers is selected for a stimulation period of 1 ms. Cooperation on the part of the patient is a prerequisite for this technique.

The distribution of the block is shown in Figure 22.4.

Dosage
Surgical
10–15 ml local anesthetic, e. g. 0.75 % ropivacaine, 0.5 % bupivacaine, 1 % prilocaine, 1 % mepivacaine.

Therapeutic (block series)
5–10 ml local anesthetic, e. g. 0.2 % ropivacaine, 0.125–0.25 % bupivacaine.

Complications
No specific complications.

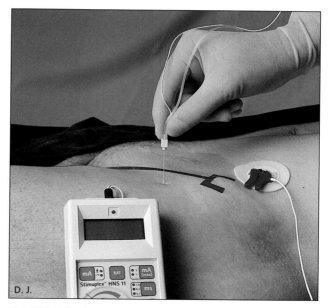

Fig. 22.3 Injection

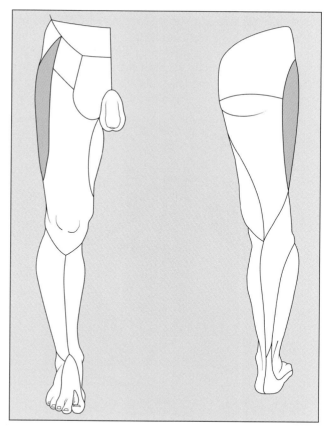

Fig. 22.4 Cutaneous innervation area of the lateral femoral cutaneous nerve

23 Obturator nerve

Definition
Block of the nerve emerging from the lumbar plexus in the obturator canal.

Anatomy (Fig. 23.1)

The obturator nerve arises from the ventral branches of the **L2–L4** spinal nerves.
The trunk runs downwards along the medial edge of the psoas muscle, passing behind the common iliac vessels to reach the lesser pelvis and the obturator canal. Within the canal, it divides into its two end branches – the anterior and posterior branches. It provides the motor supply for the obturator externus muscle and the adductors of the thigh, sends off branches to the hip and knee joints and to the femur and provides the sensory supply for a highly variable cutaneous area on the inside of the thigh and lower leg.

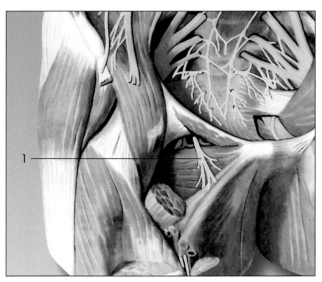

Fig. 23.1 Anatomy. (1) Obturator nerve

Indications

Surgical
For procedures in the knee joint and above the knee joint, as well as in the urological field, particularly for resections of bladder tumors in combination with blocks of neighboring nerves from the lumbar plexus and of the sciatic nerve.

Diagnostic
▨ Localization of hip joint pain.

Therapeutic
▨ Hip joint pain and elimination of adductor spasm.

Contraindications

Infection in the injection area.

Procedure

Preparations
(See Chap. 18, p. 152)

Materials (Fig. 23.2)
Fine 26-G needle, 2.5 cm long, for local anesthesia.
80 mm long, atraumatic 22-G needle (15°) with injection lead ("immobile needle", e. g. Stimuplex D, B. Braun Melsungen), or an 80 mm long, 22-G spinal needle.
Nerve stimulator (e. g. Stimuplex HNS 11, B. Braun Melsungen).
Syringes: 2, 10 and 20 ml.
Local anesthetics, disinfectant, swabs, sterile gloves and drape.

Patient positioning
Supine, with slight abduction of the leg being blocked. The patient's ipsilateral hand is under the head.

Landmarks
Anterior superior iliac spine, pubic tubercle. The pubic tubercle is located. The injection site lies about 1.5 cm lateral and 1.5 cm caudal to it.

Skin prep, local anesthesia, drawing up local anesthetic, checking patency of injection needle and correct functioning of the nerve stimulator, attaching electrodes.

> **Caution**
> The genitalia must be protected during skin prep.

Injection technique
- The injection needle is introduced perpendicular to the skin. At a depth of about 1.5–4 cm (depending on the anatomy), **bone contact** is made with the upper part of the inferior branch of the pubic bone. This depth is marked (Fig. 23.3 A, B).
- The needle is then withdrawn and advanced in a corrected direction **laterally** and slightly **caudally,** close underneath the superior branch of the pubic bone (Fig. 23.4 A, B).
- Entry into the **obturator canal** takes place after the needle has been advanced about 2–3 cm deeper than marked after bone contact with the inferior branch of the pubic bone. Paresthesias are not produced.

- When a nerve stimulator is being used, correct needle positioning is indicated when slight adductor twitches become visible after reduction of the stimulant current from 1 mA to 0.3 mA.
- Aspiration test.
- Injection of a local anesthetic is carried out on an incremental basis and in a fan shape (injection-aspiration).
- Success of the block depends directly on the amount of local anesthetic injected. A successful block is characterized by restricted adduction in the thigh.

Disadvantage
This technique is not easy to perform and the success rate is variable.
The distribution of numbness (very variable) is shown in Figure 23.5.

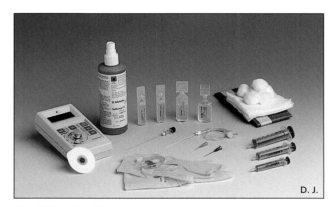

Fig. 23.2 Materials

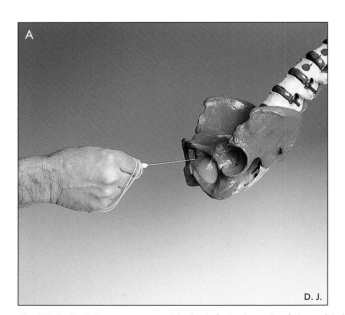

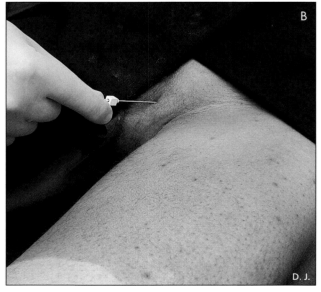

Fig. 23.3 A, B Bone contact with the inferior branch of the pubic bone. **A** In the skeleton

173

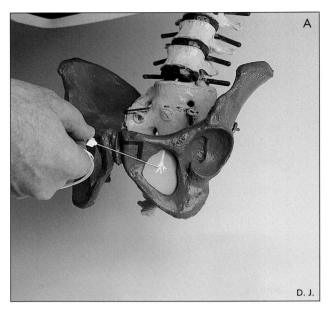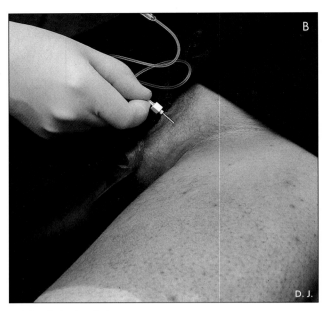

Fig. 23.4 A, B Advancing the injection needle laterally and slightly caudally. **A** In the skeleton

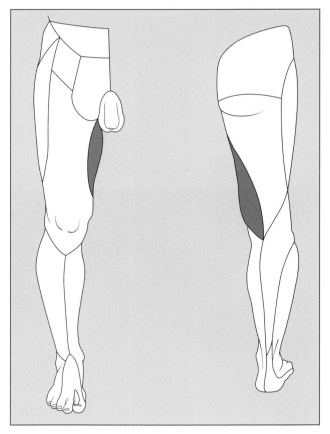

Fig. 23.5 Cutaneous innervation area of the obturator nerve

Dosage

10–15 ml local anesthetic, e. g. 0.375–0.5 % ropivacaine, 0.25–0.5 % bupivacaine, 1 % prilocaine, 1 % mepivacaine.

Complications

Complications are very rare, but possible:

▨ Intravascular injection (the injection area is very well vascularized; see Chap. 4, p. 42).
▨ Hematoma formation.
▨ Puncture of or injury to the vagina or bladder.

24 Ilioinguinal and iliohypogastric nerves

Definition
Block of these two neighboring nerves originating from the upper part of the lumbar plexus.

Anatomy (Fig. 24.1)

The **ilioinguinal** and **iliohypogastric nerves** arise from the upper branch of the first lumbar nerve in the lumbar plexus; the **genitofemoral nerve** is formed from the lower branch of the first lumbar nerve and from a small branch of the second lumbar nerve. These three nerves run parallel to the intercostal nerves, and participate in the innervation of the transversus and obliquus abdominis muscles.

The **ilioinguinal** nerve penetrates the internal oblique muscle at the level of the anterior superior iliac spine, and runs between this and the external oblique muscle in the direction of the inguinal ligament and the canal around the skin of the mons pubis, the scrotum (or lip of the pudendum in women) and the adjoining part of the femoral triangle.

The lateral cutaneous branch of the **iliohypogastric nerve** innervates the skin of the anterolateral part of the gluteal region, and ends in its anterior branch above the pubic bone.

The **genitofemoral nerve** passes through the psoas major muscle and divides into a genital branch and a femoral branch.

Indications

Surgical
- As an important part of field block in the inguinal region when carrying out herniorrhaphies.

Therapeutic
- Scar pain after herniorrhaphies.
- Post-herpetic neuralgia.

Contraindications

- Local infection.
- Anticoagulant therapy.

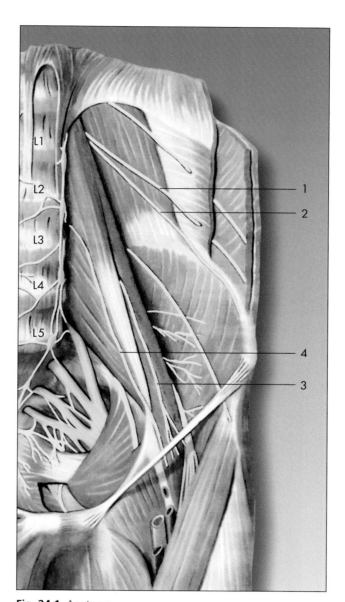

Fig. 24.1 Anatomy.
(1) Iliohypogastric nerve, (2) ilioinguinal nerve, (3) genitofemoral nerve (femoral branch), (4) genitofemoral nerve (genital branch)

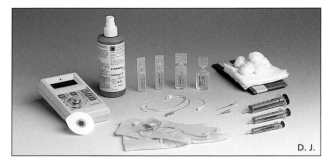

Fig. 24.2 Materials

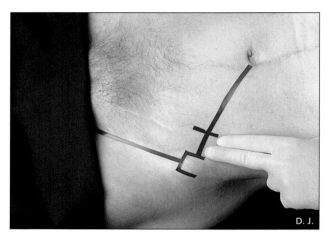

Fig. 24.3 Location

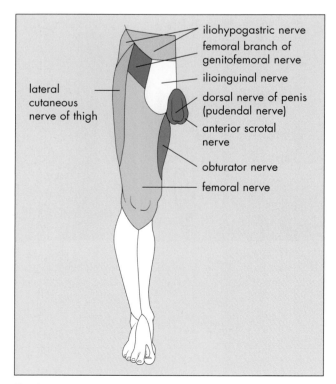

iliohypogastric nerve

femoral branch of genitofemoral nerve

ilioinguinal nerve

dorsal nerve of penis (pudendal nerve)

anterior scrotal nerve

obturator nerve

femoral nerve

lateral cutaneous nerve of thigh

Fig. 24.4 Cutaneous innervation areas in the ilioinguinal region

Procedure

Preparations
(See Chap. 18, p. 152)

Materials (Fig. 24.2)
40–50 mm long injection needle, 23–25 G. When a nerve stimulator is used, a 35–50 mm long atraumatic 22-G needle (15°) with an injection lead (e. g. Stimuplex D, B. Braun Melsungen).
Syringes: 2, 5, and 10 ml.
Local anesthetics, antiseptic, swabs, sterile gloves and drape.

Patient positioning
Supine, with the ipsilateral hand under the head.

Landmarks
A line is drawn connecting the anterior superior iliac spine and the umbilicus.
The injection site is located about 3 cm medial to the iliac spine (Fig. 24.3).
Skin prep, subcutaneous local anesthesia, covering with a sterile drape, drawing up the local anesthetic.

Injection technique
- The injection needle is introduced perpendicular and then slightly laterally until bone contact is made with the wing of the ilium. It is then withdrawn slightly, and after aspiration ca. 5 ml of the local anesthetic is injected.
- The needle is then withdrawn subcutaneously, and the direction is altered medially along the connecting line until there is penetration of the fascia of the external oblique muscle and internal and transverse oblique muscles.
- After aspiration, fan-shaped injection of 10 ml of local anesthetic.

The cutaneous innervation of the ilioinguinal region is shown in Figure 24.4.

Dosage
10–15 ml local anesthetic, e. g. 0.75 % ropivacaine, 0.5 % bupivacaine, 1 % prilocaine, 1 % mepivacaine.

Complications
- Hematoma
- Infection.

25 Blocking peripheral nerves in the knee joint region

In the distal part of the thigh, the **sciatic nerve** divides into the **tibial nerve,** which runs medially and straight and a lateral branch, the **common peroneal (fibular) nerve.** A third nerve in the area of the knee joint, the **saphenous nerve,** is the largest and thickest branch of the **femoral nerve.**

Anatomy

Sciatic nerve area

Tibial nerve (Figs. 25.1, 25.3)
Almost twice as thick as the common peroneal nerve, the tibial nerve continues the course of the sciatic nerve, running down through the middle of the popliteal fossa and lying posterior and slightly lateral to the popliteal vessels.
It then passes between the two heads of the gastrocnemius muscle to the upper edge of the soleus muscle. Between the posterior tibial muscle and the soleus muscle, it runs distally together with the posterior tibial artery through the calf musculature, as far as the center between the medial malleolus and the calcaneus, to the medial side of the foot joint.
It divides into its two end branches, the medial and lateral plantar nerves, behind the medial malleolus. These pass under the flexor retinaculum to the sole of the foot and provide it with its sensory innervation.
While in proximity to the common peroneal nerve as part of the sciatic nerve, it gives off branches for the obturator internus muscle, gemelli muscles, quadratus femoris muscle, semitendinosus muscle, semimembranosus muscle, adductor magnus muscle and long head of the biceps.

Common peroneal (fibular) nerve (Figs. 25.2, 25.3)
After separating from the tibial nerve, the common peroneal nerve runs along the medial edge of the biceps femoris muscle over the lateral head of the gastrocnemius muscle to the lateral angle of the popliteal fossa. At the neck of the fibula, it passes to the lateral surface of the bone. Before entering the longus peroneus muscle, which originates here, it divides into the mainly sensory superficial peroneal nerve and the mainly motor deep peroneal nerve.

Up to the point at which it divides, its small branches supply the short head of the biceps femoris muscle, the lateral and posterior parts of the joint capsule and the tibiofibular joint and it gives off the lateral sural cutaneous nerve. The anterior branch of this runs subcutaneously to the lateral surface of the lower leg as far as the lateral malleolus and its posterior branch runs subfascially and then subcutaneously until it unites with the medial sural cutaneous nerve from the tibial nerve.

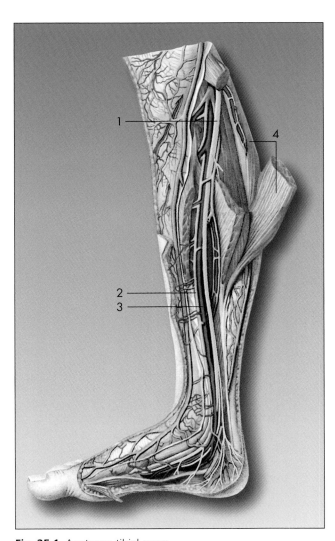

Fig. 25.1 Anatomy: tibial nerve.
(1) Tibial nerve, (2) posterior tibial vein, (3) posterior tibial artery, (4) gastrocnemius muscle

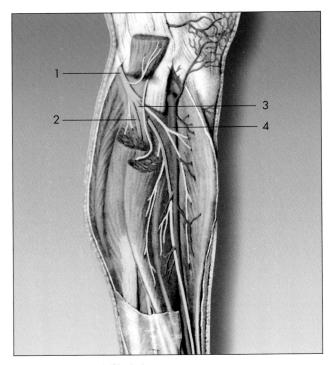

Fig. 25.2 Peroneal (fibular) nerve.
(1) Common peroneal (fibular) nerve, (2) superficial peroneal (fibular) nerve, (3) deep peroneal (fibular) nerve, (4) anterior tibial artery

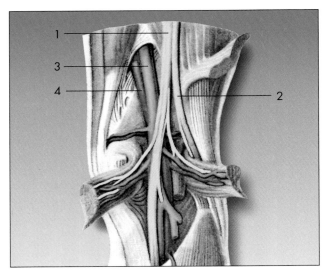

Fig. 25.3 Tibial and common peroneal (fibular) nerve in the popliteal area.
(1) Tibial nerve, (2) common peroneal (fibular) nerve, (3) popliteal vein, (4) popliteal artery

Area supplied by the femoral nerve

Saphenous nerve (Fig. 25.4)

The sensory saphenous nerve is the longest branch of the femoral nerve (see Chap. 18, Fig. 18.1). It forms the continuation of the posterior trunk, and in the thigh it lies initially on the lateral surface and further down on the anterior surface of the femoral artery. Along with the femoral vessels, it enters the adductor canal and penetrates its anterior wall and covered by the sartorius muscle runs between the vastus medialis muscle and adductor magnus muscle to the medial side of the knee. Here, at the tendon of the sartorius muscle, it passes to lie below the skin and runs up to the great saphenous vein, then down subcutaneously alongside this vein in the lower leg. Its terminal nerves supply the skin on the medial edge of the foot and medial malleolus. One branch connects with the superficial peroneal nerve in the ankle. Apart from a branch to the knee joint, it also gives off the infrapatellar branch to the skin on the medial side of the knee as far as the anterior surface of the patella and the medial crural cutaneous nerves, which supply the skin over the medial surface of the tibia and the medial calf skin.

Indications

Surgical

▓ Procedures in the lower leg (including ischemia/tourniquet) using combined blocks of all three nerves, or superficial procedures in the region of the individual nerves, without using a tourniquet.
▓ Particularly suitable for outpatient procedures.
▓ Postoperative pain therapy.
▓ Supplementation of incomplete epidural anesthesia or incomplete block of the sciatic or femoral nerves.

> **Caution**
> Care must be taken to avoid nerve injury, as paresthesias are not available as a warning signal (see Chap. 7, section on axillary block).

Contraindications

- Lesions of the nerves being blocked distal to the injection site.
- Anticoagulation treatment.
- Infection in the injection area.

Procedure

Preparations
Check that the emergency equipment is complete and in working order. Sterile precautions, intravenous access, ECG monitoring, pulse oximetry, intubation kit, ventilation facilities, emergency medication.

Materials (Fig. 25.5)
40–55 cm long atraumatic 22-G needle with injection lead ("immobile needle", e. g. Stimuplex D, B. Braun Melsungen) for block of the peroneal and tibial nerves, 40 mm long 25-G needle for block of the saphenous nerve.
Syringes: 2, 10 and 20 ml.
Local anesthetics, disinfectant, swabs, compresses, sterile gloves and drape.

Simultaneous block of the tibial and common peroneal (fibular) nerve in the popliteal area

Popliteal fossa (Fig. 25.6)
The **caudal** boundary of the popliteal fossa is determined medially and laterally by the gastrocnemius muscle, **craniomedially** by the semimembranosus and semitendinosus muscles and **craniolaterally** by the biceps femoris muscle. The two nerves lie superficially and are located at a depth of about 1.5–2 cm.

Patient positioning
Prone, with the treated leg stretched out. The person carrying out the injection stands on the side being injected.

Landmarks
The popliteal fossa is divided into a medial and a lateral triangle, the base of which is represented by the intercondylar line between the lateral and medial epicondyles. The midpoint of the base is marked and from there a line is drawn 5 cm proximally and then 1 cm laterally. This point determines the injection site (Fig. 25.7).
Skin prep, local anesthesia, covering with a sterile drape, drawing up the local anesthetic, checking the patency of the injection needle and the functioning of the nerve stimulator, attaching electrodes.

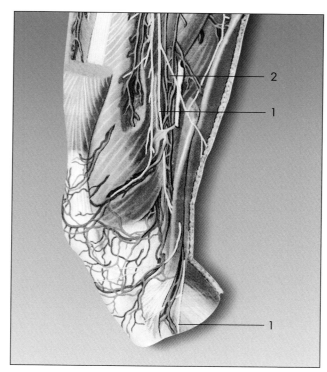

Fig. 25.4 Saphenous nerve in the popliteal area. (1) Saphenous nerve, (2) femoral artery

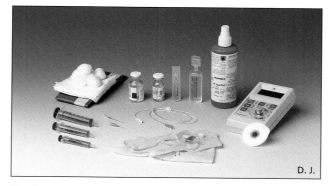

Fig. 25.5 Materials

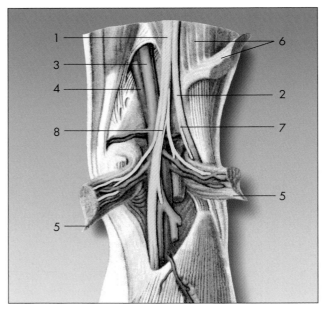

Fig. 25.6 Popliteal fossa.
(1) Tibial nerve, (2) common peroneal (fibular) nerve,
(3) popliteal vein, (4) popliteal artery, (5) gastrocnemius muscle,
(6) biceps femoris muscle, (7) lateral sural cutaneous nerve,
(8) medial sural cutaneous nerve

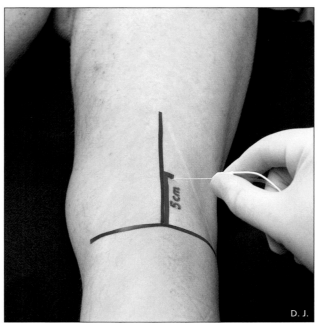

Fig. 25.7 Injection. Simultaneous block of the common
peroneal (fibular) nerve and tibial nerve

Injection technique (Fig. 25.7)
The injection needle is advanced at an angle of 45–60°
and in an anterosuperior direction. After paresthesias
have been produced at a depth of about 1.5–2 cm, incremental injection of a local anesthetic is carried out
after prior aspiration.

When a nerve stimulator is used, either plantar flexion
(as a motor response from the tibial nerve) or plantar
dorsiflexion (common peroneal nerve) are sought.

After removal of the needle, better distribution of the
local anesthetic is encouraged with pressure compression (3–5 min) and simultaneous massaging of the injection area. This also serves for hematoma prophylaxis.

Dosage
Surgical
35–40 ml local anesthetic, e. g. 0.75 % ropivacaine,
0.5 % bupivacaine, 1 % prilocaine, 1 % mepivacaine.
A combination of longer-term and medium-term local
anesthetics has proved particularly suitable for surgical
indications.

Complications
Complications are extremely rare, but possible:
▨ Neuritis and dysesthesia.
▨ Intravascular injection.
▨ Hematoma formation.

Block of the tibial nerve

Patient positioning
Prone, with the treated leg stretched out. The person
carrying out the injection stands on the side being injected.

Landmarks
Popliteal fossa. The center of the connecting line between
the lateral and medial epicondyles determines the injection point.

Injection technique (Fig. 25.8)
The injection needle is introduced perpendicular to the skin until paresthesias are produced. This normally occurs at a depth of about 1.5–3 cm. When a nerve stimulator is used, plantar flexion is noted as a motor response. After aspiration at two levels, incremental injection of local anesthetic is carried out.

Dosage
5–10 ml of local anesthetic, e. g. 0.75 % ropivacaine, 0.5 % bupivacaine, 1 % prilocaine, 1 % mepivacaine.

Complications
(See the section on simultaneous block of the tibial and common peroneal (fibular) nerves in the popliteal area, p. 180)

Block of the common peroneal (fibular) nerve

Patient positioning
Supine, with the treated leg positioned at a slight angle. The person carrying out the injection stands on the side being injected.

Landmarks
Head of the fibula, tendon of the biceps femoris muscle. The head of the fibula is palpated. The injection point lies about 2 cm below the head of the fibula.

Injection technique (Fig. 25.9)
The injection needle is advanced perpendicularly until paresthesias are produced at a depth of about 1 cm. When a nerve stimulator is used, plantar dorsiflexion is noted as a motor response. After aspiration at two levels, incremental injection of a local anesthetic is carried out behind the head of the fibula.

Dosage
5–10 ml of local anesthetic, e. g. 0.75 % ropivacaine, 0.5 % bupivacaine, 1 % prilocaine, 1 % mepivacaine.

Complications
(See the section on simultaneous block of the tibial and common peroneal (fibular) nerves in the popliteal area, p. 180)

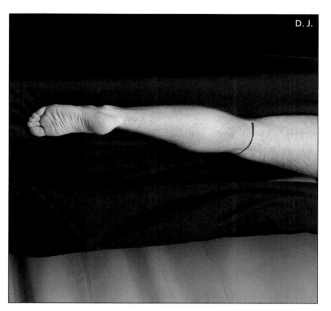

Fig. 25.8 Tibial nerve

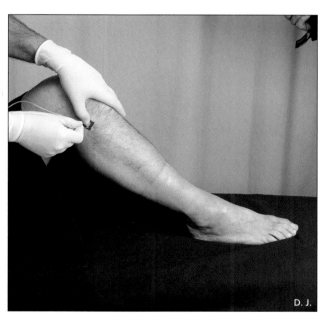

Fig. 25.9 Common peroneal (fibular) nerve

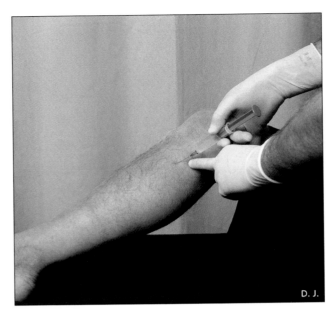

Fig. 25.10 Saphenous nerve

Block of the saphenous nerve

Patient positioning
Supine, with the treated leg positioned at a slight angle.

Landmarks
Medial condyle of the tibia, tibial tuberosity, gastrocnemius muscle.

Injection technique (Fig. 25.10)
The medial condyle of the tibia is palpated. Distal to this a subcutaneous ring-shaped infiltration of the following areas is carried out: medial condyle, tibial tuberosity and gastrocnemius muscle.

Dosage
5–10 ml of local anesthetic, e. g. 0.75 % ropivacaine, 0.5 % bupivacaine, 1 % prilocaine, 1 % mepivacaine.

Complications
No specific complications.

The areas of cutaneous innervation of the individual nerves discussed in this Chapter are illustrated in Figure 25.11.

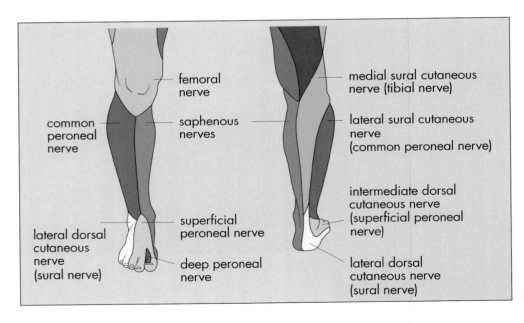

Fig. 25.11 Cutaneous innervation areas in the lower leg

26 Blocking peripheral nerves in the ankle joint region

Definition
Individual or combined infiltration anesthesia of the following nerves in the ankle joint region:

- Tibial nerve
- Superficial and deep peroneal (fibular) nerves.
- Sural nerve.
- Saphenous nerve.

Anatomy

Tibial nerve (Fig. 26.1 A, B)
The tibial nerve reaches the distal lower leg posterior to the medial malleolus. It gives off medial calcaneal branches to the heel and divides into its two end branches, the medial and lateral plantar nerves, which pass to the sole of the foot and provide it with its sensory supply.

Superficial peroneal (fibular) nerve
(Figs. 26.2, 26.3)
This nerve runs through the peroneus longus muscle, extends between the peroneus longus and brevis muscles, and penetrates the crural fascia in the distal third of the lower leg. Subcutaneously, or still at the subfascial level, it divides into the thicker medial dorsal cutaneous nerve and the smaller intermediate dorsal cutaneous nerve, providing the sensory supply for the skin on the back of the foot and the toes.

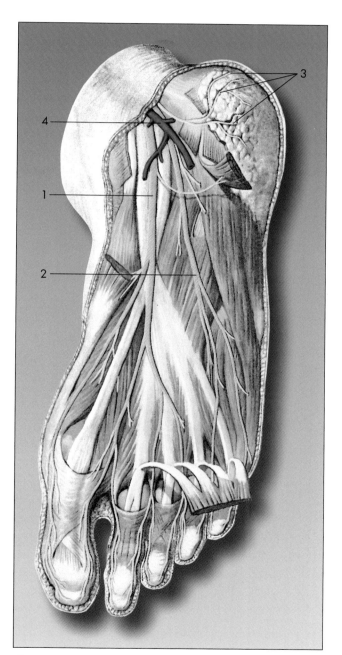

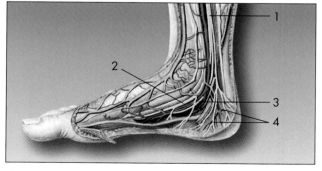

Fig. 26.1 A Tibial nerve. (1) Tibial nerve, (2) medial plantar nerve, (3) lateral plantar nerve, (4) calcaneal branches

Fig. 26.1 B Tibial nerve – sole of the foot.
(1) Medial plantar nerve, (2) lateral plantar nerve, (3) medial calcaneal branches, (4) posterior tibial artery

Deep peroneal (fibular) nerve (Figs. 26.2, 26.3)

This nerve runs between the tibialis anterior muscle and the extensor hallucis longus muscle in the direction of the ankle, where it divides into a medial and a lateral end branch. The medial end branch continues in the direction of the trunk, and passes with the dorsalis pedis artery to the first interosseous space, crossing under the tendon of the extensor hallucis brevis muscle to the distal end of the interosseous space. Here it joins with a strand of the superficial peroneal nerve and divides into the end branches for the facing sides of the backs of the first and second toes.

The lateral end branch turns laterally and supplies the extensor digitorum brevis muscle, sending off three interosseous nerves.

Sural nerve (Figs. 26.2, 26.3)

The medial sural cutaneous nerve arises in the proximal part of the popliteal area, runs down between the two heads of the gastrocnemius muscle, and joins the peroneal communicating branch to form the sural nerve. Accompanied by the small saphenous vein, the sural nerve runs behind the **lateral malleolus** and courses as the lateral dorsal cutaneous nerve along the lateral side of the foot, where it gives off a connecting branch to the intermediate dorsal cutaneous nerve and ends as the dorsalis digiti minimi nerve on the lateral edge of the back of the small toe.

Behind the lateral malleolus it sends off branches (the lateral calcaneal branches) to the skin there and at the heel. The branches for the lateral side of the ankle, for the anterior capsular wall, and for the tarsal sinus originate proximal to the malleolus.

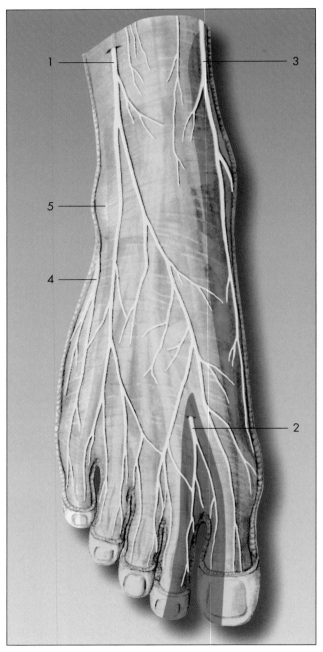

Fig. 26.3 Cutaneous innervation areas in the region of the back of the foot (from the front).
(1) Superficial peroneal (fibular) nerve, (2) deep peroneal (fibular) nerve, (3) saphenous nerve, (4) lateral dorsal cutaneous nerve (sural nerve), (5) lateral malleolus

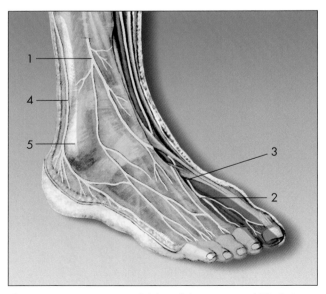

Fig. 26.2 Common, superficial, and deep peroneal (fibular) nerve, and sural nerve. Cutaneous innervation areas of the back of the foot (lateral).
(1) Superficial peroneal (fibular) nerve, (2) deep peroneal (fibular) nerve, (3) dorsalis pedis artery, (4) sural nerve, (5) lateral malleolus

Saphenous nerve (Fig. 26.3)
The saphenous nerve courses along the medial side of the lower leg and anterior to the medial malleolus, and sends off branches to the skin of the medial side of the foot. It usually ends in the metatarsal area, without reaching the big toe.

Indications

- Surgical procedures in the foot area.
- Outpatient surgery.
- Postoperative pain therapy.
- Supplementation of incomplete epidural anesthesia or an incomplete block of the sciatic or femoral nerve.

> **Caution**
> Care must be taken to avoid nerve injury, as paresthesias are not available as a warning signal (see Chap. 7, p. 76).

Contraindications

- Anticoagulant treatment.
- Infections in the injection area.

Procedure

Preparations
Check that the emergency equipment is complete and in working order; sterile precautions.

Materials (Fig. 26.4)
3 cm long 25-G needle.
Syringes: 2, 5, 10 ml.
Local anesthetics, disinfectant, swabs, sterile gloves, drape.

Skin prep, subcutaneous local anesthesia, drawing up the local anesthetic.

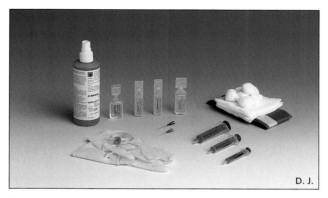

Fig. 26.4 Materials

Posterior tibial nerve

Patient positioning
Prone, with a pillow under the ankle (or the patient may be seated).

Landmarks
Medial malleolus, posterior tibial artery.

Injection technique (Figs. 26.5, 26.7)
Lateral to the palpated pulse of the posterior tibial artery, a fine 3 cm long 25-G needle is introduced at a right angle to the posterior side of the tibia and just posterior to the posterior tibial artery.
After paresthesias are elicited and after a negative aspiration test, 5 ml of local anesthetic is injected. If paresthesias cannot be elicited, then after reaching the posterior tibia the needle is withdrawn for about 1 cm, and 5–10 ml of local anesthetic is injected.
Another method is to carry out perpendicular puncture of the skin at the level of the medial malleolus, dorsal and then ventral to the posterior tibial artery, and to distribute the total dose of local anesthetic in two equal halves on each side [7].

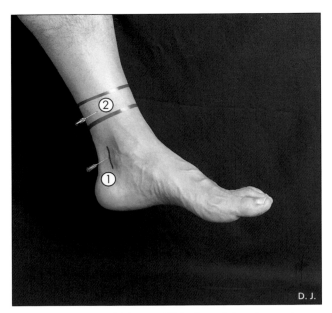

Fig. 26.5 Posterior tibial nerve (1) (red needle) and posterior tibial artery (red), (2) saphenous nerve (black needle)

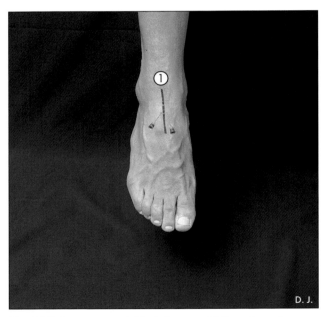

Fig. 26.6 Deep peroneal (fibular) nerve. (1) Dorsalis pedis artery

Deep peroneal nerve

Patient positioning
Supine, or sitting.

Landmarks
Dorsalis pedis artery, proximal back of the foot.

Injection technique (Fig. 26.6)
A fine 25-G injection needle, 3 cm long, is introduced perpendicular to the skin surface.
5 ml of the local anesthetic is injected on each side, first lateral to the artery and then medial to it [7].

Sural nerve and superficial peroneal nerve

Patient positioning
Supine, or sitting.

Landmarks
Lateral malleolus.

Injection technique (Fig. 26.8)
About 10 cm above the lateral malleolus, parallel to the upper ankle, fan-shaped subcutaneous infiltration of the Achilles tendon is carried out as far as the edge of the tibia, using about 10 ml of local anesthetic.

Saphenous nerve

Patient positioning
Supine, or sitting.

Landmarks
Medial malleolus.

Injection technique (Fig. 26.5)
About 10 cm above the medial malleolus, 5–10 ml of local anesthetic is injected subcutaneously around the great saphenous vein and in a fan-shaped fashion in a mediolateral direction.

The cutaneous innervation areas of the individual nerves are shown in Figure 26.9.

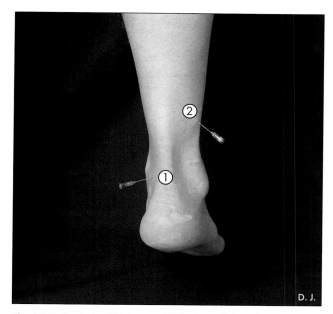

Fig. 26.7 Posterior tibial nerve (1) (red needle) and (2) sural nerve (green needle)

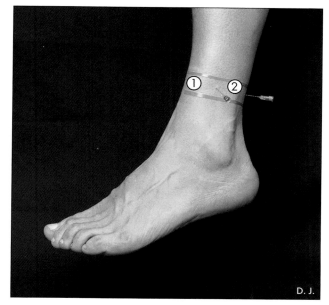

Fig. 26.8 (1) Superficial peroneal (fibular) nerve (blue needle) and (2) sural nerve (green needle)

Dosage
Tibial nerve and deep peroneal nerve
5–10 ml of local anesthetic.

Sural nerve, superficial peroneal nerve, saphenous nerve
10–20 ml of local anesthetic (subcutaneous fan-shaped infiltration).

Local anesthetics
0.5–0.75 % ropivacaine, 0.25–0.5 % bupivacaine, 1 % prilocaine, 1 % mepivacaine.

Complications
No specific complications.

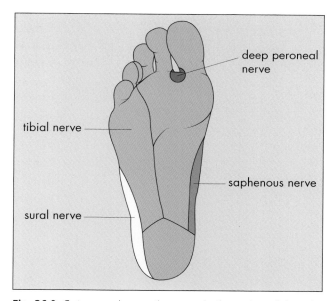

Fig. 26.9 Cutaneous innervation areas in the region of the sole of the foot

Record and checklist

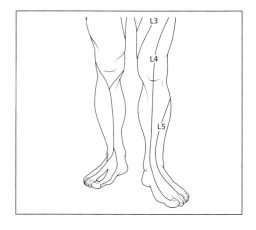

	1. h			2. h		
	15	30	45	15	30	45

mm Hg — 220 200 180 160 140 120 100 80 60 40 20

O₂

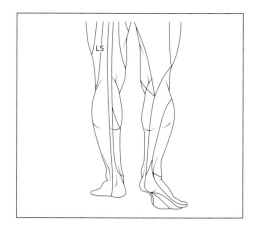

Peripheral nerve blocks – knee joint and foot

Block no.   □ Right   □ Left

Name: _____ Date: _____

Diagnosis: _____

Premedication: □ No   □ Yes

Neurological abnormalities: □ No   □ Yes _____

Purpose of block: □ Surgery   □ Diagnosis   □ Treatment

Needle: G _____ Length _____   □ Short bevel   □ Other

i. v. access: □ Yes   □ No

Monitoring: □ ECG   □ Pulse oximetry

Ventilation facilities: □ Yes (equipment checked)

Emergency equipment (drugs):   □ Checked

Patient: □ Informed   □ Consent

Knee joint region:

□ Tibial nerve/Common peroneal (fibular) nerve (simultaneous)
□ Superficial/deep peroneal (fibular) nerve □ Tibial nerve □ Saphenous nerve

Foot region:

□ Posterior tibial nerve   □ Deep peroneal nerve   □ Sural/superficial peroneal nerve
□ Saphenous nerve

Position: □ Supine   □ Prone   □ Sitting

Location technique: □ Electrostimulation   □ Paresthesias

Injection:

Local anesthetic: _____ ml _____ %
(incremental)

□ Addition to LA: _____ µg/mg

Patient's remarks during injection:

□ None   □ Paresthesias   □ Warmth   □ Pain (intraneural position?)

Neural area: _____

Objective block effect after 15 min:

□ Cold test   □ Temperature measurement before _____ °C   after _____ °C
□ Sensory   □ Motor

Monitoring after block: □ < 30 min   □ > 30 min

Complications:

□ None   □ Intravascular injection   □ Signs of toxicity
□ Hematoma   □ Neurological complications   □ Other

Subjective effects of block: Duration: _____

□ None   □ Increased pain   □ Reduced pain   □ No pain

VISUAL ANALOG SCALE

0   10   20   30   40   50   60   70   80   90   100

Special notes:

Neuraxial anesthesia

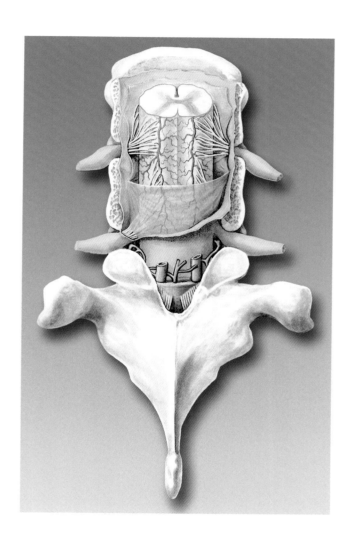

27 Neuraxial anatomy

Spine and sacrum

Spine

The spinal column consists of 33 vertebrae – seven cervical vertebrae; 12 thoracic vertebrae; five lumbar vertebrae; the sacrum, consisting of five fused sacral vertebrae; and the coccyx, consisting of four fused coccygeal segments (Fig. 27.1).

The average length of the spine in adult men is about 72 cm, while in women it is 7–10 cm shorter.

All of the vertebrae have the same basic shape, which is subject to certain variations in the individual sections of the spine. The basic shape consists of a ventral body (the body of the vertebra) and a dorsal arch (the vertebral arch), which consists of pedicles and laminae (Fig. 27.2).

The laminae of the vertebral arch join dorsally to form the spinous process. A transverse process branches off on each side of the vertebral arch, as well as a superior and an inferior articular process.

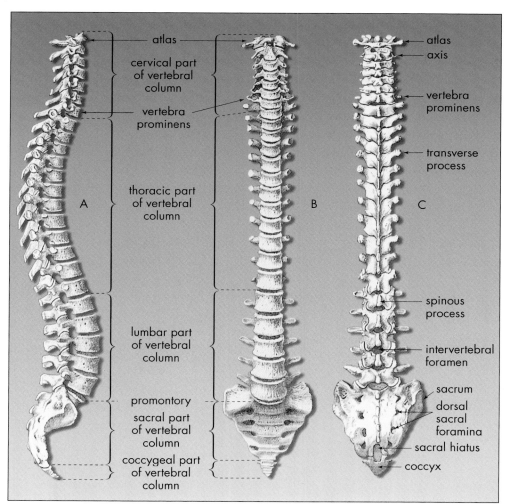

Fig. 27.1 A–C
Spine. **A** Lateral,
B Ventral, **C** Dorsal

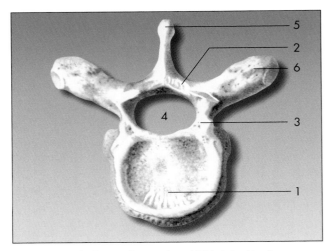

Fig. 27.2 Basic shape of a vertebra. (1) Vertebral body, (2) vertebral arch, (3) pedicle of the vertebral arch, (4) vertebral foramen, (5) spinous process, (6) transverse process

The vertebrae in the cervical region are smaller, but their size increases from cranial to caudal.

The angle of inclination of the spinous processes – important topographic signposts for neuraxial injections – varies at different levels of the spine.

The cervical spinous processes, the first two thoracic spinous processes and the lumbar spinous processes lie at the same level as their vertebrae. From T3 to L1, the spinous processes are angled caudally (particularly in the T4–T9 area) (Fig. 27.3 A–C).

The vertebral canal (which provides excellent protection for the spinal cord) and the spinal cord, with its meningeal covering, extend throughout the whole length of the spine terminating in the cauda equina.

The spinal vessels and nerves emerge laterally through openings at the upper and lower margins of the roots of the arches of the adjoining vertebrae (the intervertebral foramina).

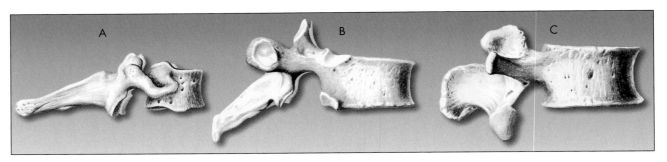

Fig. 27.3 A–C Cervical, thoracic and lumbar spinous processes.
A C7 cervical vertebra (vertebra prominens, nuchal tubercle), **B** T8 thoracic vertebra, **C** L3 lumbar vertebra

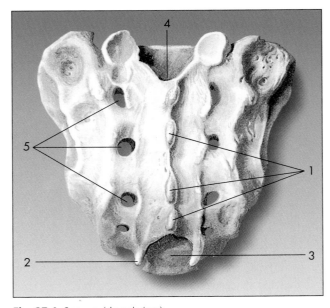

Fig. 27.4 Sacrum (dorsal view).
(1) Median sacral crest, (2) sacral horn, (3) sacral hiatus, (4) sacral canal, (5) posterior sacral foramina

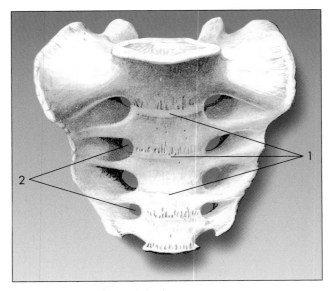

Fig. 27.5 Sacrum (ventral view).
(1) Transverse lines, (2) anterior pelvic sacral foramina

Sacrum

The sacrum is wedge-shaped and consists of five vertebrae fused together. It lies proximal to the fifth lumbar vertebra and is connected distally, with the apex of the sacrum, to the coccyx.

Dorsally, the sacrum has a convex surface, in the middle of which the **median sacral crest** stands out (Fig. 27.4).

The crest is produced by the fusion of the rudimentary spinous processes of the upper third or fourth sacral vertebrae. Normally, the arch of the fifth and occasionally also of the fourth sacral vertebra is absent, so that there is a **sacral hiatus** at this point.

The hiatus is bounded by the sacral horn as a remnant of the caudal articular process and it is used as a passage by the five small sacral nerves and by the coccygeal nerves.

Between the median sacral hiatus and the lateral sacral hiatus lie the four sacral openings (the posterior sacral foraminae), through which the dorsal branches of the sacral spinal nerves emerge.

The anterior view shows a concave aspect. Alongside the transverse lines (fused vertebrae), there are large anterior openings (the anterior pelvic sacral foramina), through which the primary anterior parts of the sacral nerves emerge (Fig. 27.5).

Spinal ligaments

The vertebrae are supported from the axis to the cranial sacrum by intervertebral disks and by various ligaments (Fig. 27.6).

The intervertebral disks lie between neighboring vertebrae and function as fixed connecting elements and pressure-absorbing buffers. The disks are at their thinnest in the area of T3–T7 and thickest in the lumbar area.

The **anterior longitudinal ligament** is attached at the anterior edge of the vertebral bodies and intervertebral disks and is at its thickest in the thoracic area.

The **posterior longitudinal ligament** is wider cranially than it is caudally and it lies behind the vertebral bodies in the medullary canal. The **supraspinous ligaments** extend as far as the sacrum along the tips of the spinous processes, with which they are connected, and continue cranially in the nuchal ligament and ventrally in the **interspinous ligament**. They become thicker from cranial to caudal. The interspinous ligaments connect the roots and tips of the spinous processes.

The **intertransverse ligaments** serve to connect the transverse processes (Fig. 27.7).

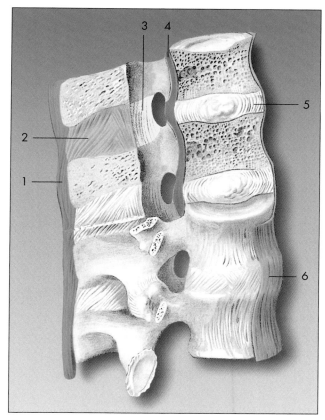

Fig. 27.6 Ligaments of the spinal cord.
(1) Supraspinous ligament, (2) interspinous ligament, (3) ligamentum flavum, (4) posterior longitudinal ligament, (5) intervertebral disk, (6) anterior longitudinal ligament

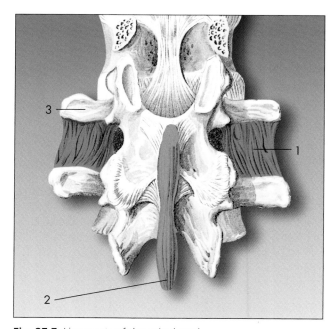

Fig. 27.7 Ligaments of the spinal cord.
(1) Intertransverse ligament, (2) supraspinous ligament, (3) transverse process

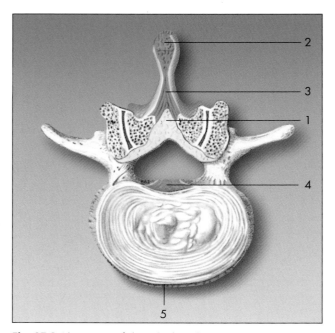

Fig. 27.8 Ligaments of the spinal cord.
(1) Ligamentum flavum, (2) supraspinous ligament,
(3) interspinous ligament, (4) posterior longitudinal ligament,
(5) anterior longitudinal ligament

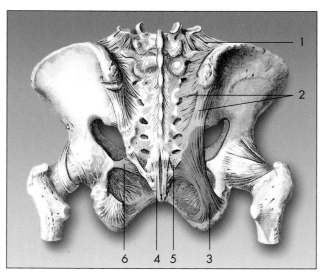

Fig. 27.9 Iliolumbosacral ligaments (dorsal view).
(1) Iliolumbar ligament, (2) dorsal sacroiliac ligament,
(3) sacrotuberous ligament, (4) superficial dorsal and deep
dorsal sacrococcygeal ligaments, (5) lateral sacrococcygeal
ligament, (6) sacrospinous ligament

The **ligamentum flavum** largely consists of yellow, elastic fibers and it connects the neighboring laminae (Fig. 27.8).

It is at its thinnest in the midline (small fissure spaces exist for the veins running from the internal vertebral venous plexus to the external vertebral venous plexus) and its thickness increases laterally. The size and shape of the ligamentum flavum vary at the various levels of the spine. Caudally, for example, it is thicker than in the cranial direction.

Iliolumbosacral ligaments

The stability of the iliolumbosacral region is ensured by lumbosacral and sacroiliac connections that transfer the entire weight of the trunk via the hip bones to the lower extremities. These ligamentous connections serve to connect the vertebrae with one another and to stabilize the sacrum.

Clinically important ligaments: interspinous, supraspinous, iliolumbar, interosseous sacroiliac, sacrospinous and sacrotuberous ligaments (Figs. 27.9, 27.10).

Spinal cord

The spinal cord (medulla spinalis), with a length of about 46 cm, is the caudal continuation of the medulla oblongata, which extends from the atlas to the medullary cone (the lower edge of the first lumbar vertebra).

The **medullary cone** continues in the threadlike median **filum terminale** as far as the posterior side of the coccyx (Fig. 27.11 A, B).

The dura mater and arachnoid and consequently the subarachnoid space as well, extend downward as far as the level of the second sacral vertebra.

Meninges

The spinal cord is surrounded and protected by the meninges (the **dura mater, arachnoid and pia mater**) and by cerebrospinal fluid, epidural fatty tissue and veins (Fig. 27.12).

The **dura mater of the spinal cord**, a fibroelastic membrane, extends as far as the second sacral vertebra, where it ends in a blind sac. It encloses the anterior and posterior spinal nerve roots.

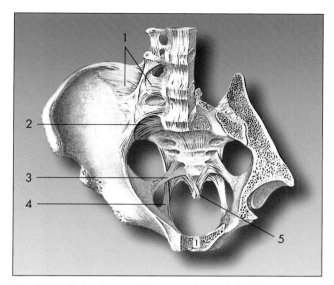

Fig. 27.10 Iliolumbosacral ligaments (ventral view).
(1) Iliolumbar ligament, (2) ventral sacroiliac ligament,
(3) sacrospinous ligament, (4) sacrotuberous ligament,
(5) ventral sacrococcygeal ligament

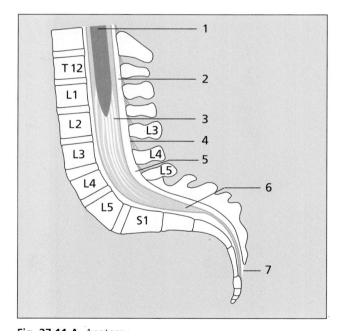

Fig. 27.11 A Anatomy.
(1) spinal cord, (2) dura mater, (3) cauda equina, (4) ligamentum
flavum, (5) epidural space, (6) subarachnoid space, (7) sacral
hiatus

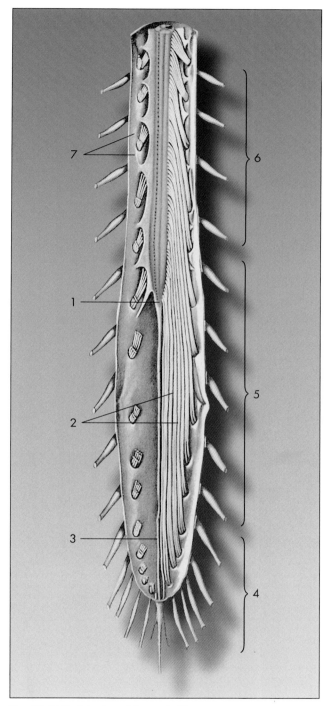

Fig. 27.11 B Spinal cord (lower half).
(1) Medullary cone, (2) cauda equina, (3) filum of spinal dura
mater (filum terminale), (4) sacral nerves, (5) lumbar nerves,
(6) thoracic nerves, (7) dura mater

Between the dura mater and the arachnoid, there is a space, the subdural space, in which a small amount of lymph-like fluid is located.

The **arachnoid of the spinal cord**, a nonvascularized membrane, also ends at the level of the second sacral vertebra. Between the arachnoid and the pia mater lies the subarachnoid space, which is filled with cerebrospinal fluid.

The **spinal pia mater** is a thin, very well vascularized membrane that tightly encloses the spinal cord. Caudal to the medullary cone, it develops into the thin filum terminale, which descends medial to the cauda equina, penetrates the final part of the dural sac and arachnoid and fuses with the connective tissue posterior to the first coccygeal segment.

The pia mater sends off 22 denticulate ligaments on either side, which attach to the dura mater and thus stabilize the spinal cord.

Spinal nerves

There are 31 pairs of spinal nerves in the human: eight cervical pairs, twelve thoracic pairs, five lumbar pairs, five sacral pairs and one coccygeal pair. These are connected to the spinal cord by a series of ventral and dorsal radicular filaments, which combine to form the nerve roots (Fig. 27.12).

The thicker dorsal (posterior) root is responsible for conducting afferent impulses (pain, temperature, touch, position). Each of the dorsal spinal nerve roots has a sensory **spinal ganglion** incorporated in it. The ventral (anterior) root is responsible for conducting efferent impulses (muscles, glands): The nerve roots in the lower segments of

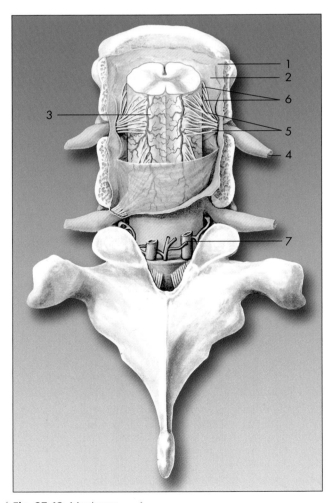

Fig. 27.12 Meninges.
(1) Dura mater, (2) arachnoid, (3) pia mater, (4) spinal nerve, (5) dorsal (posterior) root, (6) ventral (anterior) root, (7) internal vertebral venous plexus

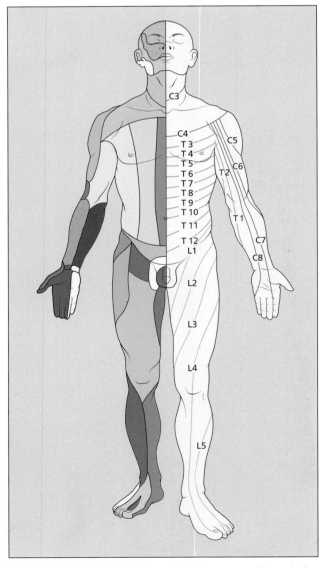

Fig. 27.13 Spinal dermatomes and their corresponding spinal cord segments

the spinal cord descend in the horsetail-shaped **cauda equina** to their exit openings.

After exiting from the subarachnoid space, the ventral and dorsal roots cross the epidural space.

In spinal anesthesia, the nerve roots are the principal targets for local anesthesia.

Spinal dermatomes

Via its branching spinal nerves, each segment of the spinal cord provides the sensory supply for a specific area of skin, known as the dermatome.

These skin areas, which often overlap, are very important for checking and verifying the spread of anesthesia (Figs. 27.13, 27.14).

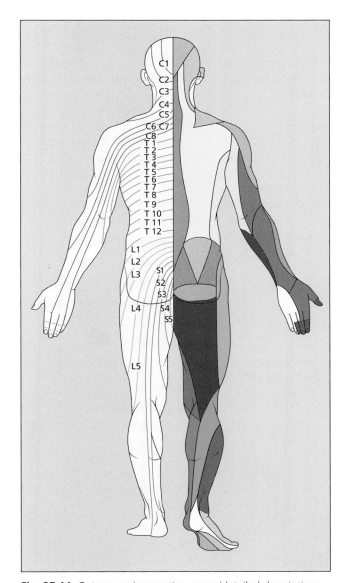

Fig. 27.14 Cutaneous innervation areas (detailed descriptions are given in the relevant chapters)

Arteries of the spinal cord

The spinal cord is supplied by numerous radicular arteries, which form the **anterior spinal artery** and **posterior spinal arteries**.

The radicular arteries branch off from the cervical vertebral artery, the thoracic intercostal arteries and the abdominal lumbar arteries (Figs. 27.15, 27.16).

The **anterior spinal artery**, which arises from the fourth segment of the vertebral arteries, accompanies the spinal cord in the midline (anterior median fissure) along its entire course.

Via the central branches and small branches of the arterial pial network, the anterior spinal artery supplies the anterior two-thirds of the spinal cord.

The cervical and first two thoracic spinal cord segments receive blood from the radicular branches of subclavian artery branches.

In the mediothoracic spinal cord region (T3–T7), there is a radicular branch at the level of T4 or T5.

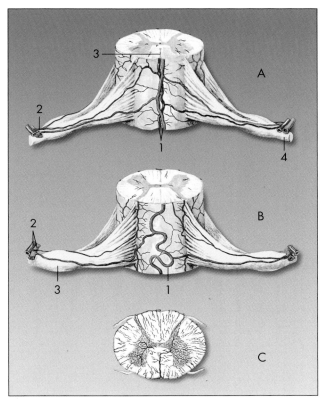

Fig. 27.15 A–C Spinal cord.
A Ventral view: (1) anterior spinal artery and vein, (2) spinal branch, (3) anterior median fissure, (4) spinal nerve.
B Dorsal view: (1) posterior spinal vein, (2) dorsal branch of the posterior intercostal artery, (3) spinal ganglion.
C Cross-section

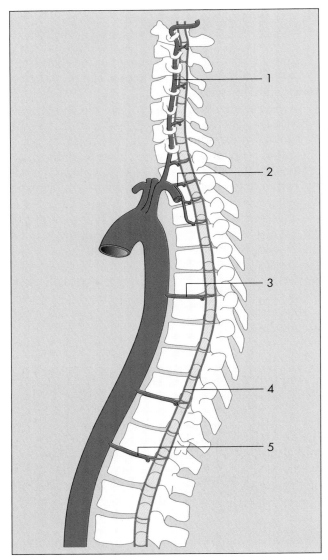

Fig. 27.16 Arteries of the spinal cord (side view).
(1) Vertebral artery, (2) deep cervical artery, (3) intercostal artery, (4) anterior and posterior spinal artery, (5) arteria radicularis magna (artery of Adamkiewicz)

The thoracolumbar segment of the spinal cord (T8 to the medullary cone) draws its arterial supply mainly from the large-caliber arteria radicularis magna (the artery of Adamkiewicz), which arises from an intercostal artery on the left side.

The cauda equina is supplied by branches of the lumbar, iliolumbar and lateral or median sacral arteries. These also supply the medullary cone.

The paired **posterior spinal arteries** arise from the fourth segment of the vertebral artery, receiving tributary flow from 10–23 posterior radicular branches and supply the dorsal third of the spinal cord.

Thin pial branches run from the spinal arteries, forming a network on the surface of the spinal cord known as the **arterial pial network**.

Veins of the spinal cord and vertebrae

The entire spinal canal is traversed by two venous plexuses, the **internal** and **external vertebral venous plexuses** (Figs. 27.17, 27.18).

Together, these form a ring around each vertebra, freely anastomosing with one another and receiving tributary flow from the vertebrae, ligaments and spinal cord.

They are largely avalvular. Pressure changes in the thoracic or cerebrospinal fluid (CSF) spaces consequently affect the blood volume in the venous plexuses.

The plexuses are most strongly developed in the anterolateral area of the epidural space. They drain not only the spinal cord and its canal, but also part of the CSF.

Cerebrospinal fluid

The production of CSF is mainly achieved by active secretion and diffusion through the epithelial cells of the **choroid plexus**, but also to a small extent in the **subarachnoid space** and **perivascularly**.

The main tasks of the cerebrospinal fluid are:
- To function as a hemodynamic buffer and protection against forces affecting the spinal cord and brain.
- To substitute for the function of the lymphatic vessels, which are absent in the central nervous system.
- To allow metabolic exchange between blood and neural tissue.

There is a selective barrier between the blood and the CSF, the **blood-brain barrier**, which is formed by capillary endothelial cells and the choroid plexus. This barrier is clinically significant, as it is impermeable to many drugs.

The total quantity of the CSF in the adult is about 120–150 ml (with about 20–35 ml below the foramen ovale and about 15 ml below T5).

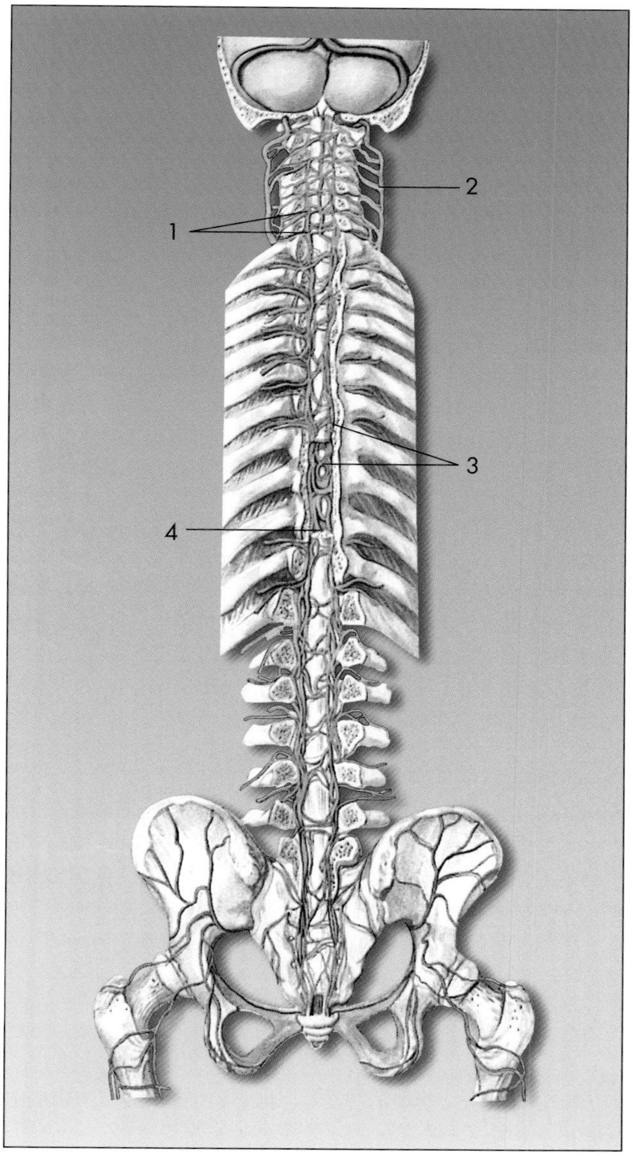

Approximately 400–450 ml of CSF is produced every day and complete exchange of the fluid takes place every 10–12 hours.

Lumbar **CSF pressure** in a supine position is about 60–100 mm H_2O and in a seated position it is about 200–250 mm H_2O.

The **specific gravity** of the CSF is 1.007 (1.003 to 1.009) and this must be taken into account in relation to the local anesthetic being used.

The **osmolarity** of CSF is comparable with that of the blood plasma (300 osmol/L) and the **pH value** is approximately the same as the physiological value.

Injected drugs mainly spread by diffusion, since CSF in the spinal canal circulates very little, if at all.

Resorption of CSF into the blood takes place via the **arachnoid granulations** and through the walls of the capillary vessels in the central nervous system and pia mater. The liquid in the CSF sheaths of the cranial nerves and in the root pockets of the spinal nerves is an exception to the above rule. This liquid can enter the extradural lymphatic vessels directly.

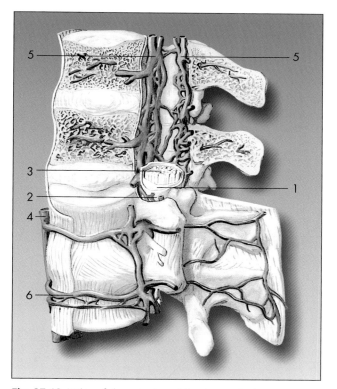

Fig. 27.17 Veins of the spinal cord.
(1) Vertebral veins, (2) deep cervical vein, (3) internal vertebral venous plexus, (4) spinal veins

Fig. 27.18 Veins of the spinal cord (lumbar region).
(1) Arachnoid, (2) dura mater, (3) cauda equina, (4) inferior vena cava, (5) internal vertebral venous plexus, (6) lumbar vein

Spinal anesthesia

28 Spinal anesthesia

Spinal anesthesia is one of the oldest, most valuable and today most frequently used regional anesthesia techniques.
The injection of a local anesthetic into the subarachnoid space leads to temporary blocking of stimulation conduction in the spinal nerve roots and paralysis of the autonomic, sensory and motor nerve fibers.
Spinal anesthesia has the following characteristics:
- It is easy to perform.
- The onset of effect is fast.
- Excellent anesthesia is produced.
- There is no systemic toxicity.

The application of spinal anesthesia depends on the following factors:
- The area of surgery.
- The type and expected duration of the procedure.
- The degree of muscle relaxation required.
- The presence of concomitant disease.
- The expected blood loss.

Indications

Surgical
Spinal anesthesia is particularly advantageous for all types of surgical procedure below the level of the umbilicus.

- Surgical procedures in the area of the lower extremities, hip joint and inguinal region.
- Vascular surgery.
- Prostate and bladder surgery.
- Gynecological and obstetric procedures.
- Surgery in the perineal and perianal region.
- Lumbar surgery, e. g. intervertebral disk operations [79].

Pain therapy
- Chemical intraspinal neurolysis with phenol in glycerine or alcohol (in advanced stages of malignant disease).

The use of spinal anesthesia has proved particularly valuable in:
- Patients with a full stomach.
- When intubation difficulties are expected.
- When there is a history of malignant hyperthermia, or a suspicion of malignant hyperthermia.
- Muscular disease.
- Cardiopulmonary disease.
- Metabolic disease.
- Renal and hepatic disease.
- Neurological diseases with a stable course.
- After high spinal cord injury.
- Geriatric patients.

Advantages:
- Very good muscle relaxation.
- Very good postoperative analgesia.
- Increased bowel motility.
- Prophylaxis against thromboembolism caused by the sympathetic block.
- Suitable for outpatient procedures.
- Highly cost-effective, with easy and safe monitoring.

Disadvantages:
- Unsuitable for upper abdominal procedures (high spinal anesthesia, e. g. T4–T6, is necessary).
- Lack of anesthetization of the vagus and phrenic nerves (leads to adverse effects such as nausea, vomiting, hiccup, pain and reduced blood pressure).

Contraindications

There are only a few contraindications to carrying out spinal anesthesia.

Specific
- Patient refusal or patients who are psychologically or psychiatrically unsuited.
- Coagulation disturbances, anticoagulant treatment.
- Sepsis
- Local infections (skin diseases) at the injection site.

- Immune deficiency.
- Severe decompensated hypovolemia, shock.
- Specific cardiovascular diseases of myocardial, ischemic, or valvular origin, if the procedure being carried out requires sensory distribution of the anesthesia as far as T6.
- Acute cerebral or spinal cord diseases.
- Raised intracranial pressure.
- A history of hypersensitivity to local anesthetic agents, without a prior intracutaneous test dose.

Specific injection-related
- CSF mixed with blood (which does not clear even after repeated aspiration).
- No free CSF flow (even after rotating the needle at various levels and repeated attempts at aspiration).

Relative

These contraindications always require a risk-benefit assessment and are more medicolegal in nature.
- Severe spinal deformities, arthritis, osteoporosis, intervertebral disk prolapse or post intervertebral disk surgery. Following spinal fusion, spinal metastases.
- Spinal canal stenosis [70].
- Repetition of spinal anesthesia with hyperbaric solutions if the block originally carried out is ineffective [30, 49] (see Chap. 29 on neurological complications, p. 218). A wait of at least 10–15 minutes should be observed; attention should be given to possible mistakes with the initial injection procedure and a maximum of half of the original dose without any addition should be administered.

Relative injection-related
- Further attempts after three unsuccessful injections.
- Inexperienced anesthetist without supervision.
- No anesthesiological expertise.

> **Caution**
> Head and back pain in the patient's history does not today represent a contraindication for carrying out spinal anesthesia, provided that small-caliber (> 25 G) "pencil point" injection needles are used and provided *only one* dural perforation is carried out.

Procedure

Preparation and materials
- Check that the emergency equipment is complete and in working order (intubation kit, emergency drugs); sterile precautions, intravenous access, anesthetic machine.
- Initiate an infusion and ensure an adequate volume supply (250–500 ml of a balanced electrolyte solution).
- Precise monitoring: ECG monitoring, BP check, pulse oximetry.
- Skin prep.
- Local anesthetic.

The use of a ready-supplied spinal intubation kit, e. g. from B. Braun Melsungen, is recommended (Fig. 28.1).

Spinal needles (Fig. 28.2)
There are two possibilities here:
- **25–29-G spinal needles with conical tips** ("pencil point"), e. g. Pencan, Sprotte, Whitacre as today's standard.
  When the dura is penetrated with these needles, the dural fibers are pushed apart to begin with and afterwards close together again. This means that the most troublesome complication – postdural puncture headache – hardly ever occurs when the dural puncture is carried out correctly.
- **Spinal needles with Quincke tip, 25–27 G**
  The opening of the needle tip should be directed laterally during the puncture, in order to pass through the dura in a longitudinal direction. A 22-G needle is only used in exceptional cases – e. g. in older patients, or when there are difficulties with positioning.

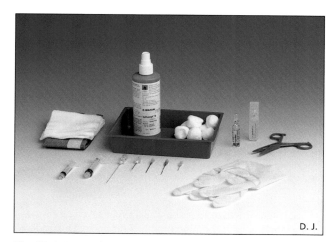

Fig. 28.1 Materials

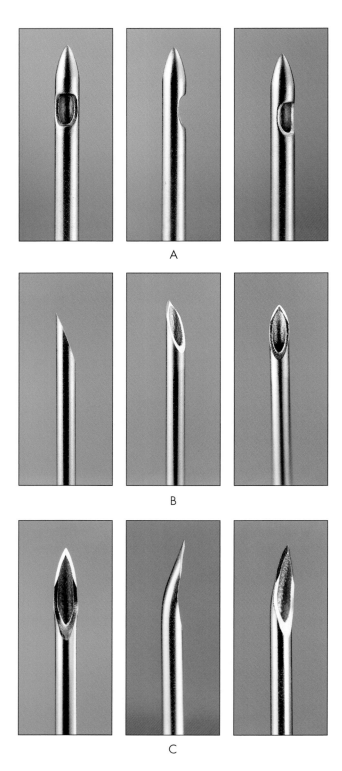

A

B

C

Fig. 28.2 A–C Spinal needles.
A Pencan: pencil point, 25 G.
B Quincke: Spinocan Quincke tip, 27 G.
C Atraucan: Atraucan Special Cut, 26 G

Patient positioning

Optimal patient positioning during puncture and during the fixation phase of the local anesthetic is a prerequisite for successful spinal anesthesia.

The following positions are possible:
- Lateral decubitus position.
- Sitting.
- Prone.

In all three positions, it is important to locate the **midline** and to follow it during the entire injection procedure. Lumbar lordosis must be relieved.

Lateral decubitus position
The assistant stands in front of the patient. If the anesthetist is right-handed, the patient is placed in the left lateral position. Legs flexed upon the abdomen and chin flexed upon the chest in order to bend the spine and allow optimal expansion of the intervertebral spaces.
It is important here for the spine to be parallel and for the intercristal line and the line connecting the two scapular tips to be perpendicular to the operating table (Fig. 28.3 A, B).

Advantages:
- More comfortable for the patient and thus particularly suitable for frail patients (risk of collapse).
- The reduction in blood pressure is less marked.
- When hyperbaric solutions are used, anesthesia concentrating on one side or unilateral anesthesia is possible.
- Can be used in pregnant patients (note the left lateral decubitus position).

Sitting
The patient is seated at the back edge of the operating table and supported by an assistant standing in front of him or her (Fig. 28.4).

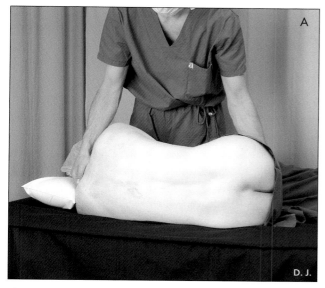 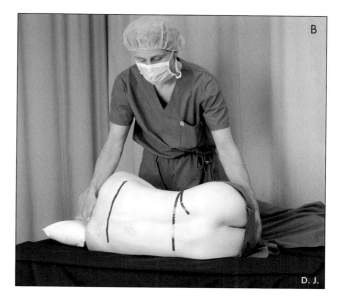

Fig. 28.3 A, B Position: lateral decubitus

Advantages:

– When palpation of the spinous processes is difficult (e. g. in obese patients or those with spinal deformities), it is easier to locate the midline.
– The position is less painful for patients with fractures of the hip or lower extremities. Particularly in older patients with femoral neck fractures, we additionally administer 4–6 mg Hypnomidate (etomidate) before the puncture, to make the short sitting phase easier.
– When anesthesia in the perineal or perianal region is required.
– The CSF flows more quickly.

Disadvantages:

– This position may lead to a drop in blood pressure (risk of collapse) and should be avoided in frail and heavily sedated patients, as well as in pregnant patients (aortocaval compression).
– An assistant is always required to support the patient.

Prone jackknife

This position is only used in the very rarely practiced hypobaric technique for spinal anesthesia (procedures in the rectum, perineum, sacrum, lower spine). An assistant and subsequent repositioning of the patient are not required (Fig. 28.5).

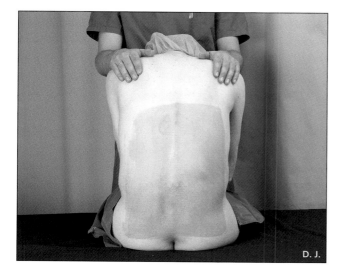 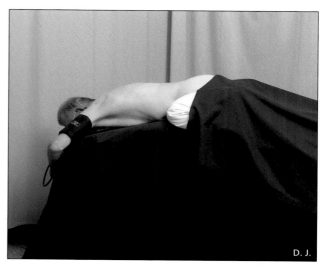

Fig. 28.4 Position: sitting

Fig. 28.5 Position: prone ("jackknife" position)

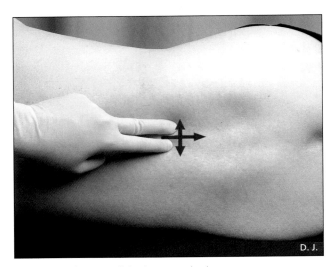

Fig. 28.6 Palpation of the intervertebral space

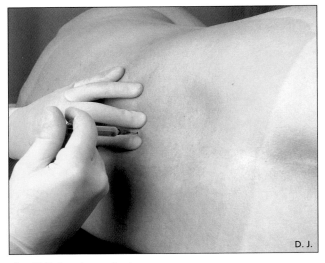

Fig. 28.7 Local anesthesia

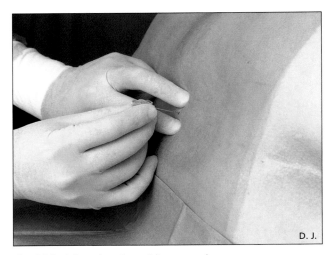

Fig. 28.8 Advancing the guiding cannula

Injection technique

Median approach (midline)

Landmarks
The injection is carried out in the midline below the L2 segment (medullary cone), usually between the spinous processes of L2/3 or L3/4 (depending on the desired level of anesthesia).
The patient is asked to draw the legs tightly up to the abdomen and to place the chin on the chest.
A line is drawn from one iliac crest to the other. This connection (Tuffier's line) crosses either the spinous process of L4 (50 %) or the intervertebral space of segments L4/L5.
The intervertebral space is palpated, the midline is located as the most important signpost and the injection site is marked with the nail of the thumb.
As this is done, the palpating fingers move in a craniocaudal direction, or side to side (Fig. 28.6).

Strict asepsis
Thorough, repeated and wide skin prep and drying and covering of the injection site with a drape.

Local anesthesia
The skin and supraspinous and interspinous ligaments are anesthetized with 1–1.5 ml of a local anesthetic (e. g. 1 % mepivacaine).
The injection is carried out between the spread index and middle fingers of the left hand (Fig. 28.7).

Injection
Advancing the guiding cannula
Without moving the spread index and middle finger of the **left** hand away from the intervertebral space, the guiding cannula is grasped between the thumb and index finger of the **right** hand and advanced parallel to the operating table and slightly cranially (10°) far enough for it to lie firmly in the interspinous ligament (Fig. 28.8). It should be ensured that the **midline position** is maintained.
After this, the guiding cannula is fixed with the thumb and index finger of the left hand, with the dorsum of the hand lying firmly on the patient's back.

Introducing the spinal needle, puncture
of the subarachnoid space
The spinal needle, held between the thumb and index finger (or middle finger) of the **right** hand, is introduced through the interspinous ligament, ligamentum flavum, epidural space and dura/arachnoid as far as the subarachnoid space. The characteristic **"dural click"** occurs when the subarachnoid space is reached (Fig. 28.9).

When a Quincke needle is used, it should be ensured that the opening of the needle tip is directed laterally, so that the dura is punctured in a longitudinal direction.

Removing the stylet
The following may occur here:

░ *CSF flows off freely*
   The injection needle is advanced 1 mm and fixed between the thumb and index finger of the **left** hand, which is supported on the patient's back. The desired amount of local anesthetic can now be injected (Fig. 28.10 A, B).
   With the single-injection technique, aspiration of CSF (0.1 ml) should be attempted immediately before and after injection of local anesthetic. The subarachnoid injection is made at the rate of 1 ml per 5 s.

░ *Blood in the CSF*
   Slightly bloody CSF, which clears quickly (spontaneously, or after aspiration) usually occurs after penetration of an epidural vein on the way into the subarachnoid space. The local anesthetic can be injected. However, when pure blood flows, it indicates that the injection needle is positioned within a vein. A new attempt at puncture must be made in a different intervertebral space.

░ *No CSF flow*
   Rotation of the needle at all four levels and careful aspiration. After positioning of the stylet, the needle is minimally advanced.
   If no CSF flows in spite of all these measures, puncture must be carried out after redirection.
   Unexpectedly deep bone contact suggests that the posterior side of the vertebra or an intervertebral disk has been reached. CSF appears in most cases after the needle has been minimally withdrawn and aspiration has been repeated.

░ *Paresthesias during puncture* (Fig. 28.11)
   These occur if the spinal needle touches a nerve root or the periosteum on its path. The direction needs to be corrected.
   When paresthesias are produced at the **subarachnoid** level, the needle must be withdrawn minimally. When paresthesias occur **during the injection**, the needle must be repositioned before any further drug is injected.

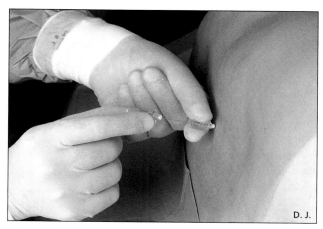

Fig. 28.9 Introducing the spinal needle. Puncture of the subarachnoid space

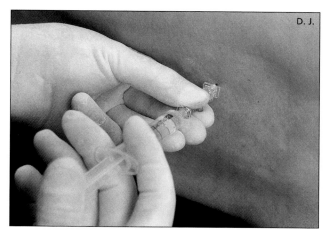

Fig. 28.10 A Removing the stylet. Subarachnoid injection

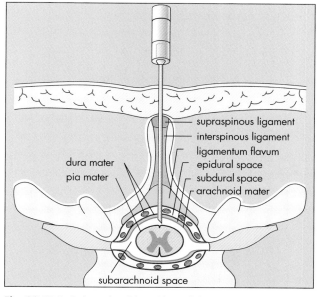

supraspinous ligament
interspinous ligament
ligamentum flavum
epidural space
subdural space
arachnoid mater

dura mater
pia mater

subarachnoid space

Fig. 28.10 B Subarachnoid position of the needle (diagram)

The local anesthetic must never be injected without evidence of CSF!
The location and distribution of paresthesias arising during the puncture procedure must be recorded.

Experience shows that failure is usually due to the following causes:
- The injection needle has left the midline.
- The cranial angle selected is too large.

Alternative access routes

Paramedian approach (Figs. 28.12., 28.14)
(Lateral, paraspinal)
In this technique, the supraspinous and interspinous ligaments are avoided, so that the ligamentum flavum is the primary target on the way to the subarachnoid space.

Procedure
This technique can be used in all the patient positions mentioned. Flexion of the spine is not required.
The caudal edge of the spinous process is marked. The injection site is located 1–1.5 cm lateral and caudal to this. The puncture is carried out in a craniomedial direction, at an angle of about 10–15°. The dura is reached after about 4–6 cm.
Most mistakes arise when the cranial angle of the injection is too large.

This access route can be used in:
- Degenerative changes in the spine.
- Older patients with marked calcification of the supraspinous and interspinous ligaments.
- Obesity.
- Fractures or other pathological conditions in which pain makes it impossible to bend the spine.

Taylor's approach (Figs. 28.13, 28.14)
This lumbosacral approach is a paramedian injection via the intervertebral space of L5 and S1, the largest interlaminar space in the spinal region.

Procedure
Lateral decubitus position, or sitting. The injection site is located about 1 cm medial and about 1 cm caudal to the posterior superior iliac crest. The injection needle is advanced in a craniomedial direction and at an angle of about 55°. If it touches the periosteum (sacrum), the needle must be withdrawn and the direction must be corrected.
The rare indications for this access route include procedures in the perineal and perianal region.

Positioning of the patient after the injection

The level of the anesthetic spread is controlled by patient positioning measures and checked with cold tests at intervals of 2–5 minutes.

Hyperbaric spinal anesthesia
Lateral decubitus position
The patient remains on the side being operated on for 10–15 minutes if a unilateral emphasis in the anesthesia is desired.
The patient is laid supine if adequate bilateral anesthesia is required.

Sitting position
The patient is immediately laid down to allow the required anesthetic to spread.
The patient remains sitting if sacral spread is desired.

Isobaric spinal anesthesia
Horizontal positioning is adequate; other positions have no significant influence on the spread of the anesthesia.

Hypobaric technique
Hypobaric spinal anesthesia is not suitable for everyday routine and is rarely used. It is mainly used for operations requiring a prone "jackknife" position, so that the patient does not need to be repositioned (Fig. 28.5).

Fixation phase

The phase immediately after injection of the local anesthetic is particularly critical and requires precise monitoring. The fixation phase lasts about 10–15 minutes.

Properties of local anesthetics in the subarachnoid space

Injecting a local anesthetic into the subarachnoid space blocks sensory and motor function. The main targets of local anesthesia are the posterior roots with the ganglia and anterior roots of the spinal nerves, the autonomic nerve fibers and mixed neural trunks.

The spread of the anesthesia should be checked at close intervals (2–5 min) and confirmed with pinpricks shortly before the start of the operation. The first sign of an effect on the spinal nerve roots is a subjective sensation of warmth in the feet. The further development of the block encompasses the sense of touch, depth sense, motor function, vibration sensitivity and positional sense.

Motor function is completely blocked at the site of greatest concentration of the local anesthetic. **Sensory**

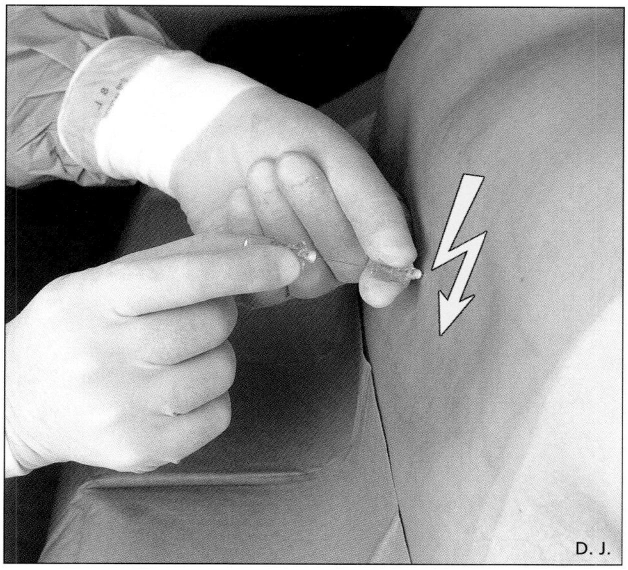

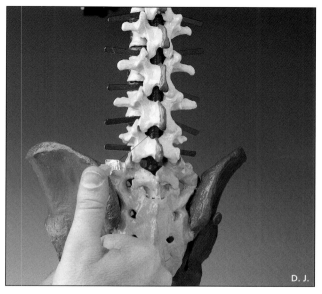

Fig. 28.11 Paresthesias during puncture

Fig. 28.12 Paramedian approach

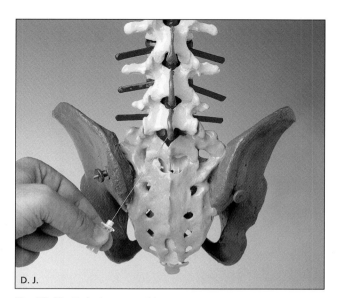

Fig. 28.13 Taylor's approach

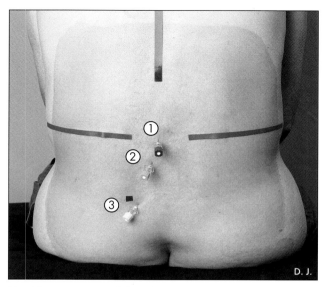

Fig. 28.14 Puncture of the subarachnoid space:
(1) median, (2) paramedian, (3) Taylor

block covers two to four segments and **sympathetic** block spread extends for a further two to four segments cranially. Subsidence of the block is marked by a return of motor function.

Elimination of local anesthetic that has been injected into the subarachnoid space takes place by subarachnoid vascular resorption (through the vessels of the pia mater and spinal cord), or epidurally [13].

Local anesthetics

The following local anesthetics are the main ones used as hyperbaric and isobaric solutions:

▨ 0.5 % **bupivacaine** as a long-term local anesthetic.
▨ 2–4 % **mepivacaine** or 2–5 % **lidocaine** as medium-term local anesthetics.
▨ 0.5–1 % **tetracaine** as a local anesthetic of the ester group.

Local anesthetics administered in the subarachnoid space reach body temperature in about 60 s.

Hyperbaric technique

This is the most frequently used and preferred technique for spinal anesthesia. Mixing a local anesthetic with glucose (5–10 %) increases its baricity in comparison with CSF and the level of anesthesia can be determined by patient positioning (Table 28.1).

Isobaric technique

In the isobaric technique, the position of the patient does not have a significant effect on the spread of the anesthesia. With a slow injection, the local anesthetic remains in the vicinity of the injection site and with a fast injection or barbotage, higher anesthesia can be achieved.

The most important parameter for the spread of the anesthesia is the volume of local anesthetic injected (Table 28.2).

Table 28.2 Dosage with isobaric local anesthetic*

Mepivacaine	2 %	3–5 ml (60–100 mg), Duration of effect: 30–90 min
Lidocaine	2 %	3–5 ml (60–100 mg), Duration of effect: 30–90 min
Bupivacaine	0.5 %	3–4 ml (15–20 mg), Duration of effect: up to 160 min

* Note the dose reduction (20–30 %) in obese patients and pregnant patients.

Factors affecting the spread and duration of spinal anesthesia [54]

▨ **Spread**
The following factors are very important:
– Dose and volume of local anesthetic solution injected.
– The injection pressure of the anesthetic solution.
– Position of the patient during and immediately after the injection.

Important factors are:
– The patient's age, weight and height.
– Anatomic configuration of spinal column.
– Volume of cerebrospinal fluid.
– Level of the injection site.
– Speed and barbotage of the injection.
– Direction of the injection needle's beveled tip.

Table 28.1 Dosage of hyperbaric local anesthetics*

Local anesthetic and concentration	0.5 % bupivacaine 5–8 % glucose		5 % lidocaine 7.5 % glucose		4 % mepivacaine 9.5 % glucose		1 % tetracaine 5 % glucose	
	ml	mg	ml	mg	ml	mg	ml	mg
Level of anesthesia								
T6 High	2.5–4.0	12.5–20.0	1.5–2.0	75–100	1.5–2.0	60–80	1.5–2.0	7.5–10.0
T10 Medium	2.0–2.5	10.0–12.5	1.0–1.5	50–75	1.0–1.5	40–60	1.0–1.5	5.0–7.5
L1 Deep	1.5	7.5	1.0–1.2	50–60	1.0–1.2	40–48	1.0–1.2	5.0–6.0
S1–S5 Saddle block	1.0	5.0	0.6–1.0	30–50	0.6–1.0	24–40	0.5–1.0	2.5–5.0
Onset of effect (min)	10–20		5–10		5–10		10–20	
Duration of effect (min)	up to 160		up to 60		up to 60		up to 150	
Prolongation of effect with vasopressors	No clinically significant effect with bupivacaine, lidocaine, or mepivacaine [20, 21, 76]						Up to about 180–240 min	

* Note the dose reduction (20–30%) in obese patients and pregnant patients.

– Intra-abdominal pressure.
– Diameter of the needle.

Less important factors are:
– CSF pressure.
– Concentration of the local anesthetic.

Duration
– Type and dosage of the local anesthetic.
– Anesthetic level achieved.
– Patient's age.
– Vasopressor addition: only in tetracaine; no clinical significance with bupivacaine or lidocaine [20, 21, 76].

Location of the procedure and required anesthetic spread (Fig. 28.15 A)

Anesthetic spread	Procedure
T4–T6	Upper abdominal procedures, Caesarean section, appendectomy, inguinal hernia (T6), testes, ovaries
T6–T8	Gynecological operations in the pelvis, ureter, renal pelvis
T10	Transurethral resections with bladder dilatation, vaginal delivery, procedures in the vaginal and uterine region, hip joint operations, knee joint and below, with ischemia
L1	Transurethral resections without bladder dilatation, thigh and lower-leg amputations
L2–L3	Knee joint and below, without ischemia
S2–S5	Perineal and perianal procedures

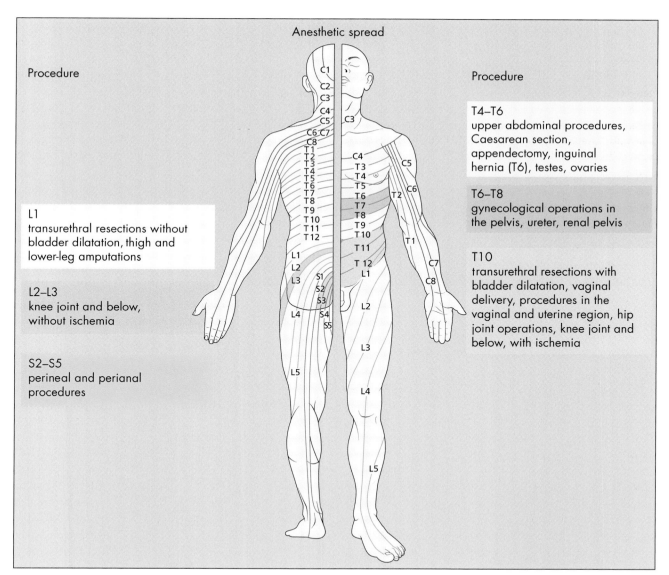

Fig. 28.15 A Location of the procedure and required sensory spread of local anesthesia

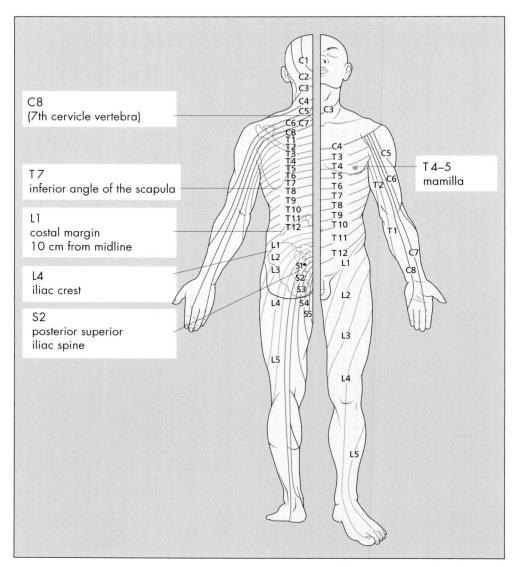

C8
(7th cervicle vertebra)

T 7
inferior angle of the scapula

L1
costal margin
10 cm from midline

L4
iliac crest

S2
posterior superior
iliac spine

T 4–5
mamilla

Fig. 28.15 B Landmarks for testing the spread of a local anesthetic after neuraxial anesthesia

Spinal anesthesia

Name: _____ Date: _____

Diagnosis: _____

Premedication: ☐ No ☐ Yes

Neurological abnormalities: ☐ No ☐ Yes _____

Purpose of block: ☐ Surgery

Needle: ☐ Pencil point G ____ ☐ Quincke G ____ ☐ Other ____

i. v. access and infusion: ☐ Yes

Monitoring: ☐ ECG ☐ Pulse oximetry

Ventilation facilities: ☐ Yes (equipment checked)

Emergency equipment (drugs): ☐ Checked

Patient: ☐ Informed ☐ Consent

Position: ☐ Lateral decubitus ☐ Sitting

Approach: ☐ Median ☐ Paramedian ☐ Taylor

Injection level: ☐ L3/4 ☐ Other

CSF: ☐ Clear ☐ Slightly blood-tainted ☐ Bloody

Abnormalities: ☐ No ☐ Yes _____

Injection:

Local anesthetic: _____ % ____ mg

☐ hyperbar ☐ isobar

Addition: _____ % ____ µg/mg

Patient's remarks during injection:

☐ None ☐ Pain ☐ Paresthesias ☐ Warmth

Duration and area: _____

Objective anesthetic effect after 15 min:

☐ Cold test ☐ Temperature measurement before ____°C after ____°C

☐ Sensory: L ____ T ____

☐ Motor

Complications:

☐ None ☐ Pain
☐ Radicular symptoms ☐ Vasovagal reactions
☐ BP drop ☐ Total spinal anesthesia
☐ Subdural spread ☐ Disturbance of breathing
☐ Drop in body temperature ☐ Muscle tremor
☐ Bladder emptying disturbances ☐ Back pain
☐ Postdural puncture headache ☐ Neurological complications

Special notes:

_____
_____
_____
_____
_____

Record and checklist

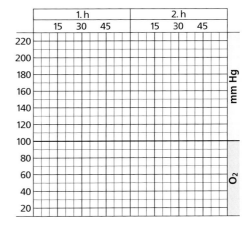

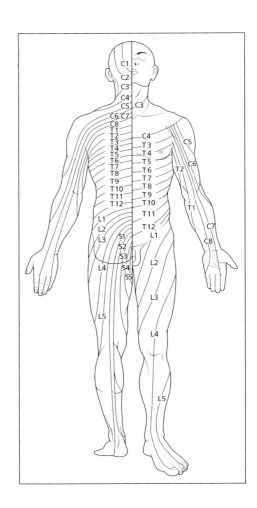

29 Complications of spinal anesthesia

Complications during the injection

Collapse (vasovagal syncope)

This is a harmless complication, which often occurs in young, nervous and anxious patients during injections in a sitting position. It involves a "neurogenic", normovolemic shock state, which requires no treatment other than laying the patient supine.

Prophylaxis
Injection in lateral decubitus position, mild sedation.

Complications immediately after the injection and during the fixation phase

Hypotension

This is the most frequent complication of spinal anesthesia. It arises due to blocking of sympathetic root fibers and is usually accompanied by bradycardia (preganglionic block of the sympathetic nerves to the heart, T1–4) and nausea.

Mechanism

Vasodilatation, postarteriolar trapping of blood, reduction in the circulating blood volume and venous return to the heart [10, 13].
The higher the spread of the spinal anesthesia or sympathetic block, the greater the reduction in arterial blood pressure.
A drop in blood pressure is also possible after the fixation period of the local anesthetic and it is often exacerbated by acute blood loss, repositioning maneuvers or quick release of the pneumatic tourniquet in ischemia.

Treatment

The aim is to increase venous return to the heart and to raise cardiac output, using the following physiological and pharmacological measures:
- Volume supplementation.
- Oxygen administration.
- Raise the legs to increase central blood volume.
- Place the patient in a slight Trendelenburg position (10°).
- Atropine when there is bradycardia.
- Small intravenous doses of vasopressor may also be needed (e. g. ephedrine 5–10 mg increments).

Prophylaxis

- Before spinal anesthesia is administered any deficits in intravascular volume should be corrected and an additional volume of at least 500 ml of a balanced electrolyte solution should be infused.
- Accurate assessment of the patient's level of cardiovascular risk.
- In pregnant patients, as well as older or obese patients: reduced dose of the local anesthetic, opioid or combination.

Prophylactic administration of a vasopressor is not recommended!

High and total spinal anesthesia

Causes

- Overdosage of the local anesthetic.
- Positioning error.
- Undesired spinal anesthesia when attempting to carry out epidural anesthesia (most frequent cause!)

The clinical picture has a dramatic course, characterized by restlessness, breathing difficulties, a severe drop in blood pressure and loss of consciousness. It is life-threatening and requires immediate treatment.

Therapy

- Immediate intubation (thiopental 1–2 mg/kg b. w., routinely ca. 150 mg i. v.); succinylcholine if appropriate, since the masticatory muscles are not affected [54].
- Ventilation with 100 % oxygen.
- Raise legs to increase central blood volume.
- Slight Trendelenburg position.
- Fast volume administration.
- Atropine.
- Vasopressor.
- Dopamine infusion.
- Precise cardiovascular monitoring.
- In cases of cardiac arrest, the usual cardiopulmonary resuscitation.

Subdural spread of the local anesthetic

Subdural injection can never be excluded with certainty. It may occur slightly more frequently after spinal anesthesia or myelography than after epidural anesthesia. The subdural space is at its widest in the cervical region, particularly dorsolaterally. It does not end at the great foramen like the epidural space, but continues cranially.

Warning signs

An unusually high sensory block, which develops very slowly (even after 20 minutes) and much less marked motor block.
The clinical picture resembles that of total spinal anesthesia and is characterized by moderate hypotonia, breathing difficulties with retained consciousness and often involvement of the cranial and cervical nerves:

Trigeminal nerve: trigeminal nerve palsy, with accompanying paresthesias in the area supplied by the nerve and transient weakness of the masticatory muscles with simultaneous Horner's syndrome, has been observed particularly after high epidural anesthesia or subdural spread [26, 36, 74, 77].

Horner's syndrome: Horner's syndrome is produced after neuraxial anesthesia with a high spread of the injected local anesthetic and block of very sensitive sympathetic nerve fibers in the areas of segments T4–C8 [43, 69]. Most often, Horner's syndrome is seen after high spinal or epidural anesthesia in obstetrics and when there is subdural spread of the local anesthetic [23, 28]. Relatively rapid resolution of the symptoms is characteristic.

Differential diagnosis

Total spinal anesthesia – dramatic course, blood pressure not measurable, respiratory arrest, longer time required for symptoms to resolve.

Prophylaxis

- Individual dosage and dose reduction in older patients, pregnant patients, obese patients and those with diabetes mellitus or arteriosclerosis.
- Incremental injection in epidural anesthesia.

Respiratory disturbances

These only arise after spread of the local anesthetic above segment T8. They result from block of the intercostal nerves and accompanying paralysis of the intercostal muscles. Resting ventilation is largely unaffected, thanks to compensatory diaphragmatic movement.

Therapy

- Mild sedation.
- Oxygen administration.
- Reassure the patient.

Gastrointestinal tract disturbances

Due to blocking of sympathetic inhibition, disturbances of bowel tone and motility may occur, becoming manifest as nausea or more rarely in vomiting. These disturbances are very often associated with a drop in blood pressure and bradycardia.

Reduced body temperature

Particularly in cool surroundings and when there is intraoperative blood loss, sympathetic block and the associated vasodilatation can lead to a drop in body temperature.

Complications in the early postoperative phase

Urinary retention

This affects 14–56 % of patients, mainly older ones and results from autonomic dysfunction caused by block of the parasympathetic segments from S2 to S4, which recover last after spinal anesthesia.

Clinical symptoms

Patients complain of severe lower abdominal and back pain, radiating up to the nape and this is often accompanied by an increase in blood pressure.

Therapy

If physical measures, early mobilization or administration of carbachol (Doryl, i. m.) are not successful, a single catheterization can lead to rapid improvement in the symptoms.

Late complications

Late complications are usually caused by the technique or spinal anesthesia. They manifest as:
- Postdural puncture headache.
- Back pain.
- Neurological complications.

Postdural puncture headache (PDPH)

This is a very unpleasant complication after spinal anesthesia, diagnostic lumbar puncture, myelography or diagnostic or therapeutic sympathetic block [51]. It usually develops after 24–48 hours or even later.

Frequency

0.2–24 % [13] up to 76.5 % [26, 29, 83] after puncture with large-diameter needles.

Mechanism

PDPH is thought to represent a multistep phenomenon initiated by dural puncture and resultant CSF leakage. Two proposed mechanisms for PDPH pain have been discussed in the literature. The first theory proposes that a decrease in CSF pressure produces traction on structures within the cranium, resulting in the generation of pain. The second hypothesis suggests that decreased CSF pressure leads to intrathecal hypotension and painful vasodilatation of the intracranial blood vessels (a so-called "intracranial vascular response" [16, 83]). Mainly when the patient is in a standing position, painful areas dilate (meninges, tentorium, vessels) and there is further pain transmission via the cerebral nerves and upper cervical nerves.

Etiology

Postdural puncture headache occurs frequently in younger patients and women, particularly during pregnancy. Repeated dural perforation, puncture with large-diameter needles and in particular accidental spinal anesthesia when attempting to carry out epidural anesthesia, are liable to lead to postdural puncture headache.

Location

Usually occipitofrontal (occipital: 25 %, frontal: 22 % or occipitofrontal: 25 %) [12, 83].

Clinical symptoms

Position-dependent headache, which is more severe when sitting and standing, coughing or straining, with marked relief when lying down.

Associated symptoms

Pain in the nape of the neck, stiffness in the neck, nausea, vomiting, sensitivity to light, smells and noise, auditory disturbances, tinnitus, loss of appetite, depressive mood. Patients whose headaches persist for any length of time feel miserable, tearful, bedridden and dependent.

CSF hypotension syndrome and involvement of the cranial and cervical nerves

All of the cranial nerves, with the exception of the olfactory nerve, glossopharyngeal nerve and vagus nerve, can be affected by low CSF pressure. The abducent nerve and vestibulocochlear nerve are most frequently affected (Fig. 29.1).
- Abducent nerve
  The long intracranial course of this nerve leads to traction and consequent irritation of the nerve when there are changes in intracranial pressure. The patient complains of double vision, with parallel horizontal images and difficulties in focusing on objects [6, 28, 80].
- Vestibulocochlear nerve
  When precise audiometric examinations are carried out, unilateral or bilateral hypacusis can be observed in 0.4–40 % of patients with CSF hypotension syndrome [28]. The prognosis is good.

Differential diagnosis

- Migraine.
- Tension headache.
- Cervical myofascial pain, particularly in the sternoclei-domastoid muscle, with what is known as "pseudo-spinal headache" [33].
- CNS infections (bacterial meningitis).
- Sinus thrombosis (in the second half of pregnancy or in the puerperium, frequently in preeclampsia).
- Pneumocephalus (after accidental dural perforation in attempted epidural anesthesia when using the loss-of-resistance technique with air [40]).

Therapy

When there is a diagnosis of postdural puncture headache, various treatment approaches are possible.

Noninvasive conservative therapy
This is used initially and includes traditional symptomatic measures such as:
- Bedrest (compulsory).
- Analgesics.
- Sedatives.
- Antiemetics.

The majority of patients experience marked improvement in the symptoms or complete recovery after five to seven days with this form of treatment [83]. In ca. 80 % of patients, the symptoms improve spontaneously within two weeks without any treatment ("tincture of time" [19]).

> **Caution**
> Treatment measures recommended in the past, such as massive fluid intake or obligatory 24-hour bedrest after puncture, are unnecessary.

Caffeine sodium benzoate is often used as part of noninvasive conservative treatment, with considerable success (> 85 %) [12, 16, 34, 41, 47, 73, 74]. The substance leads to cerebral vasoconstriction and a reduction in cerebral blood flow [72].

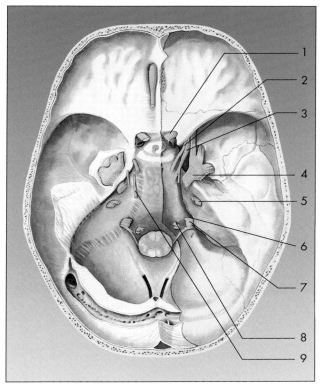

Fig. 29.1 Cranial nerves:
(1) optic nerve, (2) oculomotor nerve, (3) trochlear nerve, (4) trigeminal nerve, (5) vestibulocochlear nerve, (6) glosso-pharyngeal nerve, (7) vagus nerve, (8) hypoglossal nerve, (9) abducent nerve

The following infusion is used most frequently: 2 liters of liquid are administered over 2 hours, with the first liter containing 500 mg caffeine sodium benzoate. When there is residual pain, the treatment can be repeated after 4 hours [47].
Mild CNS stimulation and dizziness have been observed as side effects. Caffeine sodium benzoate can also be administered orally or intramuscularly [16, 40].
This form of treatment is particularly indicated in immune-suppressed patients, when there is a risk of infection, when there are difficulties in performing epidural puncture ("blood patch") and in postdural puncture headache after thoracic or cervical puncture.
Other alternatives that have been reported in the area of noninvasive conservative treatment of postdural puncture headache include administering adrenocorticotropic hormone (ACTH) [5] or sumatriptan (serotonin type Id receptor agonist) [17].

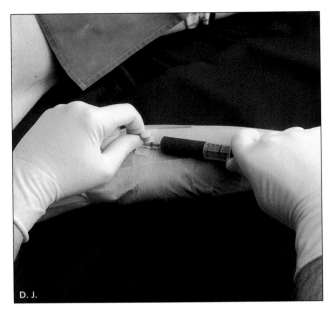

Fig. 29.2 Sterile withdrawal of blood

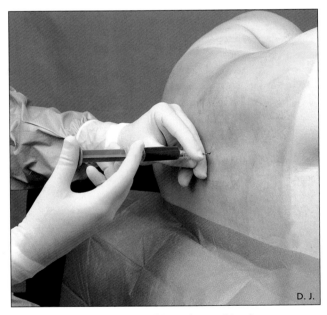

Fig. 29.3 Epidural injection of homologous blood

> **Caution**
> None of the conservative treatment approaches remove the cause of postdural puncture headache; they merely bridge the period until the dural leak closes naturally.

Invasive therapy
The method of choice in treatment-resistant postdural puncture headache is administration of a "blood patch" at the dural perforation site.

Prerequisites
- Correct diagnosis.
- Exclusion of all contraindications.
- Informing the patient.
- Experienced anesthetist.

> **Caution**
> This procedure should never be carried out without a correct diagnosis!

Procedure
A quantity of 10–20 ml of blood, taken from the patient under sterile conditions (Fig. 29.2), is reinjected epidurally. The injection is carried out at the same level as the original spinal anesthesia procedure or one segment deeper (Fig. 29.3).

The injection is carried out slowly (1 ml in 3–4 seconds). After the injection, the patient remains lying supine for ca. 30–60 minutes.

This procedure can be repeated after 24 hours. The patient is recommended to maintain bedrest for ca. 24 hours.

Using magnetic resonance imaging, Beards et al. [9] followed the spread of the extradurally injected homologous blood. The maximum compression effect on the dura was seen after an interval of 30 minutes to three hours, encompassing four to five neighboring segments. After about 7 hours, this effect subsided.

Other authors [18] have observed a spread over six segments above and three segments below the puncture site after extradural injection of radioactively marked blood.

Extradurally injected blood also spreads in the subarachnoid area [7] and particularly in the subcutaneous fatty tissue in the region of the lumbar spine. This is under discussion as a possible cause of postinjection back pain.

Complications

Back pain (35.9 %), pain in the nape of the neck (0.9 %), increased temperature (5 %) and dizziness are temporary phenomena and do not require treatment [13]. The treatment has a 95 % success rate.

> **Caution**
> Epidural injection of homologous blood is normally not painful. If injection pain occurs, the procedure should be interrupted.

Potential complications
- Inadvertent subarachnoid injection.
- Hematoma formation, with compression of the spinal cord.
- Risk of infection.
- Persistent back pain.
- Radicular pain.
- Facial palsy [64].
- Neural injury [12, 47].

Alternative methods
Epidural dextran patch [78, 83].
  Initially, a test dose of 20 ml Promit (dextran 1) is injected intravenously, to avoid potential allergic reactions.
  Then, at the level of the dural perforation site, a slow epidural injection of 20–25 ml dextran 40 is carried out. The viscosity and high molecular weight of dextran 40 lead to very slow resorption from the epidural space, so that a longer period of compression of the dural defect is achieved.

Infusion of isotonic saline via an epidural catheter 150–200 ml/day [7, 26, 42]. This method represents a temporary solution of the problem.

Prophylaxis against postdural puncture headache

- Use thin pencil-point spinal needles: 25–29 G, e. g. Pencan, Sprotte, Whitacre.
- If needles with a Quincke tip are being used, the angle of the tip should be placed parallel to the mainly longitudinally coursing dural fibers.
- Atraumatic technique: avoid multiple perforations of the dura.
- Experienced anesthetist.

> **Caution**
> When these prerequisites are observed, spinal anesthesia can also be carried out in patients with a history of headache and in young patients.

Back pain

This complication is a frequent occurrence after spinal anesthesia (2–25%), but it is no more frequent than after general anesthesia. Prior diseases of the spine make this complication more likely.

Mechanism
- Tissue trauma after multiple attempts at puncture.
- Position-dependent pressure during surgery on bones, joints and ligaments in the lumbar region.

Treatment
Symptomatic.

Neurological complications (see also Chap. 33, p. 249)

Neurological complications occur extremely rarely after spinal anesthesia.

> **Caution**
> If there is the slightest suspicion, an immediate neurological consultation should be carried out!

Etiology [50]

- Traumatic lesions of neural structures by the direct action of the injection needle or catheter or due to intraneural injection of the local anesthetic.
- Toxic effects of the injected local anesthetic (see "Cauda equina syndrome", below).
- Hemorrhage into the spinal canal, particularly in coagulation disturbances (subarachnoid or subdural hemorrhage, epidural hematoma).
- Vascular causes (thrombosis and spasm in the anterior spinal artery).
- Infection in the form of bacterial meningitis, which may be caused by inadequate asepsis or hematogenic or lymphatic bacterial transmission.
- Chemical irritation by substances used for skin prep at the puncture site.
- Introduction of foreign bodies.

- Exacerbation of latent prior neurological diseases (e. g. multiple sclerosis, tabes, tumor, latent viral infections).
- Injury due to inadequate surgical positioning.
- Psychogenic causes: e. g., as initiating factor in paraplegic symptoms [22, 38].

Neurological complications manifest as arachnoiditis, myelitis, spinal or epidural abscess, cauda equina syndrome or anterior spinal artery syndrome (see also Chap. 33, section on complications, p. 249).

Cauda equina syndrome (CES)

Cauda equina syndrome is an extremely rare complication [27], which can occur both after intrathecal and after epidural techniques (single-shot or continuous techniques).

Clinical symptoms
Peripheral paralysis, often asymmetric, of both legs, "saddle-like" sensory disturbances of all types in the lumbar and sacral segments, pain, absence of spontaneous bladder or rectal emptying, impotence.

Diagnosis
MRI, CT and/or myelography [46, 65].

Nerves of the cauda equina
The nerves of the cauda equina, located in a poorly vascularized distal area of the dural sac, possess only a weak protective layer [46, 48, 49].

Consequently, they react particularly sensitively to:
- The effects of local anesthetics [49, 62], depending on the type, dose, baricity and duration of exposure, particularly when an epidural dose is inadvertently administered intrathecally. Injurious effects of various local anesthetics (chloroprocaine [66] and hexylcaine [81]) have been reported in the past. Since the 1990s, there have also been reports that hyperbaric lidocaine can damage the nerves of the cauda equina [71], particularly after intrathecal administration via microcatheters [49, 70, 71].
Bupivacaine has proved to be safe, although there have also been individual reports of CES after intrathecal administration of hyperbaric solutions or after continuous epidural administration [49].
- Direct trauma caused by the puncture needle or by a catheter, particularly microcatheters (see Chap. 30, p. 219).
- Chemical irritation due to bacterial contamination.

Risks
Repetition of spinal anesthesia with a hyperbaric solution when the original block is incomplete represents a potential risk (see Chap. 28, section on relative contraindications, p. 201). In patients with a diagnostically manifest spinal canal stenosis, caution should be exercised due to potential accumulation or incorrect spread of the local anesthetic [30, 31, 49, 70].

Major prophylactic measures [45]
- Always choose the lowest possible concentration of a local anesthetic and inject it on a incremental basis.
- Caution should be exercised when using hyperbaric solutions (5 % lidocaine in particular should be avoided).
- Advance the spinal catheter a maximum of 2–3 cm beyond the needle tip (see Chap. 30, p. 219).

Anterior spinal artery syndrome

This syndrome can be caused by direct trauma to the vessel or by ischemia in the anterior two-thirds of the lower spinal cord [50].
Injury to the artery is expressed in a clearly definable clinical syndrome: motor disturbances and loss of pain and temperature sensitivity below the level of the lesion, with preserved positional sense and vibration sensitivity [62].

30 Continuous spinal anesthesia (CSA)

Continuous spinal anesthesia requires placement of a catheter in the subarachnoid space. Continuous administration of a local anesthetic or opioid, or a combination of the two, is carried out via the catheter, to produce adequate intraoperative and postoperative analgesia.

History of continuous spinal anesthesia

1907 H. P. Dean reported the first use of CSA via an intrathecal spinal needle during surgery.

1944 E. Tuohy: an N4 urethral catheter was introduced through a 15-G needle (PDPH > 30 %).

1964 D. Bizzari, J. G. Giuffrida: 27-G catheter through a 21-G needle.

1983 D. D. Peterson used standard epidural instruments (18-G Hustead needle with 20-G plastic catheter).

1989 Introduction of the microcatheter technique (by Boom in the USA), 28-G spinal microcatheter through a 22-G needle.

1992 Reports on cauda equina syndrome (14 per 50 000). The Food and Drug Administration (FDA) banned the use of the spinal microcatheter in the USA. Suspected causes:
 – Overdosage with hyperbaric 5 % lidocaine or 1 % tetracaine.
 – Extremely slow injection, required by the narrow-lumen catheter, leading to "sacral pooling" of the local anesthetic.
 – Caudal migration of the spinal microcatheter.

1993 In Germany, the BGA confirmed the above causes, but the use of the spinal microcatheter for CSA continued to be permitted.

1994 Development of a new "over-the-needle" CSA macrocatheter system (analogous to the indwelling venous catheter): lower risk of PDPH.

CSA is characterized [18, 45, 54] by:
- Fast onset of effect.
- Lowest possible dose of the local anesthetic or opioid through careful titration.

- Low cardiovascular and respiratory risks.
- Allows anesthesia to be prolonged as required.
- Shorter recovery times.
- Postoperative pain therapy.

Advantages over "single-shot" spinal anesthesia
- Injection of a local anesthetic only after placing the patient in the surgical position, with consequent reduction in cardiopulmonary risk.
- Better checking and control of the spread of anesthesia due to careful titration.
- Prolongation of anesthesia for as long as required.
- Precise control and short recovery time, due to injection of medium-term local anesthetics.
- At the end of the operation, the transition to additional opioid administration for postoperative pain therapy is made easier.

Advantages over continuous epidural anesthesia
- Easier identification of the subarachnoid space, and thus higher success rates, particularly when there are anatomical difficulties.
- Easy preoperative confirmation of subarachnoid positioning of the catheter.
- Only about 10 % of the usual epidural dose is needed, so that the risk of toxic reactions is very low.
- Faster onset of effect.
- Reliable block.
- Shorter recovery time.
- Lower risk in catheter migration.

Advantages over combined spinal and epidural anesthesia (CSE)
- Easy preoperative confirmation of subarachnoid positioning of the catheter.
- Reliable implementation of the anesthesia and postoperative pain therapy using only a single technique ("all-in-one system").
- Continuity and better control with fast-working subarachnoid top-ups.
- Test dose to check the catheter position is unnecessary.

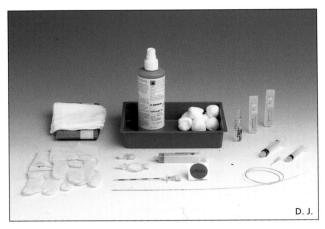

Fig. 30.1 Materials

Indications

- More prolonged surgical procedures with subsequent postoperative pain therapy.
- Older patients and high-risk patients.
- Anatomical difficulties.
- Use in vascular surgery, orthopedics, urology, gynecology and obstetrics, and in postoperative pain therapy.

Contraindications

These are the same as the general contraindications for neuraxial anesthesia (see Chap. 28).

Procedure

> **Caution**
> Continuous spinal anesthesia (CSA) should only be carried out by experienced anesthetists.

Preparations and materials
- Check that the emergency equipment is complete and in working order (intubation kit, emergency drugs).
- Strict asepsis.
- Intravenous access, anesthetic machine.
- Ensure adequate volume supplementation with a balanced electrolyte solution (250–500 ml).
- Precise monitoring: ECG monitoring, BP control, pulse oximetry.

The use of a ready-supplied set is recommended (Fig. 30.1).

Classic technique – through-the-needle system
Standard 18-G epidural Tuohy needle, with a 20-G epidural catheter (e. g. Perifix, B. Braun Melsungen) or a standard spinal needle (25–26 G), with a 32-G microcatheter or 22-G pencil-point spinal needle with a 28-G microcatheter.

Over-the-needle system (spinal needle lying in the catheter)
22-G or 24-G Spinocath, epidural guiding needle with a 30° beveled tip, smoothly moving, catheter connector, flat epidural filter (0.2 mm, antibacterial), B. Braun Melsungen.

Patient positioning
The lateral decubitus position is preferred, but paramedian approach, which offers the best angle for catheter placement, is also often used.

Injection technique
Classic technique – through-the-needle system
- The opening in the needle tip (Quincke, Tuohy or pencil-point) is first directed cranially.
  Shortly before the ligamentum flavum is reached, the needle is rotated 90° or directed laterally (Quincke, Tuohy), in order to puncture the dura after penetrating the ligamentum flavum. When the subarachnoid space has been reached, the opening in the needle tip is rotated cranially.
- After removal of the stylet and free flow of CSF, the injection needle is advanced by 1–2 mm.
  The catheter is then carefully advanced into the subarachnoid space up to a maximum of 2–3 cm beyond the needle tip, to avoid neural irritation or vascular puncture.
- Once the catheter has been placed in the desired position, the puncture needle is slowly withdrawn over the positioned catheter.

- The catheter connector and bacterial filter are then attached, with the catheter being fixed in the same way as an epidural catheter.
- Careful aspiration of CSF (in microcatheters, aspiration can be very difficult or even impossible).

> **Caution**
> If there are technical difficulties, the catheter and injection needle are always removed simultaneously. A catheter must never be withdrawn through a positioned injection needle.

The patient is then placed in the position required for the operation, and the drugs for subarachnoid administration are prepared (diluted with 0.9 % NaCl when appropriate).

Over-the-needle system
- **Epidural** puncture is carried out using the loss-of-resistance technique, with a needle that has a 30° bevel on the tip. This serves as the **guiding needle** for the Spinocath catheter system. The stylet is withdrawn (Fig. 30.2).
- The catheter and internal spinal needle are grasped with the thumb, index finger, and middle finger at the end of the needle, ensuring safe fixation of the spinal needle in the catheter for the dural puncture (Fig. 30.3).
- Dural puncture with the spinal needle and catheter tip (advance about 5 mm). The dural click and dilatation of the dura by the catheter tip are usually easily felt.
- CSF appears at the end of the spinal needle (lateral eye of the spinal needle) within about 3–6 s (22 G) or 6–10 s (24 G).
- The catheter is grasped with one hand about 3 cm behind the guiding needle, and the pull-out wire is grasped at its end and stretched with the other hand (Fig. 30.4).
- Advance the catheter over the spinal needle maximally 2–3 cm into the spinal space (technique analogous to indwelling venous catheters).
- Withdraw the spinal needle from the catheter completely on the pull-out wire (Fig. 30.5).
- Remove the epidural guiding needle, fixing the spinal catheter in the usual way.
- The connector and flat filter are then attached.

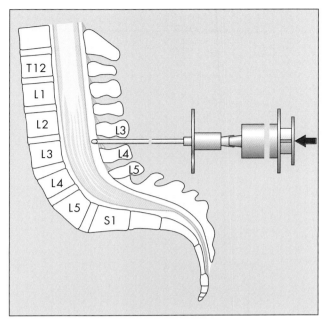

Fig. 30.2 Guiding needle. Epidural puncture using the loss-of-resistance technique

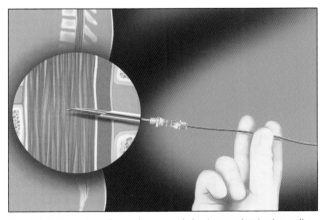

Fig. 30.3 Grasping the catheter and the internal spinal needle

Advantages
Easy puncture, secure positioning, little puncture trauma, gentle dilatation with the cone-shaped catheter tip, immediate sealing, no initial CSF loss and thus a reduced risk of postdural puncture headache.

Problem situation with the two techniques
Intrathecal positioning of the catheter – cranial or caudal?

221

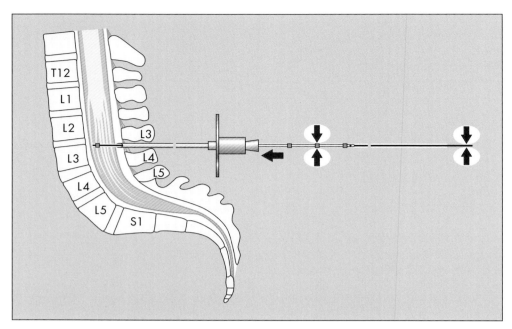

Fig. 30.4 Advance the catheter about 2–3 cm over the spinal needle (keeping the catheter stretched with the other hand on the withdrawal cord as this is done)

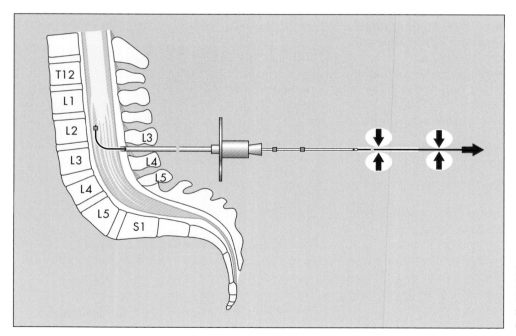

Fig. 30.5 Fix the catheter in position with one hand. Using the other hand, the spinal needle is withdrawn on its cord

Dosage

Surgical
Local anesthetic
0.5 % bupivacaine (isobaric): 1–1.5 ml = 5–7.5 mg (± 0.2 ml) after careful titration.
0.5 % bupivacaine (hyperbaric) for unilaterally accentuated anesthesia [59].

Combination
0.5 % bupivacaine 2.5–5 mg and sufentanil 7.5–10 µg.
0.5 % bupivacaine 2.5–5 mg and fentanyl 25 µg.

Postoperative pain therapy [58]
Intermittent intrathecal administration:
0.25 % bupivacaine (isobaric) – 1 ml every 4 h.
When there is inadequate analgesia, an additional injection of 0.5 ml 0.25 % bupivacaine is given every 30 minutes (maximum dose 2.5 ml/4 h).

Continuous intrathecal infusion:
0.25 % bupivacaine (isobaric) – 10 ml/24 h.
When there is inadequate analgesia, an additional injection of 1 ml 0.25 % bupivacaine is administered initially; a maximum of 1 ml 0.5 % bupivacaine can be given subsequently.

Disadvantages and complications (see also Chap. 29)
Postdural puncture headache
The aim is to reduce the frequency of postdural puncture headache through the use of microcatheters (e. g. a 32-G microcatheter through a 26-G injection needle or a 28-G catheter through a 22-G pencil-point injection needle) or the Spinocath catheter system. It is assumed that an inflammatory reaction occurs in the area of the puncture site, which allows sealing of the dural perforation site and thus reduces or prevents CSF loss [45]. The initial CSF loss after catheter placement is in theory avoided when the Spinocath system is used.

Cauda equina syndrome (CES)
The etiology of the cauda equina syndrome is probably multifactorial. The microcatheter technique (intramural positioning of the catheter with direct damage caused by the injection pressure) and subarachnoid injection of hyperbaric lidocaine or tetracaine have been linked to the development of CES [31, 71].
The causes are thought to be high doses and sacral pooling of the injected local anesthetic, due to the high injection resistance in the microcatheter. It is still unclear whether the neurological damage is caused by direct toxic effects of the local anesthetic or by indirect ischemic effects in the cauda equina area, which has a poor blood supply [45, 48].
It should also be emphasized that the subarachnoid space is very sensitive to any accidental injection of unintended medications – in contrast to the epidural space, which is very robust and "more forgiving" [11].

Shearing off of the catheter
This rare complication can occur during catheter placement and catheter removal (particularly with the microcatheter technique).

Prophylaxis
– When technical difficulties arise, never withdraw a spinal catheter through a positioned injection needle.
– A catheter should always be removed with extreme care. The patient is placed in the lateral position, with the back extended in order to stretch the ligamentum flavum [3].
– Never use force to pull the catheter, particularly against elastic resistance.
– If difficulties arise, wait until the patient is able to stand.
– Subsequent inspection of the catheter to check that it is complete, and keeping a record of the removal, are obligatory.

Opioid side effects
(See Chap. 41, additions to local anesthetics, section on opioids, p. 309)

Record and checklist

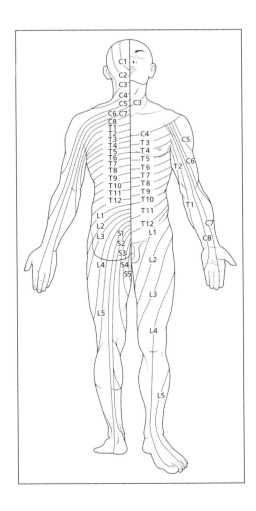

Continuous spinal anesthesia

Name: _____ Date: _____

Diagnosis: _____

Premedication: ☐ No   ☐ Yes

Neurological abnormalities: ☐ No   ☐ Yes _____

Purpose of block: ☐ *Surgery*   ☐ *Treatment (postoperative)*

☐ **Needle:** *G* ____ *Tip* ____ ☐ *Spinal catheter* ____ *G (micro, macro)* ____

i. v. access and infusion: ☐ *Yes*

Monitoring: ☐ *ECG*   ☐ *Pulse oximetry*

Ventilation facilities: ☐ *Yes (equipment checked)*

Emergency equipment *(drugs)*:   ☐ *Checked*

Patient: ☐ *Informed*   ☐ *Consent*

Position: ☐ *Lateral decubitus*   ☐ *Sitting*

Approach: ☐ *Median*   ☐ *Paramedian*

Puncture level: ☐ *L3/4*   ☐ *Other* _____

Technique: ☐ *Through-the-needle*   ☐ *Over-the-needle*

Subarachnoid space: ☐ *Identified*

Catheter: ☐ *Advanced 2–3 cm*

Aspiration test: ☐ *No*   ☐ *Yes*

Bacterial filter: ☐ *No*   ☐ *Yes*

Abnormalities: ☐ *No*   ☐ *Yes* _____

Injection:

☐ *Local anesthetic (isobaric, hyperbaric):* _____ *mg* ____ *%*
    (incremental)

☐ *Opioid* _____ *(μg)*   ☐ *Other* _____ *μg/mg/ml*

☐ *Subsequent injection of* _____ *ml* _____ *%*

Patient's remarks during injection:

☐ *None*   ☐ *Pain*   ☐ *Paresthesias*   ☐ *Warmth*

Duration and area: _____

Objective block effect after 20 min:

☐ *Cold test*   ☐ *Temperature measurement before* _____ *°C after* _____ *°C*

☐ *Sensory: L* _____ *T* _____

☐ *Motor*

Complications:

☐ *None*   ☐ *Pain*

☐ *Radicular symptoms*   ☐ *Vasovagal reactions*

☐ *BP drop*   ☐ *Total spinal anesthesia*

☐ *Subdural spread*   ☐ *Disturbance of breathing*

☐ *Drop in body temperature*   ☐ *Muscle tremor*

☐ *Bladder emptying disturbances*   ☐ *Back pain*

☐ *Postdural puncture headache*   ☐ *Neurological complications*

Special notes:

_____

_____

31 Continuous spinal anesthesia (CSA) in obstetrics

The first reports on the use of CSA in obstetrics were published in 1951. However, due to the high incidence of postdural puncture headache, use of the procedure was very limited until the 1980s. The development of improved technical systems, as well as the introduction of opioids for subarachnoid and epidural applications (particularly lipid-soluble sufentanil, fentanyl and pethidine), encouraged the wider use of this method.

However, further experience is still needed before this valuable method could be used routinely in obstetric anesthesia [3].

Patient selection

Candidates for continuous epidural anesthesia in obstetrics are also suitable for continuous spinal anesthesia.

Advantages

- Easy identification of the subarachnoid space.
- Higher success rate.
- Lowest possible dosage of local anesthetic, opioids, or a combination of the two and thus low rate of cardiotoxic effects.
- Faster onset of effect of anesthesia/analgesia.
- Bilateral spread.
- Particularly suitable in high-risk patients [1, 14, 44].

Procedure

Preparation and materials
- Check that the emergency equipment is complete and in working order (intubation kit, emergency drugs). Intravenous access, anesthetic machine.
- Strict asepsis.
- Ensure adequate volume supplementation with a balanced electrolyte solution (250–500 ml).
- Precise monitoring: ECG, BP control, pulse oximetry.
- Antacid administration (see Chap. 35, p. 260).
- Prepare the drugs, diluting them with 0.9 % NaCl when appropriate.

Patient positioning and injection

Puncture is carried out with the patient in the left lateral decubitus position, followed by placement of the spinal catheter, fixing of the catheter in position and placement of a bacterial filter.

Injection of a local anesthetic or opioid is always carried out on an incremental basis and at the lowest possible dosage, with precise monitoring (ECG, pulse oximetry; blood pressure monitoring: every 3 minutes during the first 30 minutes).

> **Caution**
> In obstetrics, it is recommended that the spinal catheter should not be left in place for more than 24 hours (risk of an increased PDPH rate).

Dosages [3, 61]

In addition to local anesthetics (bupivacaine), opioids can also be administered subarachnoidally – particularly lipid-soluble sufentanil, fentanyl and pethidine.

> **Caution**
> Injection of the local anesthetic should only be carried out once the patient is in an optimal position and with careful titration.

Local anesthetics for vaginal delivery
Initial dose: 1 ml 0.25 % bupivacaine.
If this dose is inadequate, it can be supplemented with 0.5 % bupivacaine, titrated in small portions of 0.25 ml each [3].

Opioids for vaginal delivery
Sufentanil: 7.5–10 µg.
Fentanyl: 25 µg.
In contrast to fentanyl, sufentanil (10 µg) is faster and more effective [52].

Table 31.1 Vaginal delivery: dosage and duration of effect of subarachnoidally administered drugs [3, 61]

Drug	Dose	Onset of effect	Duration of effect	Notes
Sufentanil	10 µg	2–10 min	60–180 min	Better analgesia than with fentanyl
Fentanyl	25–50 µg	2–10 min	30–120 min	
Pethidine	10–20 mg	2–10 min	60–180 min	Has sedative effects (higher dosage), more frequent vomiting
Morphine *)	0.2–2 mg	30–60 min	8–24 h	Respiratory depression
Bupivacaine	2.5–5 mg	15–20 min	30–60 min	Frequent tachyphylaxis

*) Doses ≥ 2.5 mg are often accompanied by itching, nausea and vomiting.

Caesarean section
Local anesthetics:
0.5 % bupivacaine (isobaric or hyperbaric), 2 ml increments = 10 mg (the maximum dose of 20 mg is rarely necessary) [3, 59].

Combination of opioids and local anesthetics
Initial dose: 1.5 ± 0.2 ml 0.5 % bupivacaine, hyperbaric, with the addition of 10 µg sufentanil.
Sufentanil and pethidine are more effective than fentanyl. All three opioids can lead to a slight decrease in blood pressure (not greater than 15 % of the baseline). The Apgar score in neonates remains normal [3].

Opioid side effects [3]
(See Chap. 41, section on opioids, p. 309)

Other complications
When CSA is used in obstetrics, the same complications must be expected as described earlier for continuous spinal anesthesia (see Chap. 30, p. 223) and continuous epidural anesthesia in the obstetric field (see Chap. 35, p. 259).
The occurrence of cauda equina syndrome after CSA in obstetrics has not so far been reported [3].
Various postpartum neuropathies (e. g. of the femoral nerve or obturator nerve), the duration of which is limited, must not be confused with cauda equina syndrome.

32 Chemical intraspinal neurolysis with phenol in glycerine

Chemical intraspinal neurolysis of the posterior spinal cord roots allows transient selective blocking of pain without any significant effect on cutaneous sensibility or proprioception [37, 54, 57].

Neurolytic substances at appropriate concentrations (phenol in glycerine, alcohol and chlorocresol) are used to destroy the thin C fibers, A-delta fibers and A-gamma fibers, while only having a slight effect on the thicker motor fibers [37] (Fig. 32.1).

At low doses of phenol, there is neither permanent motor weakness nor long-term loss of sensibility. Glycerine is used as the carrier substance for phenol. Phenol not only has destructive neurolytic effects, but also acts as a local anesthetic.

Indications

- Pain at the advanced stages of malignant disease (e. g. rectum, prostate, bladder, gynecological tumors). This method is particularly valuable for tumor-related pain in the rectal area.
- When opioids are ineffective in the terminal stages (method of choice in poor prognoses and poor general condition).
- When the patient declines neurosurgical pain-relief procedures.
- Spastic paraplegia with no hope of functional recovery (spasticity, hyperreflexia and pain).

Contraindications

- The general contraindications for spinal anesthesia apply (see Chap. 28, p. 200).
- No anesthesiological expertise.

Procedure

Preparations and materials
- Check that the emergency equipment is complete and in working order (intubation kit, emergency drugs); sterile precautions, intravenous access, anesthetic machine.
- Commence intravenous infusion and ensure adequate volume supplementation (250–500 ml of a balanced electrolyte solution).
- Precise monitoring: ECG, BP control, pulse oximetry.
- Spinal needle with Quincke tip, 22 G (due to the high viscosity).
- 1-ml tuberculin syringe.
- 2-ml syringe with 1–2 ml 0.9 % NaCl.
- Ampoule with 5 % or 10 % phenol in glycerine (Fig. 32.2).

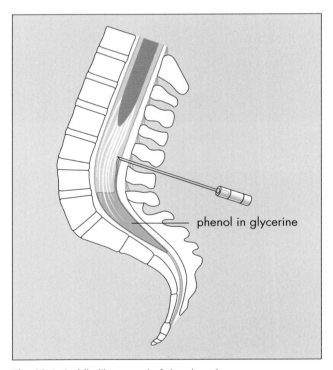

phenol in glycerine

Fig. 32.1 Saddle-like spread of the phenol

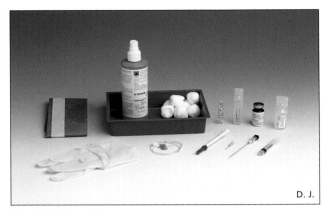

Fig. 32.2 Materials

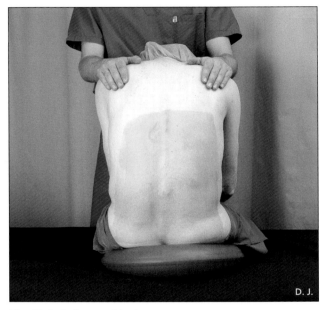

Fig. 32.3 Patient positioning

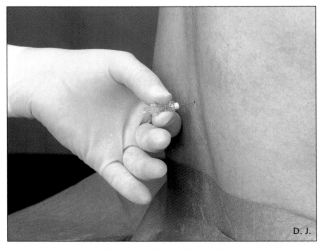

Fig. 32.4 Free CSF flow (proof) in all four planes

Warm the phenol ampoule to body temperature to reduce the viscosity [54] and then draw it up into the tuberculin syringe.

Prerequisites
The prerequisite for a neurolytic injection is a prior prognostic spinal block with a local anesthetic (e. g. with hyperbaric 4 % mepivacaine).
This is the only way to identify the correct dose and avoid giving patients with central pain an injection that is not indicated.
– Very experienced anesthetist.
– No analgesics and no premedication on the day of the block, so that the effect of the neurolytic can be more easily assessed.

Positioning and injection technique
▨ The patient is placed in a sitting position, since the aim is to achieve saddle block anesthesia. In cases of rectal carcinoma, sitting is almost impossible due to severe "fireball" pain in the anal region. A rubber ring is very helpful in such cases (Fig. 32.3).
▨ Puncture with a 22-G spinal needle in the region of the L5/S1 segment.
▨ Free CSF flow must be demonstrated in all four planes (rotate the needle and bevel) (Fig. 32.4). There is a risk of necrosis if phenol is inadvertently injected into the neighboring tissue.
▨ Very slow injection of phenol (0.5 ml over 30 min) (Fig. 32.5). The correct dosage is based on the test block with local anesthetic. Normally, symptoms improve quickly after the administration of 0.1–0.2 ml phenol, so that the patient ceases to feel any pain while sitting. If this improvement does not occur, it is usually because the phenol concentration selected was too low. 10 % solution is preferred by the authors.
▨ Constant checking of sensation by the assistant during the injection: pin-prick method (Fig. 32.6).
▨ After injecting the required amount of neurolytic (0.5–0.6 ml per session), the spinal needle is cleared of residual phenol with 1 ml 0.9 % NaCl and withdrawn (Fig. 32.7).
▨ The patient remains seated for the following 2–3 hours. After this, only 5 % of the phenol is still bound to the glycerine and an optimal saddle block is achieved.

To minimize the risks and achieve better distribution of the phenol, spread the total dose of 1–1.2 ml over two successive days.

Observations after the block

– Transient numbness in the calf region often occurs on the day of the injection.
– The first injection rarely produces adequate pain reduction.
– A repeat block is possible when the pain recurs.
– The average duration of pain reduction is about two to three months, although in the author's experience the duration of effect is difficult to assess in advance. It can range from one or two days to six months.

Caution
Opioids should not be abruptly discontinued. Instead, they should if possible be reduced step by step to a lower dose.

Complications

Complications are rare and transient [57].
Sensory and motor supply to the urinary bladder and rectum originates in the lumbosacral segments. If the procedure is not carried out carefully, there is therefore a possibility of loss of sphincter function in the bladder and rectum. In the extensive literature over the last 40 years, the frequency of this complication is reported to be 3–5 %. The loss of function is transient and usually limited to 4–6 weeks, depending on the recovery period required by the nerve fibers affected by the neurolytic. The patient must be made aware of this potential complication.

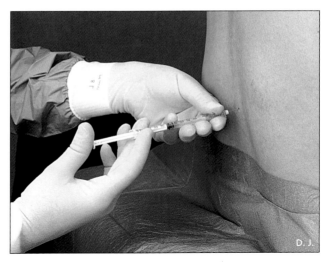

Fig. 32.5 Slow injection of phenol in glycerine

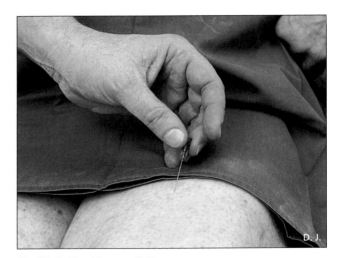

Fig. 32.6 Checking sensibility

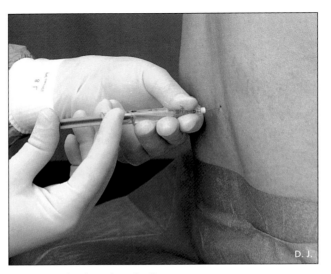

Fig. 32.7 Injection of 1 ml saline

Record and checklist

Neurolysis with phenol in glycerine

Name: _____ Date: _____

Diagnosis: _____

Premedication: ☐ No   ☐ Yes

Neurological abnormalities: ☐ No   ☐ Yes _____

Purpose of block: ☐ *Treatment*

Needle: ☐ *22-G Quincke*

i. v. access and infusion: ☐ *Yes*

Monitoring: ☐ *ECG*   ☐ *Pulse oximetry*

Ventilation facilities: ☐ *Yes (equipment checked)*

Emergency equipment *(drugs):*   ☐ *Checked*

Patient: ☐ *Informed*   ☐ *Consent*

☐ *Prognostic spinal anesthesia carried out*

Position: ☐ *Sitting*

Approach: ☐ *Median*

Puncture level: ☐ *L5–S1*   ☐ *Other* _____

Free CSF flow: ☐ *At all 4 levels*

CSF: ☐ *Clear* ☐ *Slightly blood-tainted* ☐ *Bloody*

Abnormalities: ☐ *No* ☐ *Yes* _____

Injection:

Phenol in glycerine: _____ ml ☐ *5 %* _____ ml ☐ *10 %*

Injection time: _____ *min*

☐ *Sensory and motor function checked during injection*

Patient's remarks:

☐ *During the injection:* _____

After phenol administration:

Injection of 1 ml 0.9% NaCl through the spinal needle:

☐ *Yes*   ☐ *No*

Complications:

☐ *None*   ☐ *Bladder emptying disturbances*

☐ *Bowel emptying disturbances* ☐ *Postdural puncture headache*

☐ *Back pain*   ☐ *Neurological complications*

Subjective effects of block:

☐ *None*   ☐ *Reduced pain*

☐ *Increased pain*   ☐ *No pain*

VISUAL ANALOG SCALE

0 10 20 30 40 50 60 70 80 90 100

Special notes:

_____
_____
_____

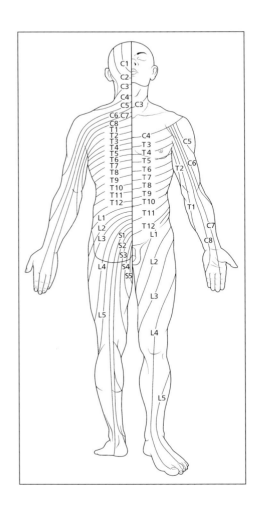

Epidural anesthesia

33 Lumbar epidural anesthesia

In epidural anesthesia, drugs are injected into the extradural space in order to interrupt conduction in the somatic and autonomic nerve fibers.

In addition to local anesthetics, opioids, steroids and homologous blood, other substances can also be used, mainly as adjuvants – e. g., the alpha-2-adrenoceptor agonist clonidine, vasopressors or ketamine.

Anatomy

The epidural space (cavum epidurale) lies between the widely separated laminae of the meninges – the thin periosteal lamina (lamina externa, endorrhachis), which covers the spinal cord and the lamina interna, the spinal dura mater to be precise.

Laterally, the epidural space is bounded by periosteum and by the intervertebral foramina. Ventral and dorsally, it is enclosed by the anterior longitudinal ligament of the vertebrae and the ligamentum flavum (Fig. 33.1). In the cervical region, the ligamentum flavum is much thinner and not very elastic.

The ligamentum flavum is most strongly developed in the midline in the lumbar region. The distance between the skin and the epidural space is about 4 cm in some 50 % of patients and between 4 cm and 6 cm in 80 % of patients. The range extends from less than 3 cm (in slim individuals) to more than 8 cm (in obese patients).

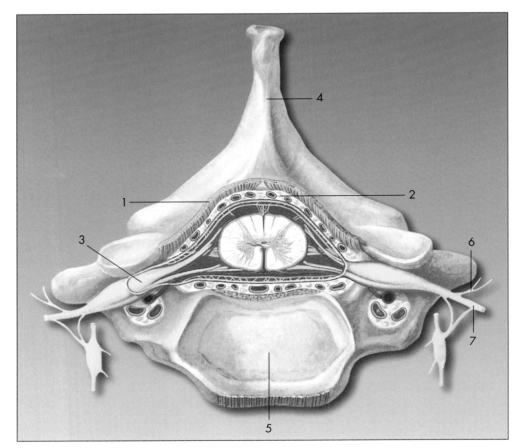

Fig. 33.1 Cross-section of the epidural space. (1) Ligamentum flavum, (2) epidural space with venous plexus, (3) spinal ganglion, (4) spinous process, (5) body of vertebra, (6) dorsal branch of spinal nerve, (7) ventral branch of spinal nerve

The distance between the ligamentum flavum and the dura mater varies from 2–3 mm cervically to up to 5–6 mm in the mid-lumbar region [22].

The volume of the epidural space, with a capacity of about 118 ml (up to 150 ml), is not as large as that of the subarachnoid space [10]. The epidural space extends from the great foramen to the sacrococcygeal ligament. It is connected via the intervertebral foramina with the paravertebral space. It has an indirect transdural link to the CSF. The substantial epidural venous network is connected to the azygos vein and to the pelvic, abdominal and thoracic veins [10, 22].

In addition to fat and connective tissue, the epidural space contains lymph, the internal and external vertebral venous plexuses and the roots of the spinal nerves. The width of the epidural space is 4–7 mm in the lumbar region, 3–5 mm in the thoracic region and 3–4 mm in the cervical region (C7–T1). There is negative pressure in the epidural space in some 80–90 % of patients. However, the negative pressure is not equally strong at all levels and it depends on intrathoracic respiratory pressure variations as well as on the patient's posture. The negative pressure increases in the sitting position, while in the supine position it is reduced. It is also reduced in pulmonary diseases (emphysema, asthma) and during heavy coughing or straining.

Indications

The use of epidural anesthesia has proved particularly valuable in the following groups of patients:
- Those with a full stomach.
- Those in whom intubation difficulties are expected.
- Those with a history or suspicion of malignant hyperthermia.
- Muscle disease.
- Cardiopulmonary disease.
- Metabolic disease.
- Renal and hepatic disease.
- Neurological diseases with a stable course.
- Geriatric patients.

Surgical indications
- Procedures in the area of the lower extremities, hip joints and inguinal region.
- Vascular surgery.
- Upper abdominal and thoracic procedures, in combination with basic general anesthesia.
- Urological procedures (prostate, bladder).
- Gynecological and obstetric procedures.
- Procedures in the perineal and perianal region.
- Interventional radiology.

Postoperative and post-traumatic pain therapy
Usually in combination with local anesthetics and opioids.

Therapeutic block with injection of depot corticoids
Caudal, lumbar or cervical.

Epidural injection of homologous blood or dextran
In postdural puncture headache.

Contraindications

Specific
- Patient refusal or patients who are psychologically or psychiatrically unsuited.
- In patients under general anesthesia.
- Abnormalities of coagulation, anticoagulant treatment.
- Sepsis.
- Local infections (skin diseases) at the injection site.
- Immune deficiency.
- Severe decompensated hypovolemia, shock.
- Specific cardiovascular diseases of myocardial, ischemic or valvular origin, if the procedure being carried out requires sensory spread as far as T6.
- Acute diseases of the brain and spinal cord.
- Raised intracranial pressure.
- A history of hypersensitivity to local anesthetics, without a prior intracutaneous test dose.

Relative
These contraindications always require a risk-benefit analysis and are more medicolegal in nature:
- Chronic disorders of the brain and spinal cord.
- Severe spinal deformities, arthritis, osteoporosis, intervertebral disk prolapse or pain after discoidectomy.
- After spinal fusion, spinal metastases.

Injection-related
- Additional attempts after three unsuccessful punctures.
- Inexperienced anesthetist without supervision.
- No anesthesiological expertise.

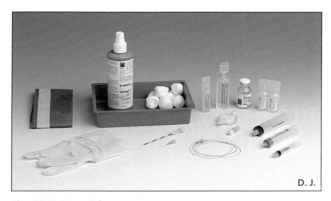

Fig. 33.2 Materials

■ Puncture should always be carried out below the level of L2 (medullary cone). Puncture above the L2 segment must only be carried out by a technically highly skilled anesthetist and must be strictly indicated [12].

■ Any severely radiating pain occurring during the puncture is a warning signal. The injection needle must not be advanced any further.

■ Epidural puncture in patients under general anesthesia, particularly above the L2 segment, should generally be avoided, except in the hands of the most skilled anesthetists. One exception to this rule is epidural puncture in pediatric patients, which must be left to experienced pediatric anesthetists [12, 51].

▨ Place the infusion and ensure adequate volume supplementation (250–500 ml of a balanced electrolyte solution).

▨ Precise monitoring: ECG, BP control, pulse oximetry.

The use of a ready-supplied kit for epidural anesthesia is recommended (e. g. from B. Braun Melsungen) (Fig. 33.2).

▨ Disinfectant.

▨ Local anesthetic.

Procedure

Preparations and materials

▨ Check that the emergency equipment is complete and in working order (intubation kit, emergency drugs); sterile precautions, intravenous access, anesthetic machine.

Epidural needles
Tuohy, Hustead, Crawford or Weiss (Fig. 33.3).

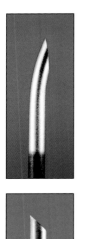
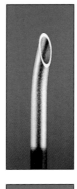
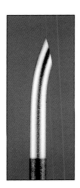
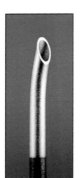

A B

C D

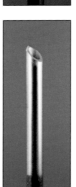
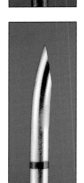
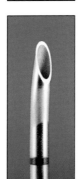

Fig. 33.3 A–D Epidural needles.
A Tuohy, **B** Hustead, **C** Crawford, **D** Weiss

233

Single-shot technique

Patient positioning
Optimal positioning of the patient during the injection and fixation phase of the local anesthetic is the prerequisite for success. Lumbar epidural anesthesia can be carried out with the patient in the lateral decubitus position (preferred) or sitting.

> **Caution**
> It is important with both positions to relieve lumbar lordosis and to locate the midline and follow it throughout the entire puncture procedure.

Injection technique

Median approach
Landmarks
The injection is carried out in the midline below the L2 segment (medullary cone), usually between the spinous processes of L3/4. The intervertebral space is palpated and the midline is located to serve as the most important signpost. In the midline, the ligamentum flavum is at its thickest, the epidural space is widest and the relative thickness of the vessels is at its lowest. The injection site is marked with the nail of the thumb (Fig. 33.4).

Strict asepsis
Thorough, repeated and wide skin prep, drying and covering of the injection site with a drape.

Local anesthesia
Anesthetization of the skin and supraspinous and interspinous ligaments is carried out between the spread index and middle fingers of the left hand, using 1–1.5 ml of a local anesthetic (e. g. 1 % mepivacaine) (Fig. 33.5).

Skin incision
Using a hemostylet or a large-diameter needle (Fig. 33.6).

Puncture of the supraspinous and interspinous ligaments and ligamentum flavum
Without moving the spread index and middle fingers of the left hand from the intervertebral space, an epidural needle is fixed between the thumb of the right hand and the index and middle finger (shaft) and advanced through the skin incision (Fig. 33.7).
After passing the supraspinous ligament, which is about 1 cm thick, the needle (with its opening directed laterally) is advanced a further 2–3 cm (depending on the anatomy), until it rests firmly in the interspinous ligament. The stylet is removed and a smoothly moving syringe is attached (Fig. 33.8).

> **Caution**
> Care should be taken to ensure that the midline position is maintained.

Inadvertent deviation from the midline leads to the needle passing the supraspinous ligament, with a slanting entry into the interspinous ligament with only brief resistance and a subsequent false loss of resistance. This type of puncture (oblique approach) ends in the paravertebral musculature and is accompanied by local pain.

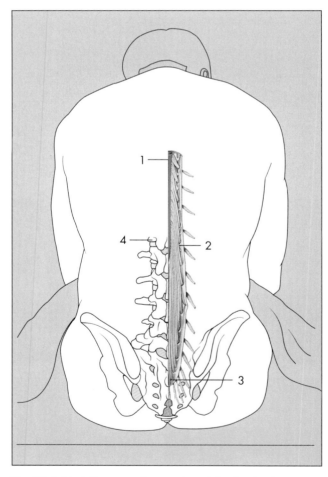

Fig. 33.4 Medullary cone (lower edge of the first lumbar vertebra). (1) Medullary cone, (2) cauda equina, (3) dural sac, (4) L1 segment

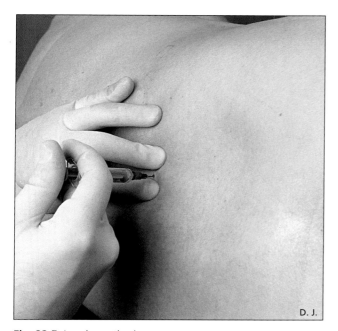

Fig. 33.5 Local anesthesia

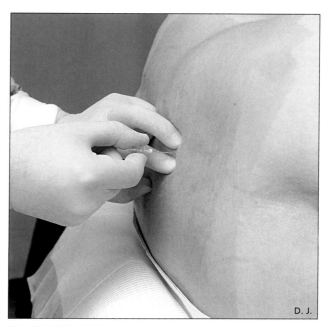

Fig. 33.6 Skin incision

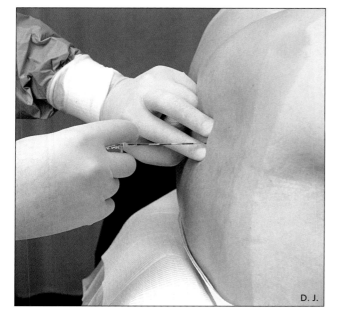

Fig. 33.7 Introducing the epidural needle

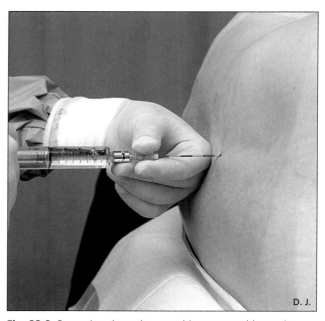

Fig. 33.8 Removing the stylet, attaching a smoothly moving syringe

The laminae and superior and inferior articular processes of the vertebrae may also be affected. Puncture trauma is accompanied by severe localized ipsilateral back pain, spasm of the paravertebral muscles and pain radiating into the leg. This type of pain is often confused with radicular pain.

Caution
After passing the interspinous ligament, the needle must be advanced millimeter by millimeter in the direction of the ligamentum flavum.

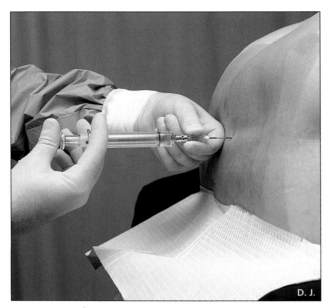

Fig. 33.9 Identifying the epidural space (loss of resistance)

Puncturing the epidural space
The thumb and index finger of the left hand, which is resting with the back of the hand firmly against the patient's back, secure the needle, advance it millimeter by millimeter and at the same exercise a braking function. The thumb of the right hand applies pressure on the syringe plunger. Loss of resistance indicates that the epidural space has been reached. The contents of the syringe are easily injected. Identification of the epidural space is carried out using the **loss-of-resistance technique** (Fig. 33.9).
The following variations on this technique can be applied:

Technique using saline or air
Saline: after the interspinous ligament has been reached, the stylet is removed and a smoothly moving syringe filled with a saline solution and with a small air bubble in it, serving as a visual indicator, is attached. When the ligamentum flavum is encountered, the air bubble is compressed by pressure on the syringe plunger (Fig. 33.10 A); when the epidural space is reached, the bubble returns to its normal, looser shape (Fig. 33.10 B).

Air: this technique is not suitable for inexperienced anesthetists or in punctures associated with technical difficulties [76, 78].

Advantage:
When the epidural space has been reached, there is no fluid dropping. Any CSF that emerges is therefore more easily identified.

Disadvantages:
The loss of resistance is not as clear and the dura is not pushed aside from the needle tip in the same way as it is using the saline injection. Complications have been reported [76] – e. g., pneumocephalus, compression of the spinal cord and nerve roots by air collecting in the epidural space, air embolism, subcutaneous emphysema.

"Hanging drop" technique
After the interspinous ligament has been reached, a drop of saline is placed within the hub of the needle (Fig. 33.11 A). After the ligamentum flavum has been passed and the epidural space has been reached, the drop is "sucked in" by the vacuum that is usually present during the inspiration phase (Fig. 33.11 B).

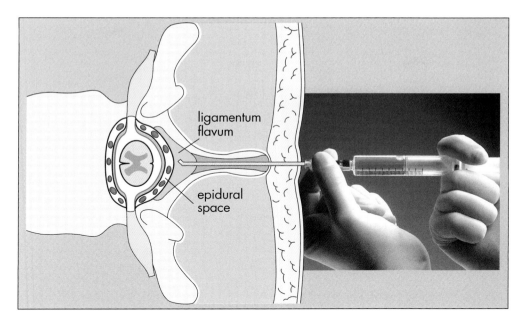

Fig. 33.10 A Loss-of-resistance technique with saline. The air bubble is compressed by pressure on the syringe plunger (diagram)

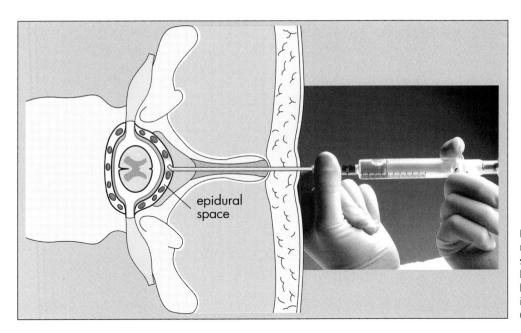

Fig. 33.10 B Loss-of-resistance technique with saline. The epidural space has been reached. The air bubble has returned to its normal, loose shape (diagram)

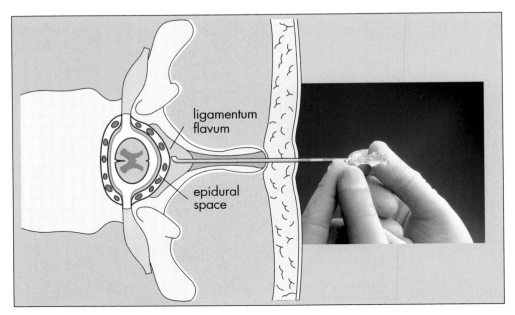

Fig. 33.11 A "Hanging drop" technique. The catheter is positioned in the ligamentum flavum (diagram)

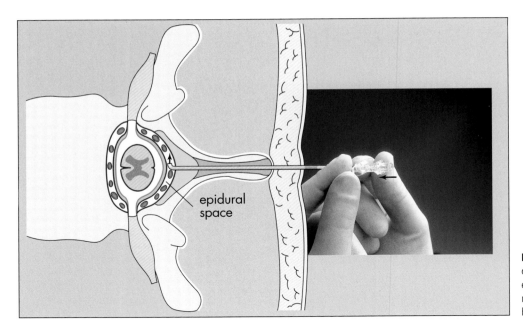

Fig. 33.11 B "Hanging drop" technique. The epidural space has been reached. The drop is sucked back in (diagram)

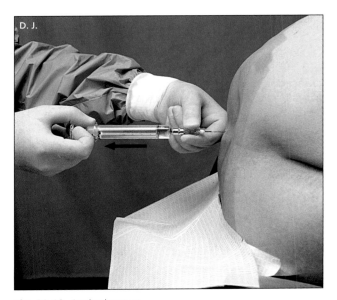

Fig. 33.12 Aspiration test

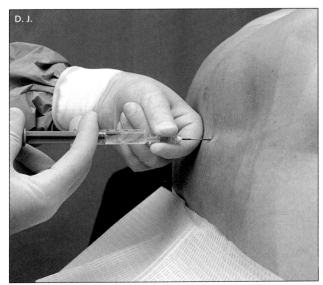

Fig. 33.13 Test dose

Aspiration and injection of a test dose
Careful aspiration is carried out in a minimum of two planes (Fig. 33.12). The needle continues to be secured by the thumb and index finger of the left hand, resting with the back of the hand firmly against the patient's back.

After a negative aspiration test, a test dose of 3–4 ml of local anesthetic mostly with epinephrine added can be injected. This allows easier detection of possible intravascular injection if tachycardia occurs (Fig. 33.13).

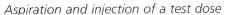

Caution
The addition of epinephrine can lead to unreliable results in the following groups of patients [59]:
– Patients taking β-blockers [40, 58].
– Patients under general anesthesia [28, 54, 90].
– Older patients [41].
– Pregnant patients [18].

Caution when adding epinephrine is required in:
– Pregnant patients (transitory fetal bradycardia due to reduced uterine perfusion [53]).
– Older patients with coronary heart disease.
– Arteriosclerosis, hypertonia, diabetes.

Contraindications to the addition of epinephrine are:
– Glaucoma (with closed iridocorneal angle).
– Paroxysmal tachycardia, high-frequency absolute arrhythmia.

The test dose should be allowed five minutes to take effect. During this period, the needle should be rotated at various levels at one-minute intervals (Fig. 33.14). Five minutes after administration of the test dose, the spread of the anesthesia is checked to exclude inadvertent subarachnoid injection. The patient is asked whether there is a sensation of warmth or numbness in the lower extremities. The following points are important in this phase:
– Maintaining constant verbal contact with the patient.
– Precise cardiovascular monitoring.

If the course is normal, a local anesthetic can be injected.

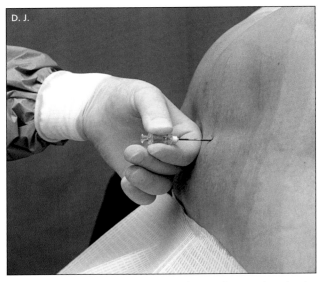

Fig. 33.14 Waiting period: rotating the needle at various levels

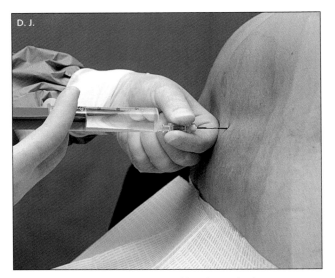

Fig. 33.15 Incremental injection of local anesthetic

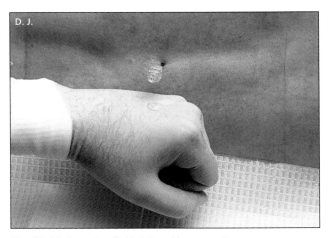

Fig. 33.16 Escaping fluid: is it cold or warm?

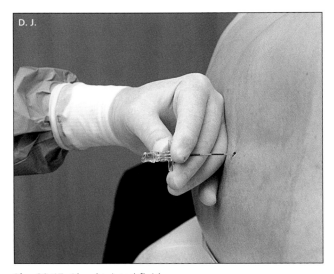

Fig. 33.17 Blood-tainted fluid

Injection of a local anesthetic (Fig. 33.15)
After aspiration has been repeated, incremental administration of a local anesthetic is carried out. In a "single-shot" injection, half of the planned dose is initially injected at a speed of < 0.3–0.5 ml/s; the syringe is disconnected again, a check is made for any escaping fluid and only then is the remainder of the dose administered. After aspiration has been repeated shortly before the end of the injection, the needle is withdrawn and the patient is placed in the desired position.

> **Caution**
> The hand securing the needle must remain constantly resting on the patient's back during puncture, aspiration, injection of the test dose, the waiting period and during injection of the local anesthetic.

Problem situations
Escaping fluid
After the epidural space has been identified or after administration of the test dose, a few drops of fluid may still drip from the positioned needle. This phenomenon often worries inexperienced anesthetists.
Procedure:
- During an attempt at aspiration, the viscosity of the fluid should be noted.
- The patient is asked to breathe in and out deeply. If the needle is positioned epidurally, there is synchronous movement of the fluid drop.
- A few drops of fluid can be tested on the back of the hand to check whether they are cold or warm: colder and slowly dripping fluid suggests saline, whereas warmer and quickly dripping fluid suggests CSF (Fig. 33.16).
- Carry out a glucose test.

Escaping blood (Fig. 33.17)
The following steps are possible:
- Renewed attempt at puncture, one segment higher or lower.
- Carry out general anesthesia.
- In all other indications, e. g. therapeutic blocks, it is advisable to abandon the procedure.

Escaping CSF

▨ The method of choice in surgical procedures is to carry out spinal anesthesia when the CSF is clear.

▨ Renewed attempt at puncture. It should be taken into account that an epidural dose of local anesthetic can spread subarachnoidally through the existing dural leak (larger puncture needles, 16–18 G) and can lead to total spinal anesthesia.

▨ Carry out general anesthesia.

▨ In all other indications, e. g. therapeutic blocks, it is again advisable to abandon the procedure.

▨ Patients must be informed about the possibility of postdural puncture headache.

> **Caution**
> The following measures have proved valuable for reducing risks of complications: aspiration, test dose of a local anesthetic containing epinephrine and incremental administration of the local anesthetic.

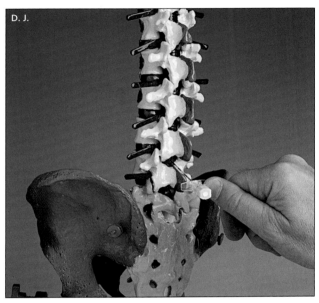

Fig. 33.18 Paramedian puncture

Paramedian (paraspinal) approach (Fig. 33.18)
This technique, which is independent of lumbar lordosis or the ability of the spine to bend, avoids puncture of the supraspinous ligament and the frequently ossified interspinous ligament. The puncture site is located in the selected intervertebral space, about 1.5–2 cm lateral from the upper edge of the lower spinous process. Fan-shaped local anesthesia identifies the depth of the vertebral arches (laminae), which are marked visually (4–6 cm). The epidural needle (usually 18-G Crawford) is introduced in a craniomedial direction at an angle of about 15° to the sagittal level and about 35° to the skin surface, so that it passes the laminae and slides into the interlaminar fissure. The only ligament that needs to be penetrated on the way to the epidural space is the ligamentum flavum. Reaching this is characterized by a "leathery" resistance. The most important step in this technique is to identify the depth of the ligamentum flavum. The stylet is then removed from the puncture needle and identification of the epidural space is carried out in the same way as described for the single-shot technique.

Record and checklist

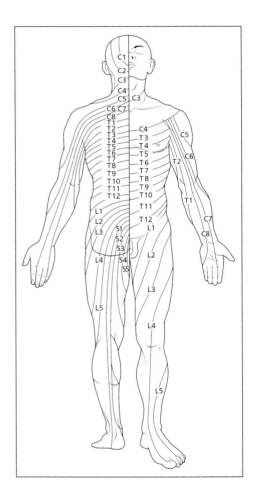

Lumbar epidural anesthesia

Name: _____ Date: _____

Diagnosis: _____

Premedication: ☐ No   ☐ Yes

Neurological abnormalities: ☐ No   ☐ Yes _____

Purpose of block: ☐ *Surgery*   ☐ *Treatment*   ☐ *Diagnosis*

Needle: ☐ ___ *G Tuohy*   ☐ *Other*

i. v. access and infusion: ☐ *Yes*

Monitoring: ☐ *ECG*   ☐ *Pulse oximetry*

Ventilation facilities: ☐ *Yes (equipment checked)*

Emergency equipment *(drugs)*:   ☐ *Checked*

Patient: ☐ *Informed*   ☐ *Consent*

Position: ☐ *Lateral decubitus*   ☐ *Sitting*

Approach: ☐ *Median*   ☐ *Paramedian*

Puncture level: ☐ *L3/4*   ☐ *Other* _____

Puncture technique: ☐ *Loss of resistance*   ☐ *Other* _____

Epidural space: ☐ *Identified*

Aspiration test: ☐ *Carried out*

Test dose: _____ Epinephrine added: ☐ *Yes* ☐ *No*

Checking of motor and sensory function after 5 min: ☐ *Carried out*

Abnormalities: ☐ *No*   ☐ *Yes* _____

Injection:

☐ Local anesthetic: _____ ml _____ %
   (incremental)

☐ Addition: _____ µg/mg

Patient's remarks during injection:

☐ *None*   ☐ *Pain*   ☐ *Paresthesias*   ☐ *Warmth*

Duration and area: _____

Objective anesthetic effect after 20 min:

☐ *Cold test* ☐ *Temperature measurement before* _____°C *after* _____°C

☐ *Sensory: L* _____ *T* _____

☐ *Motor*

Complications:

☐ *None*   ☐ *Pain*
☐ *Radicular symptoms*   ☐ *Vasovagal reactions*
☐ *BP drop*   ☐ *Dural puncture*
☐ *Vascular puncture*   ☐ *Intravascular injection*
☐ *Massive epidural anesthesia*   ☐ *Total spinal anesthesia*
☐ *Subdural spread*   ☐ *Respiratory disturbance*
☐ *Drop in body temperature*   ☐ *Muscle tremor*
☐ *Bladder emptying disturbances* ☐ *Postdural puncture headache*
☐ *Back pain*   ☐ *Neurological complications*

Special notes:

_____

_____

Continuous catheter epidural anesthesia

Procedure

The identification of the epidural space is carried out in the same way as in the single-shot injection. After the epidural space has been reached and loss of resistance has been confirmed, the aspiration test is carried out in two planes. Before the catheter is introduced, the needle bevel should be directed cranially.

The thumb and index finger of the left hand secure the epidural needle, with the back of the hand lying firmly on the patient's back. The catheter is advanced cranially, using the thumb and index finger of the right hand, by a maximum of 3–4 cm (Fig. 33.19).

Advancing it further than this can lead to lateral deviation of the catheter, with accompanying paresthesias or subsequent node formation.

Caution
If technical difficulties are experienced, the catheter and puncture needle must always be removed simultaneously. The catheter must never be withdrawn through the positioned puncture needle.

After placement of the catheter in the desired position, the puncture needle is slowly withdrawn (Fig. 33.20 A), while at the same time the thumb and index finger of the left hand secure the catheter at the injection site (Fig. 33.20 B).

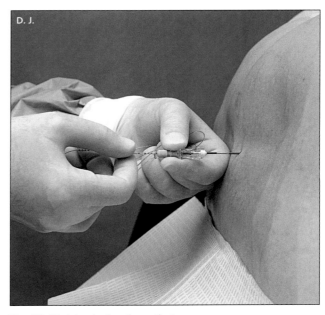

Fig. 33.19 Introducing the catheter

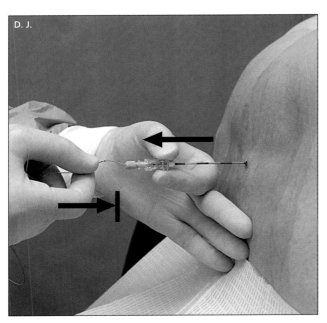

Fig. 33.20 A Withdrawing the puncture needle

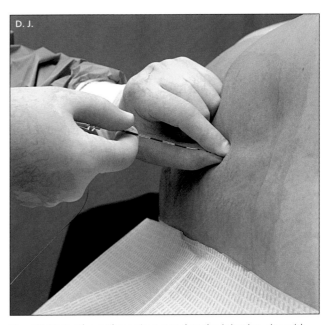

Fig. 33.20 B The catheter is secured at the injection site with the thumb and index finger

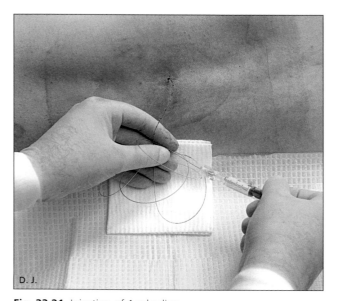

Fig. 33.21 Injection of 1 ml saline

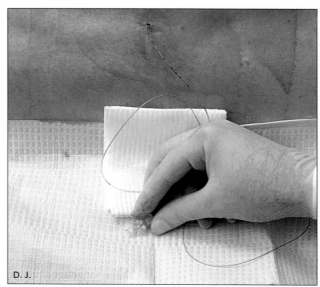

Fig. 33.22 The end of the catheter is placed below the puncture site

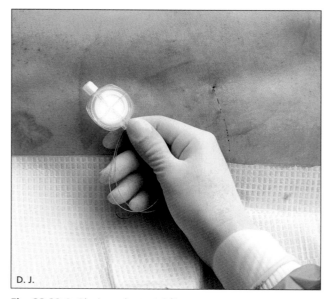

Fig. 33.23 A Placing a bacterial filter

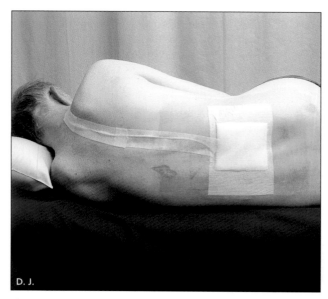

Fig. 33.23 B Securing the catheter and dressing

An adapter is attached to the end of the catheter. The patency of the catheter is tested by injecting 1–2 ml saline (Fig. 33.21). After aspiration, the syringe is disconnected and the open end of the catheter is placed on a sterile drape below the puncture site. Attention must be given to any escaping fluid (CSF or blood) (Fig. 33.22). A bacterial filter is then attached (Fig. 33.23 A) and the catheter is secured with a skin suture and a dressing (Fig. 33.23 B).

The patient is placed in the desired position and a test dose is administered, as with the single-shot injection. During the waiting period, it is important to maintain verbal contact with the patient and check the spread of the anesthesia, to exclude the ever-present risk of inadvertent subarachnoid injection. A subdural injection cannot always be excluded with absolute certainty, in spite of all precautions.

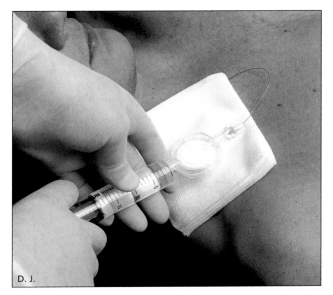

D. J.

Fig. 33.24 After the test dose – incremental injection of local anesthetic

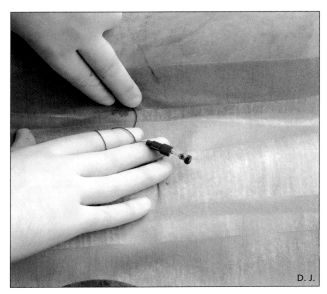

D. J.

Fig. 33.25 Blood in the catheter

After five minutes, the remainder of the dose, adjusted for the individual patient, can be administered on an incremental basis (max. 5 ml each injection) until the desired level of anesthesia is reached (Fig. 33.24).

Problem situations
Blood in the catheter (Fig. 33.25).
The catheter is withdrawn 0.5–1 cm and rinsed with 2–3 ml saline. After waiting and subsequent aspiration, a test dose can be given if no further blood is observed. If blood is still present, the catheter must be withdrawn.

Escaping CSF
When subarachnoid positioning of the catheter is demonstrated, the following steps are possible:
- Inject a spinal dose and then remove the catheter.
- Carry on with continuous spinal anesthesia.
- Remove the catheter and initiate general anesthesia.

The patient must be informed about the possibility of postdural puncture headache.

Caution
Monitoring an epidural catheter
Continuous pain therapy using an epidural catheter also requires continuous monitoring and checking of efficacy. This includes the following points in particular:
- Daily checking of the catheter position, so that intravascular or subarachnoid positioning can be recognized early.
- Changing the bacterial filter and dressing every two days, with careful checking of the puncture site, to minimize the risk of bacterial colonization and associated infection.
- Continuous monitoring of efficacy and – if necessary – adjustment of the dose of local anesthetic, opioid or other adjuvant substance.
- Records must be kept.

Record and checklist

Lumbar catheter epidural anesthesia

Name: _____ Date: _____

Diagnosis: _____

Premedication: ☐ No   ☐ Yes

Neurological abnormalities: ☐ No   ☐ Yes _____

Purpose of block: ☐ *Surgery*   ☐ *Treatment (postoperative)*

Needle: ☐ ____ *G Tuohy*   ☐ *Other*

i. v. access and infusion:: ☐ *Yes*

Monitoring: ☐ *ECG*   ☐ *Pulse oximetry*

Ventilation facilities: ☐ *Yes (equipment checked)*

Emergency equipment *(drugs)*: ☐ *Checked*

Patient: ☐ *Informed*   ☐ *Consent*

Position: ☐ *Lateral decubitus*   ☐ *Sitting*

Approach: ☐ *Median*   ☐ *Paramedian*

Puncture level: ☐ *L3/4*   ☐ *Other* _____

Puncture technique: ☐ *Loss of resistance*   ☐ *Other* _____

Epidural space: ☐ *Identified*

Catheter: ☐ *Advanced 3–4 cm cranially*

Aspiration test: ☐ *Carried out*

Catheter connector: ☐ *Positioned lower than the puncture site*

Bacterial filter: ☐

Test dose: _____ Epinephrine added: ☐ *Yes* ☐ *No*

Checking of motor and sensory function after 5 min: ☐ *Carried out*

Abnormalities: ☐ *No* ☐ *Yes* _____

Injection:

☐ Local anesthetic: _____ ml ____ %
  (incremental)

☐ Addition: _____ µg/mg

☐ Additional injection (incremental): _____ ml ____ %

Patient's remarks during injection:

☐ *None*   ☐ *Pain*   ☐ *Paresthesias*   ☐ *Warmth*

Duration and area: _____

Objective anesthetic effect after 20 min:

☐ *Cold test*   ☐ *Temperature measurement before* _____ °C *after* _____ °C

☐ *Sensory: L* _____ *T* _____   ☐ *Motor*

Complications:

☐ *None* ☐ *Radicular symptoms* ☐ *BP drop* ☐ *Vascular puncture* ☐ *Massive epidural anesthesia* ☐ *Subdural spread* ☐ *Drop in body temperature* ☐ *Bladder emptying disturbances* ☐ *Back pain* ☐ *Pain* ☐ *Vasovagal reactions* ☐ *Dural puncture* ☐ *Intravascular injection* ☐ *Total spinal anesthesia* ☐ *Respiratory disturbance* ☐ *Muscle tremor* ☐ *Postdural puncture headache* ☐ *Neurological complications*

Special notes:

_____

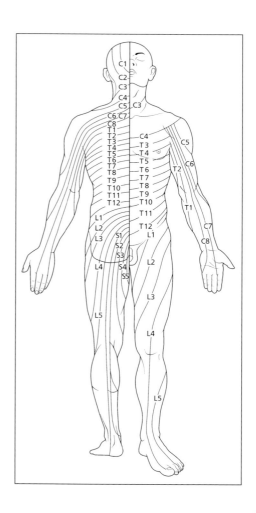

	1. h			2. h		
	15	30	45	15	30	45
220						
200						
180						
160						
140						
120						
100						
80						
60						
40						
20						

mm Hg

O₂

Effects of local anesthetics in the epidural space

Local anesthetic in the epidural space may take three routes.

- Resorption into the circulation via the epidural venous plexus.
- Transdural diffusion into the cerebrospinal fluid.
- Lateral perfusion through the intervertebral foramina and associated paravertebral block of the spinal nerves.

The targets of epidural injection of local anesthetic are the intradurally located roots of the spinal nerves, which are reached by diffusion through the dura.

The spread of the injected local anesthetic is influenced by the following factors:

- Volume and concentration have the greatest influence.
- The speed of injection has a minimal influence on the quality of the anesthesia. Too fast an injection can lead to dangerous cerebrospinal and cardiotoxic complications.
- The positioning of the patient is much less important than in spinal anesthesia.
- Location of the injection and diameter of the nerve roots: In injections in the lumbar region, the local anesthetic tends to spread more cranially, so that (particularly when injecting lipophilic local anesthetics such as etidocaine) block of segments L5–S2 is markedly delayed and they are incompletely anesthetized – probably due to the larger diameter of the nerve roots (S1 about 3.8 mm, S2 about 3.4 mm). For the same reasons, the upper thoracic and lower cervical segments show resistance to the effect of local anesthetics.
- Injection level: the closer the injection site is, the shorter the latency period.
- Anatomic relationships: Spinal deformities or operations near the spinal cord often lead to alterations of relationships in the epidural space and consequently affect the spread of local anesthetics.

- Height:
  Bromage's recommendation for patients aged between 20 and 40 has been widely accepted for clinical routine in the lumbar area [22]. The dose of the local anesthetic (2 % lidocaine) is between 1 ml and 1.6 ml per segment. For a basic height of 150 cm, 1 ml per segment is used and for each further 5 cm of body height an additional 0.1 ml per segment is added: 150 cm = 1 ml, 160 cm = 1.2 ml, 170 cm = 1.4 ml, 180 cm = 1.6 ml, 190 cm = 1.8 ml of local anesthetic.

> **Caution**
> The dose of local anesthetic in the thoracic region and in various groups of patients (e. g. pregnant patients, obese patients, elderly patients as well as in those with diabetes or arteriosclerosis) is reduced by 15–30 %.

The temporal sequence of an epidural block is as follows:

- Sympathetic block with vasodilatation.
- Block of temperature perception and depth pain.
- Loss of sensitivity to surface pain, pressure and touch.
- Block of motor functions.

Dosages

Surgical anesthesia

Medium-term amide local anesthetics (Table 33.1)

These local anesthetics are characterized by their low molecular weight, low lipophilia, moderate protein binding and high dissociation constant. At concentrations of 1.5–2 %, they produce rapid and good analgesia and a low motor block.

Table 33.1 Medium-term amide local anesthetics

Local anesthetic	Epidural dose	Onset of effect	Maximum dose	Duration of effect
1.5–2 % lidocaine with epinephrine	15–30 ml	10–30 min	300 mg 500 mg	80–120 min 120–180 min
1.5–2 % mepivacaine with epinephrine	15–30 ml	10–30 min	300 mg 500 mg	90–140 min 140–200 min
1.5–2 % prilocaine with epinephrine	15–30 ml	12–16 min	400 mg 600 mg	ca. 100 min ca. 140 min

Long-term amide local anesthetics (Table 33.2)

Table 33.2 Long-term amide local anesthetics

Local anesthetic	Epidural dose	Onset of effect	Maximum dose	Duration of effect
0.75 % ropivacaine	15–25 ml	10–20 min	250 mg (300)	180–300 min
1 % ropivacaine	15–20 ml	10–20 min	250 mg (300)	240–360 min
0.5–0.75 % bupivacaine	15–30 ml	18–30 min	150 mg	165–240 min
1 % etidocaine	15–30 ml	10–15 min	300 mg	150–280 min

Incomplete epidural anesthesia

In incomplete epidural anesthesia (failure to spread to specific segments or inadequate motor block), it is recommended that an additional injection be carried out after a delay of about 30 minutes for safety. The additional injection into the epidural catheter should be half of the initial dose, e. g. 2 % lidocaine with added epinephrine.

Diagnostic and therapeutic blocks

Medium-term amide local anesthetics (Table 33.3)

Table 33.3 Medium-term amide local anesthetics

Block	Sympathetic	Sensory	Motor
Lidocaine	0.5 %	1 %	2 %
Mepivacaine	0.5 %	1 %	2 %
Prilocaine	0.5 %	1 %	2 %

Long-term amide local anesthetics (Table 33.4)

Table 33.4 Long-term amide local anesthetics

Block	Sympathetic	Sensory	Motor
Ropivacaine	0.2 %	0.375 %	0.75–1 %
Bupivacaine	0.125 %	0.25 %	0.5–0.75 %

Postoperative or post-traumatic pain therapy

Continuous epidural infusion
▨ Local anesthetics
0.2–0.3 %   Speed:
ropivacaine   **6–14 ml/h (usually 10 ml/h)**
0.125 %   Speed:
bupivacaine   **8–18 ml/h (usually 10–14 ml/h)**
0.25 %   Speed:
bupivacaine   **4–16 ml/h (usually 8–10 ml/h)**

> **Caution**
> Individual adjustment of the dosage and duration
> of treatment is absolutely necessary.

▨ Opioids (see Chap. 41, section on opioids, p. 307)
Sufentanil: 30–50 µg
Fentanyl: 50–100 µg
Morphine: 2–5 mg

▨ Combination of local anesthetic and opioid
Bolus injection:
e. g. 10–15 ml 0.75 % ropivacaine with 1–2 µg/ml
sufentanil.
Continuous infusion starting after 60 minutes:
0.2 % ropivacaine with 0.75 µg/ml sufentanil.
Speed: 5 ml/h.

Bolus injection:
e. g. 10 ml 0.25 % bupivacaine with 1–2 µg/ml sufentanil.
Continuous infusion starting after 30 minutes:
0.125–0.0625 % bupivacaine with 0.2–0.3 µg/ml
sufentanil.
Speed: 6–10 ml/h.

Or

Bolus injection:
e. g. 10 ml 0.25 % bupivacaine with 50 µg fentanyl.
Continuous infusion starting after 30 minutes:
0.125–0.0625 % bupivacaine with 1–2 µg/ml fentanyl.
Speed: 10 ml/h.

▨ Epidural administration of clonidine (see Chap. 41,
section on clonidine, p. 309).
Bolus injection:
5–10 µg/kg b.w.
Epidural infusion:
20–50 µg/h.

Complications (Fig. 33.26)

Early complications

During puncture or when introducing the catheter
▨ Collapse (vasovagal reaction).
▨ Dural perforation.
▨ Catheter shearing.
▨ Spinal cord injury.
▨ Trauma to a nerve root.

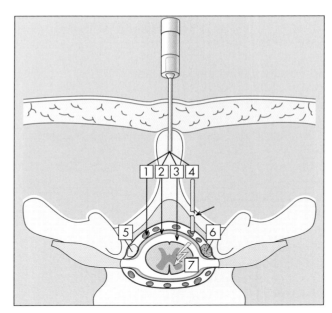

Fig. 33.26 Complications:
(1) intravascular injection, (2) subdural injection, (3) subarachnoid injection, (4) catheter shearing, (5) epidural abscess,
(6) epidural hematoma, (7) injury to the spinal cord and nerve
roots

After identifying the epidural space and administering a test dose
▨ Subarachnoid injection.
▨ Intravascular injection.

During and after injection of the full dose of a local anesthetic, during the fixation phase
▨ Massive epidural anesthesia.
▨ Total spinal anesthesia.
▨ Subdural spread.
▨ Intravascular injection, with toxic reactions.

During the surgical procedure
▨ Drop in blood pressure.
▨ Respiratory disturbance.
▨ Drop in body temperature.
▨ Muscle tremor.

Complications in the early postoperative phase

▨ Difficulty with micturition.

Late complications

▨ Postdural puncture headache.
▨ Back pain.
▨ Neurological complications.

Complications that can develop at any time with an epidural catheter in position

▨ Dural perforation.
▨ Total spinal anesthesia.
▨ Subdural injection.
▨ Intravascular injection.
▨ Retention of urine.
▨ Infections.
▨ Catheter shearing when removing the catheter.
▨ Neurological complications.

Inadvertent dural perforation

This is caused by incorrect puncture technique. As epidural puncture needles have a large diameter (16–18 G), the probability of developing postdural puncture headache is very high (70–80 %) (see Chap. 29, p. 214). Depending on whether or not the inadvertent dural puncture is noticed, various possible steps can be taken.

Dural perforation is noticed:
▨ Administer a spinal dose and carry out spinal anesthesia.
▨ New attempt at puncture.
▨ Switch to general anesthesia.

Dural perforation is not noticed:
▨ Accidental subarachnoid injection of an epidural dose leads to total spinal anesthesia, with very serious sequelae (see Chap. 29, section on high and total anesthesia, p. 212).

> **Caution**
> The patient should be informed immediately and made aware of the possible complications.

Prophylaxis
▨ Stay in midline during the puncture procedure.
▨ Always advance the puncture needle millimeter by millimeter after passing the ligamentum flavum.
▨ Aspiration test.
▨ Test dose.
▨ At every additional injection into the positioned epidural catheter, observe the same safety measures as with the single-shot injection.
▨ Maintain constant verbal contact with the patient.
▨ Check the spread of anesthesia frequently.
▨ Precise monitoring.

Therapy
(See Chap. 29, section on postdural puncture headache, p. 215)

Massive epidural anesthesia

Massive epidural anesthesia arises due to overdosage of local anesthetic and its resorption at the injection site. The condition develops more slowly than with an intravascular injection and in extreme cases it can lead to generalized tonic-clonic seizures (see Chap. 4).

Subdural spread of local anesthetic
(See Chap. 29, p. 213)

Intravascular injection

This can occur during the administration of a test dose, during a single-shot injection or during the injection of a local anesthetic through the positioned catheter and it can lead to severe toxic reactions (see Chap. 4, pp. 42, 43).

Prophylaxis
Before any single-shot injection or injection through the positioned catheter:
▨ Aspiration test.
▨ Test dose of a local anesthetic containing epinephrine.

Involvement of cranial and cervical nerves

High spread of an epidurally injected local anesthetic or a sudden increase in CSF pressure can lead to the following complications, which are mostly transient: hearing loss caused by transfer to the cochlear perilymph space; visual defects (in the most severe cases, retinal bleeding or even blindness); trigeminal nerve palsy, with weakness in the masticatory muscles; facial palsy (see Chap. 29, blood patch injection, p. 216); the development of Horner's syndrome.

Catheter shearing

Shearing of the catheter can occur both when it is being introduced and when it is being removed.

Prophylaxis
When placing the catheter
When technical difficulties occur during puncture, the catheter and the spinal needle are always removed simultaneously. A catheter must never be withdrawn through the puncture needle.

During catheter removal
When the catheter is being removed, any elastic resistance should be noted. Force should never be used when pulling. If necessary, wait until the patient is able to stand up and pull the catheter during bending or slight extension of the back.
After the catheter has been removed, it should be checked to ensure the tip has not broken off. A record must be kept.
If shearing occurs, the patient must be informed immediately. Neurological monitoring is obligatory, but surgery is very rarely indicated.

Neurological complications

Injury to the spinal cord and nerve roots
This is an extremely rare complication, since most punctures are carried out below the medullary cone. Neurological injuries can occur in all forms of neuraxial regional anesthesia.

Prophylaxis
▨ Advance the puncture needle with the utmost care.
▨ Interrupt the procedure immediately if pain occurs
 – during puncture
 – while introducing the catheter
 – during the injection (intraneural positioning).
▨ A catheter should be advanced at most 3–4 cm into the epidural space (risk of nodule formation).
▨ Puncture should be avoided at all costs in adult patients under general anesthesia, particularly above the L2 segment.

Bacterial meningitis

Strict asepsis is absolutely necessary when carrying out the block. A block is contraindicated when there is septic disease or infection in the area of the injection site.

Epidural abscess

The main cause of epidural abscess is *Staphylococcus aureus* [23]. The symptoms, which develop slowly (high fever, high-grade cervical or cervicothoracic and/or lumbar pain) require diagnostic clarification as quickly as possible (erythrocyte sedimentation rate, blood culture, CSF measurement, myelography, CT, MRI). Immediate surgical treatment (laminectomy, drainage) within 12 hours is important to reduce complications.
Epidural abscesses are extremely rare and usually arise spontaneously. Earlier mentions of them in the literature refer to continuous caudal blocks in which the necessary sterility was ignored. However, numerous studies [1, 2, 11, 23, 38, 72, 87] report evidence of a connection between prior septic disease and the development of abscesses after epidural anesthesia.
Systemic and local infections at the injection site are therefore an absolute contraindication to epidural anesthesia.

Epidural hematoma

This is an extremely rare, but feared, complication. It is characterized by rapid development of the classic symptoms, although these are not necessarily all evident in the reported forms in every patient affected: initial loss of consciousness, severe pain, substantial neurological disturbances, a lucid interval with normalization of the neurological status, headache and increasing clouding of consciousness, simultaneous pupillary dilatation, Cheyne-Stokes respiration, bradycardia, unconsciousness.

Any complaints by the patient regarding pain, fever or radicular symptoms must be immediately investigated. Maintaining constant contact with the patient, particularly after an outpatient procedure, is absolutely necessary. Immediate diagnostic clarification (myelography, CT, MRI) and immediate neurosurgical treatment within the first 12 hours are decisive for the prognosis. Among the risk factors reported in the literature [42, 86, 96] are trauma, vascular disease, coagulation disturbances and anticoagulant treatment.

Cauda equina syndrome
(See Chap. 29, p. 218)

34 Thoracic epidural anesthesia

Epidural injection or placement of a catheter for continuous epidural administration of a local anesthetic, opioid, or combination of the two in the region of the thoracic spine.

Advantages
The injection of local anesthetic is carried out directly at the selected thoracic segment. This allows a lower dosage per segment (e. g. 0.5–0.8 ml), with better-targeted anesthesia of the surgical area – without affecting sensory or motor function in the pelvis and lower extremities, or bladder function.
In addition, the risk of toxic reactions is reduced.

Disadvantage
Potential traumatic puncture of the spinal cord. A specific good indication is therefore necessary.

Prerequisite
Very experienced, technically skilled anesthetist.

Anatomy (Figs. 34.1, 34.2)

The thoracic spinous processes form varying angles with their vertebral bodies. At the upper and lower boundaries of the thoracic spine with the cervical spine (C7, T1–3) and lumbar spine (T10–12, L1), the spinous processes are almost parallel to the sagittal plane. The angle of puncture when locating the epidural space is thus almost identical to that in the lumbar region. It should also be noted that in the region of the lower thoracic spine (T10–12, L1) the distance from the skin to the spinal canal is slightly less, due to the shorter spinous processes.
In the central area of the thoracic spine (T4–9), the spinous processes have a very caudal angle and the laminae of the vertebral bodies are slanted. The ligamentum flavum becomes constantly thinner over its lumbar to cranial course and the epidural space becomes constantly narrower: 6 mm in the lumbar spine, 3–5 mm in the thoracic spine and 2–3 mm in the cervical spine.
These anatomic facts determine the puncture technique.

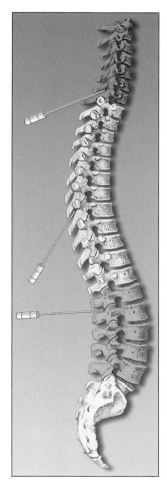

Fig. 34.1 Anatomy: cervical, thoracic and lumbar spine

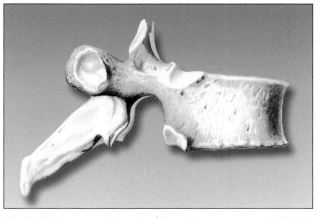

Fig. 34.2 Steep caudal angle of the spinous processes in T4–9

Indications

Surgical indications
- Upper abdominal, thoracic and two-cavity procedures in combination with basic general anesthesia, with subsequent continuation of continuous postoperative pain therapy with local anesthetics, opioids, or a combination of the two.

Indications for pain therapy
- Fractures to a series of ribs.
- Post-herpetic neuralgia.
- Acute pancreatitis.
- Cancer pain.

Contraindications

- The contraindications are the same as those for lumbar epidural anesthesia (see Chap. 33, p. 232).
- Puncture is absolutely contraindicated in adult patients under general anesthesia.

Procedure

Preparation and materials
- Check that the emergency equipment is complete and in working order (intubation kit, emergency drugs); sterile precautions, intravenous access, anesthetic machine.
- Commence intravenous infusion and ensure adequate volume supplementation (250–500 ml of a balanced electrolyte solution).
- Precise monitoring: ECG monitoring, BP control, pulse oximetry.
- Skin prep.
- Local anesthetic.

Epidural needles
18-G Tuohy or Crawford (see Chap. 33, p. 233, Fig. 33.3).

Access routes

Puncture of the epidural space is carried out on the same principles as in the lumbar region.

The sharp puncture angle in the T4–T9 region should be noted. Puncture can be carried out in the midline (median) or laterally (paramedian), with the patient sitting or in the lateral decubitus position. For a median puncture, the cervicothoracic transition (C7, T1–3) or the lower thoracic region (T10–12) are suitable. A paramedian puncture can be used at all levels of the thoracic spine, particularly in the central area from T4 to T9.

Median puncture in sitting position
The sitting position is helpful, as it increases the negative pressure in the epidural space, particularly during inspiration.

The patient sits relaxed and leaning slightly forward, with the neck flexed and the arms crossed, supported by an assistant. The patient must be aware of the importance of sitting steadily and calmly during the puncture procedure.

Location, skin prep, local anesthesia, skin incision
After thorough skin prep (strict asepsis), a sterile drape is placed on the puncture area and the puncture site in the selected intervertebral space is anesthetized with 1.5–2 ml 1 % mepivacaine. During infiltration with a 3 cm-long needle, the puncture angle is calculated. A skin incision with a hemostylet or large-lumen needle follows.

Puncture of the supraspinous and interspinous ligament and ligamentum flavum
An 18-G Tuohy needle with the opening directed cranially, or a Crawford needle with a caudally directed opening, is introduced at an angle of about 45° up to a depth of about 2.5 cm, until it is lying firmly in the interspinous ligament. The stylet is then removed.

> **Caution**
> Advancing the needle further after leaving the interspinous ligament must be carried out millimeter by millimeter and sensitively, towards the ligamentum flavum.

Puncturing the epidural space
Identification of the epidural space can be carried out using the "hanging drop" technique or the loss-of-resistance technique with saline.

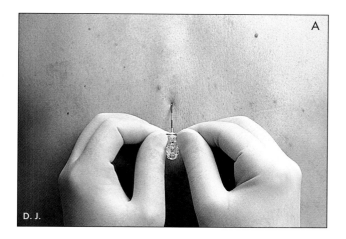

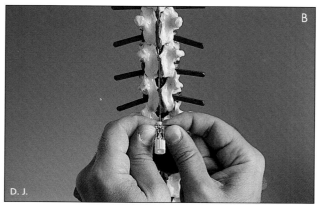

Fig. 34.3 A, B Median puncture. "Hanging drop" technique

"Hanging drop" technique (Fig. 34.3 A, B)
(See Chap. 33, p. 238, Fig. 33.11 A, B)
With this technique, high negative pressure in the thoracic epidural space during inspiration is helpful. After removal of the stylet from the puncture needle, a drop of the saline or local anesthetic is placed within the hub of the needle and the needle is advanced toward the ligamentum flavum.

The thumb and index finger of both hands secure the puncture needle and advance it millimeter by millimeter, with both thumbs firmly supported on the patient's back providing a braking function. The anesthetist's eyes are fixed on the "hanging drop".

When the epidural space is reached, the drop is sucked in during the inspiration phase and a loss of resistance in the tissue is felt.

Loss-of-resistance technique (Fig. 34.4) (see Chap. 33, p. 237, Fig. 33.10 A, B)

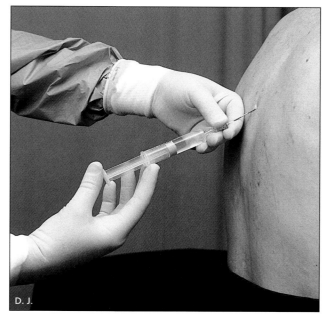

Fig. 34.4 Median puncture. Loss-of-resistance technique

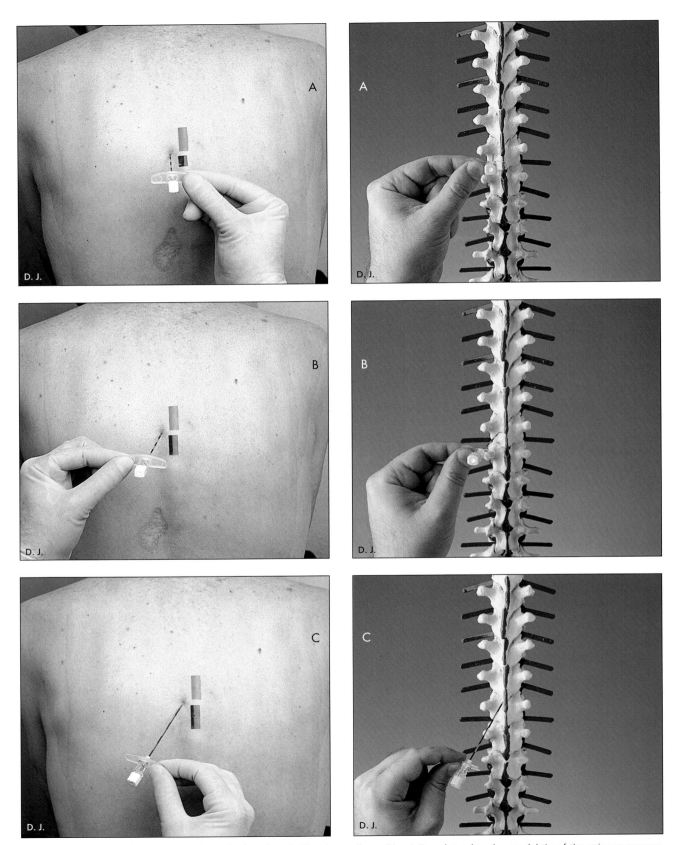

Fig. 34.5 A–C Paramedian puncture. Steps for location. **A** Step 1: needle position 1.5 cm lateral to the caudal tip of the spinous process. **B** Step 2: angle of 15° to the sagittal plane. **C** Step 3: angle of 55–60° to the skin surface

Paramedian puncture

This access route circumvents the sharply angled spinous processes and the supraspinous and interspinous ligaments.

Local anesthesia is applied about 1.5 cm lateral to the caudal tip of the spinous process in the selected puncture segment. This fan-shaped anesthesia allows the depth of the laminae to be measured and visually marked. The epidural needle is advanced alongside the spinous process at an angle of 15° to the sagittal plane and 55–60° to the skin surface or long axis of the spine (Fig. 34.5 A–C). After the ligamentum flavum has been passed, identification of the epidural space is carried out using the loss-of-resistance technique with saline.

Dosages

The dosage of local anesthetic in the thoracic region is 15–30 % lower than in the lumbar region, at about 0.5–0.8 ml per segment.

Local anesthetics
Ropivacaine
Incremental bolus injection: 0.75 %, 5–15 ml
                               (depending on the
                               injection site).
Epidural infusion: 0.2 %, 8–10 ml/h.

Bupivacaine
Incremental bolus injection: 0.25–0.5 %, 4–6 ml
                               (for two to four
                               thoracic segments).
Epidural infusion: 0.125 %, 5–10 ml/h.

Combination of local anesthetics and opioids
Bupivacaine and sufentanil
Bolus injection: Bupivacaine (0.25 %),
                               5 ml + 1 µg/ml
                               sufentanil.
Epidural infusion: Bupivacaine
                               (0.125–0.0625 %)
                               + sufentanil
                               0.2–0.3 µg/ml.
                               Speed: 6–10 ml/h.

Bupivacaine and fentanyl
Bolus injection: Bupivacaine
                               (0.25–0.5 %),
                               5 ml + 50 µg fentanyl.
Epidural infusion: Bupivacaine (0.125 %)
                               + 1–2 µg/ml fentanyl.
                               Speed: 6–10 ml/h.

Administration of opioids via the epidural catheter: lumbar or thoracic?
Lipid-soluble opioids
The precise mechanism involved in epidurally administered lipid-soluble opioids is a matter of controversy. According to a number of more recent investigations, the blocking of pain by lipid-soluble opioids after epidural administration is more the result of systemic uptake than a direct effect on spinal opioid receptors. The positioning of the epidural catheter would therefore be of secondary importance.

As some studies have reported [4, 46, 56, 70], opioid infusions via a lumbar epidural catheter have been used successfully for pain relief after thoracotomies. The authors conclude that the generally less familiar and potentially more dangerous thoracic access route is not justifiable.

Morphine as a hydrophylic substance
Morphine is hydrophilic and spreads quickly in the CSF and it is therefore able to produce analgesia in thoracic procedures even when it is injected into the caudal epidural space. Several studies have shown that lumbar administration of epidural morphine for pain relief after thoracotomies or after high abdominal surgery is just as effective as thoracic administration [8, 32, 70].

Specific complications

Spinal cord injury is among the extremely rare complications with this procedure (see Chap. 33, p. 251).

Record and checklist

Thoracic catheter epidural anesthesia

Name: _____ Date: _____

Diagnosis: _____

Premedication: ☐ No   ☐ Yes

Neurological abnormalities: ☐ No   ☐ Yes _____

---

	1. h			2. h		
	15	30	45	15	30	45

220
200
180
160
140
120
100
80
60
40
20

mm Hg

O₂

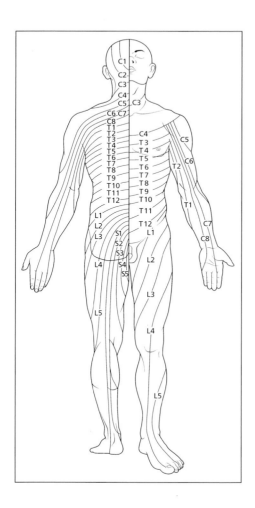

Purpose of block: ☐ *Surgery*   ☐ *Treatment (postoperative)*

Needle: ☐ ___ *G Tuohy*   ☐ *Other*

i. v. access and infusion: ☐ *Yes*

Monitoring: ☐ *ECG*   ☐ *Pulse oximetry*

Ventilation facilities: ☐ *Yes (equipment checked)*

Emergency equipment *(drugs):*   ☐ *Checked*

Patient: ☐ *Informed*   ☐ *Consent*

Position: ☐ *Lateral decubitus*   ☐ *Sitting*

Approach: ☐ *Median*   ☐ *Paramedian*

Puncture level: ☐ *T* _____

Puncture technique: ☐ *Loss of resistance*   ☐ *Other* _____

Epidural space: ☐ *Identified*

Catheter: ☐ *Advanced 3–4 cm cranially*

Aspiration test: ☐ *Carried out*

Catheter end positioned lower than the puncture site   ☐

Bacterial filter: ☐

Test dose: _____ Epinephrine added: ☐ *Yes* ☐ *No*

Checking of motor and sensory function after 5 min: ☐ *Carried out*

Abnormalities: ☐ *No*   ☐ *Yes* _____

Injection:

☐ Local anesthetic: _____ *ml* _____ *%*
   (incremental)

☐ Addition: _____ *µg/mg*

☐ Additional injection (incremental): _____ *ml* _____ *%*

Patient's remarks during injection:

☐ *None*   ☐ *Pain*   ☐ *Paresthesias*   ☐ *Warmth*

Duration and area: _____

Objective anesthetic effect after 20 min:

☐ *Cold test*   ☐ *Temperature measurement before* _____ *°C*   *after* _____ *°C*

☐ *Sensory: L* _____ *T* _____   ☐ *Motor*

Complications:

☐ *None*   ☐ *Radicular symptoms*   ☐ *BP drop*   ☐ *Vascular puncture*   ☐ *Massive epidural anesthesia*   ☐ *Subdural spread*   ☐ *Drop in body temperature*
☐ *Bladder emptying disturbances*   ☐ *Back pain*   ☐ *Pain*   ☐ *Vasovagal reactions*
☐ *Dural puncture*   ☐ *Intravascular injection*   ☐ *Total spinal anesthesia*
☐ *Respiratory disturbance*   ☐ *Muscle tremor*   ☐ *Postdural puncture headache*
☐ *Neurological complications*

Special notes:

_____

_____

35 Epidural anesthesia in obstetrics

The goal of epidural anesthesia in normal births is sensory block of the desired segments (first stage: T10–11, L1; second stage: L2–S4/5), with the lowest possible concentrations of a local anesthetic, opioid, or combination of the two.

In Caesarean sections, the aim is to achieve adequate anesthesia (T4–6) at higher dosages.

Anatomic and physiological changes during pregnancy

Anatomic changes

▨ During pregnancy, the epidural space narrows due to venous dilatation, since some of the blood from the lower extremities is transported via epidural veins to the upper caval vein (see Chap. 27, p. 199, Fig. 27.18).
The local anesthetic must therefore be administered at a lower dosage in pregnant patients.

▨ There is loosening of the vertebral ligaments and marked pooling of fluid in the tissues.
This makes it more difficult to identify the epidural space and there is an increased risk of dural puncture. Particularly during uterine contractions, the negative pressure in the epidural space is lost.

Physiological changes

Respiratory tract
Shifting of the diaphragm in the cranial direction increases the respiratory minute volume by 40 %. This causes hyperventilation, with increased oxygen consumption (+ 20 %), with peak values during birth (+ 40 % in the first stage, up to + 100 % during the second stage).

Cardiovascular system
The increase in cardiac frequency and the resulting rise in cardiac output reach a maximum of up to 40 % by the 34th gestational week.
This increase is achieved with particular involvement of the uteroplacental unit and kidneys. By contrast, arterial blood pressure does not increase.

Gastrointestinal tract
The stomach shifts cranially, resulting in increased intragastric pressure, with a tendency toward reflux, reduced tone, reduced motility and the resultant delay in gastric emptying. The risk of aspiration is increased during intubation for anesthesia.

Blood volume
The volume of blood increases by about 30 %.

Labor pain

Two types of labor pain are distinguished, depending on the stage of labor (Fig. 35.1).

First stage
Pain in the first stage of labor primarily results from dilation of the cervix and lower uterine segment and distension of the body of the uterus (10–12 hours in a primipara, 6–8 hours in a multipara) is characterized by painful uterine contractions.
Visceral dilatation pain is caused by uterine contractions and dilatation of the cervix and lower segment of the uterus.

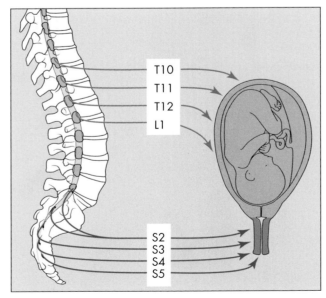

Fig. 35.1 Segmental spread of labor pain

This pain is conducted via unmyelinated C-fibers, which enter the spinal cord through the posterior roots of the spinal nerves – in the early stage at T11–12 and in the later stage at T10 and L1.

The pain radiates into the lower abdomen, groin, inside of the thighs and dorsally into the lumbar region, hip region and sacrum.

Second stage

This pain covers the period between full dilatation of the cervix (10 cm) and birth of the child. This period lasts 30–40 minutes in a primipara and 20–30 minutes in a multipara.

The pain is caused by dilatation of the vagina, vulva and pelvic floor.

Somatic perineal pain in the area innervated by the pudendal nerve is conducted via myelinated A-delta fibers and also includes segments T10 to L1 and L2 to S4–5 (Fig. 35.1).

Specific risks in obstetric anesthesia

Increased risk of aspiration during intubation for anesthesia

Caution
All patients in late pregnancy are regarded as having a full stomach.

Prophylaxis
- 30 ml sodium citrate (0.3 mol/l) about 30 minutes before the start of anesthesia.
- 400 mg cimetidine p. o. (200 mg i. v.) or ranitidine.
- 10 mg metoclopramide i. v.

Aortocaval compression syndrome

At the end of pregnancy, there is pressure from the dilated uterus on the inferior vena cava and lower abdominal aorta when the patient is in the supine position.

Mechanism

A reduction in venous return to the heart, with a decrease in cardiac output and a drop in arterial blood pressure caudal to the compression area. Since the perfusion of the uterine vessels is directly correlated with arterial blood pressure, in untreated cases there may be a risk to the mother or a risk of fetal asphyxia due to reduced circulation in the uteroplacental unit.

Compensatory mechanism

The collateral circulation is stimulated via the azygos vein system and sympathetic tone is increased to stimulate venous return to the heart. If the collateral circulation is not sufficient, or if sympathetic tone is canceled out by epidural anesthesia, a dangerous drop in cardiac output and/or arterial blood pressure may occur, with symptoms of shock.

The critical threshold for a drop in blood pressure is 70–80 mmHg, but values between 90 and 100 mmHg over a period of 10–15 minutes can also threaten the fetus in untreated cases.

Clinical symptoms

Nausea, faintness, pallor, sweating, breathing difficulty.

Prophylaxis
- *Left lateral position* or at a 15° angle to the left (with a wedge-shaped cushion under the right hip (Fig. 35.2), or using the palm of the hand to move the uterus to the left (Fig. 35.3).

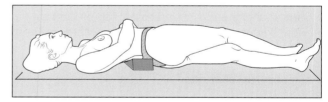

Fig. 35.2 Wedge-shaped cushion under the right hip

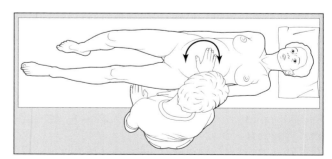

Fig. 35.3 Shifting the uterus to the left

- *Adequate volume supplementation* prior to anesthesia (1000 ml in vaginal delivery, 1500–2000 ml of a balanced electrolyte solution in Caesarean section).
- *Oxygen supply.*
- *Vasopressor administration* – provided the intravascular volume is adequate. The drug of choice is ephedrine 10–20 mg i. v.

Hypotension

A drop in maternal blood pressure is the most frequent complication of epidural anesthesia. In untreated cases, it leads to reduced perfusion of the uteroplacental unit or fetal asphyxia.

Prophylaxis
- Infusion of a balanced electrolyte solution 20 minutes before the start of anesthesia.
- Prevention of the aortocaval compression syndrome.

Treatment
- Increase in fluid supply.
- Slight Trendelenburg position (10°)
- Oxygen supply.
- Vasopressor.

Indications [77]

Maternal
- Labor pain.
- Pulmonary disease (e. g. asthma, upper airway infection).
- Cardiovascular disease.
- Metabolic disease (e. g. diabetes mellitus).
- Neurological diseases (e. g. epilepsy, aneurysms of the cerebral vessels, arteriovenous malformations).
- Preeclampsia.

Fetal
- Premature birth.
- Growth retardation.
- Breech presentation.
- Multiple pregnancy.

Obstetric
- Protracted birth or arrested birth.
- High-risk birth.
- Induction of birth with oxytocin.
- Uncoordinated uterine activity (dystocia).

Anesthesiological
- Anticipated intubation difficulties.
- Obesity.
- Suspicion or history of malignant hyperthermia.

Contraindications

General
(See Chap. 33, p. 232)

Specific
- Placenta previa.
- Prolapse of the umbilical cord.
- Acute fetal asphyxia.

Relative
- Prior Caesarean section (overlooked uterine rupture).
- Premature detachment of the placenta (absence of pain).

Procedure

Caution
- Puncture should only be carried out during a pause in labor (the negative epidural pressure is lost during uterine contractions and there is therefore a risk of dural perforation).
- The oxytocin drip should be interrupted during administration of a local anesthetic. Oxytocin administration can only be resumed 15 minutes after the last major dose of a local anesthetic and when the cardiotocogram is normal.
- An amniotomy should not be carried out within 30 minutes before or after administration of a major dose of local anesthetic.
- Placement of an epidural catheter and administration of a local anesthetic can only be carried out if the cervix has opened 5–6 cm in a primipara or 3–4 cm in a multipara.

Preparation and materials
- Check that the emergency equipment is complete and in working order (intubation kit, emergency drugs).
- Strict asepsis.
- Intravenous access, anesthetic machine.
- Ensure adequate volume supplementation with prior administration of a balanced electrolyte solution (500–1000 ml).

- Precise monitoring: ECG monitoring, BP monitoring, pulse oximetry.
- Monitoring of bladder function (atonic bladder during epidural anesthesia!)
- Continuous fetal monitoring.

The use of a pre-prepared set for epidural anesthesia is recommended.

Patient positioning
The patient is usually placed on the left side; more rarely, a sitting position is adopted – e. g., in obese patients or in those with severe spinal deformities.

Location, skin prep, local anesthesia, skin incision
Location and marking of the puncture site (L2/3 or L3/4) is followed by thorough skin prep, covering with a drape, local anesthesia and skin incision using a hemostylet.

Puncturing the epidural space

Puncture is carried out in the midline using a Tuohy needle (16–18 G) with the angled tip directed cranially. The loss-of-resistance technique is used to identify the epidural space (10-ml LOR syringe, filled with saline and with a small air bubble; advance with constant pressure on the plunger as far as the epidural space).
The catheter is advanced a maximum of 3–4 cm cranially in the epidural space.
After aspiration, the open end of the catheter is placed below the puncture site on the sterile drape and any escaping fluid (CSF or blood) is noted.

Administration of a test dose

3–4 ml 0.5 % ropivacaine, or 0.25 % bupivacaine, or 1 % mepivacaine with epinephrine added.
The addition of epinephrine in obstetrics is controversial, as it can lead to false-positive reactions and reduced uteroplacental perfusion in about 27 % of pregnant patients. In patients who are receiving β-blockers, there may be an increase in blood pressure without an increase in the pulse frequency. As spontaneous pulse and blood pressure increases often occur spontaneously during birth, a false-positive reaction is possible. Many authors therefore recommend only using epinephrine-containing test doses in unclear situations [18, 53, 59]. During the waiting period of five minutes, verbal contact with the patient must always be maintained and the spread of the anesthesia must be monitored.

Incremental administration of local anesthetic

If there is no evidence of intravascular or subarachnoid injection, incremental administration of a local anesthetic is now carried out (5 ml each in several test doses), until the anesthesia has reached the desired level. During this phase, particular attention should be given to the patient's position (not supine).
During the following 20–30 minutes, the spread of the sensory block must be monitored.

Caution
- Repeated aspiration.
- Use a test dose.
- Select the lowest possible dosage.
- Always inject on an incremental basis (with several test doses).
- Maintain verbal contact.
- Conduct precise monitoring.

Local anesthetic and opioids in obstetrics

Local anesthetics

Due to their physicochemical properties, local anesthetics pass the placenta easily. Independent of the site of injection, amide local anesthetics appear very quickly in the maternal and fetal circulation and produce higher plasma levels.
The concentrations in the umbilical blood after the injection of ropivacaine, bupivacaine, or etidocaine are lower (high protein binding of over 90 % in maternal blood) than those of lidocaine and mepivacaine (50–70 % binds to plasma proteins).
The elimination half-lives in the newborn are 3 hours for lidocaine, 9 hours for mepivacaine, 8 hours for bupivacaine and 6.5 hours for etidocaine.

Most important local anesthetic in obstetrics

Ropivacaine
Ropivacaine is structurally similar to bupivacaine and it has a similar profile of activity, but it has a much lower cardiotoxic potential.
According to studies of plasma in neonates and their mothers, it has a stable and high level of maternal protein binding (94 %), so that placental transmission is limited.
In relation to analgesia and motor block, ropivacaine is equivalent to bupivacaine. The onset of effect, duration of effect and anesthetic quality are also comparable to those of bupivacaine [3, 29].

The concentrations used vary from 0.5 % to 0.75 % (Caesarean section) up to 0.2 % (vaginal delivery).
Ropivacaine produces a very good differential sensori-motor block (good analgesic quality with largely preserved motor function – up to 80 % of patients have no measurable motor block on the Bromage scale). At a concentration of 2 mg/ml, ropivacaine is thus the agent of choice for epidural obstetric and postoperative analgesia.

Single-shot injection
Five minutes after administration of the test dose, 10–20 ml 0.2 % ropivacaine (20–40 mg) is injected on an incremental basis. Onset of effect after 10–15 minutes, duration of effect 30–90 minutes.

Intermittent epidural analgesia
10–15 ml 0.2 % ropivacaine (20–30 mg).

Continuous-infusion epidural analgesia (CIEA)
0.2 % ropivacaine, speed 6–10 ml (12–20 mg)/h.

Bupivacaine

Bupivacaine has been used successfully in obstetrics for many years as a long acting amide local anesthetic. The concentrations used vary from 0.5 % (Caesarean section) to 0.25 % (vaginal delivery) up to 0.125–0.0625 %, usually in combination with opioids.
Low-dose bupivacaine (0.125 %) leads to effective analgesia in some 70 % of mothers giving birth. Higher concentrations (0.5 %) are often associated with a motor block that is not desirable in a normal birth.
Higher concentrations (0.75 %) should be avoided in obstetrics. The cardiotoxicity of bupivacaine must be regarded as a considerable disadvantage [77].

Single-shot injection
After a test dose of 3–4 ml 0.25–0.5 % bupivacaine (or 3 ml of a 1 % epinephrine-containing mepivacaine solution), 15 ml 0.5 % or 20 ml 0.375 % bupivacaine (3–5 ml) are injected on an incremental basis.

Intermittent epidural analgesia
After a test dose of 3–4 ml 0.25–0.5 % bupivacaine (or 3 ml of a 1 % epinephrine-containing mepivacaine solution), injection of an initial dose of 5–8 ml 0.25 % (or 0.125 %) bupivacaine (titrated in smaller portions) is given until the level of segment T10 is reached.

Additional injections:
Intermittent administration is continued with additional injections of 0.125 % (8–16 ml) or 0.25 % (5–8 ml) bupivacaine at intervals of 60–90 minutes, or as required.
During the first stage of labor, the local anesthetic dose is injected with one half in the right and left lateral positions, or the full dose with the patient supine (persistent left shift of the uterus).
During the second stage, the patient's trunk should be raised by about 30–60° in order to reach lower segments.

> **Caution**
> Every new bolus of a drug involves the same risks as the initial bolus. It is possible to confuse overdosage with underdosage.

Continuous-infusion epidural analgesia (CIEA)
Five minutes after the administration of the test dose, 5–8 ml 0.25 % bupivacaine is injected in smaller increments.
After 30 minutes, when the course is normal, the continuous infusion can be started: 6 ml 0.25 % or 10–15 ml 0.125 % bupivacaine per hour.
Precise monitoring of the circulation and checking of the anesthetic spread must be carried out.

Lidocaine

Lidocaine is rarely used for epidural anesthesia in obstetrics, as it produces a marked motor block even at relatively low doses. The duration of effect is 60–90 minutes. Due to its rapid onset of effect, lidocaine is very suitable for short-term intensification of epidural anesthesia (10–15 ml of a 1.5–2 % solution; see also p. 248).

2–3 % chloroprocaine

Chloroprocaine is a fast-working local anesthetic that is certainly one of the safest of the ester type and it has proved its value particularly in emergency situations [77]. It is hydrolyzed to inactive metabolites very quickly even at high dosages (short duration of effect of about 30–60 minutes) and has hardly any effect on the neonate's condition. Chloroprocaine is a very good supplement to bupivacaine, particularly if large amounts of bupivacaine have already been used during a Caesarean section.

Single-shot injection
2 % chloroprocaine: 10–15 ml, onset of effect after 4–6 minutes, duration of effect 30–45 minutes.
3 % chloroprocaine: 10 ml, onset of effect after 4–6 minutes, duration of effect 45–60 minutes.
The analgesic effect of an opioid injected subsequently (fentanyl) is reduced by antagonism caused by chloroprocaine at the opiate receptor [21].

Opioids

When opioids alone were used in obstetric anesthesia, adequate analgesia was only achieved in the treatment of visceral pain in the first stage of labor. Somatic pain in the second stage was more difficult to influence [70, 77].
The fast-working lipophilic opioids sufentanil and fentanyl, which have a duration of effect of two to three hours, have replaced the hydrophilic morphine (duration of effect 8–24 hours).
The agents of choice are low-dose sufentanil or fentanyl in combination with low-dose bupivacaine in the form of an epidural infusion.

Advantages
- Faster onset of effect.
- Longer duration of analgesia.
- Lower total dose of local anesthetic and opioid (about 20–25 %).
- Reduced motor block.
- No significant side effects on the mother or child.

Continuous-infusion epidural analgesia (CIEA) [33, 70]

Sufentanil and bupivacaine
After administering a test dose and bolus administration of 10 ml 0.125–0.0625 % bupivacaine and 1–2 µg/ml sufentanil (10–20 µg), a continuous infusion can be started after about 30 minutes:
0.0625–0.03125 % bupivacaine and 0.2–0.3 µg/ml sufentanil. Speed: 6–10 ml/h.

Fentanyl and bupivacaine
After administering a test dose and bolus administration of 10 ml 0.25 % bupivacaine and 50 µg fentanyl, a continuous infusion can be started after about 30 minutes:
0.0625 % bupivacaine and 1–2 µg/ml fentanyl. Speed: 10 ml/h.

Patient-controlled epidural analgesia (PCEA) (on-demand analgesia) [33, 70]

Sufentanil and bupivacaine
After administering a test dose and bolus administration of 5–10 ml 0.125 % bupivacaine and 10–30 µg/ml sufentanil, a continuous infusion can be started:
0.0625 % bupivacaine and 1 µg/ml sufentanil.
Basic setting: Speed 5 ml/h (5 µg sufentanil)
                    Bolus dose 5 ml (5 µg sufentanil)
                    Injection lock 20 min

Fentanyl and bupivacaine
After administering a test dose and bolus administration of 6–10 ml 0.125–0.25 % bupivacaine and 10 µg fentanyl, incremental until segment T10 is reached, a continuous infusion can be started:
0.125 % bupivacaine and 0.0001 % fentanyl [77].
Basic setting: Speed 4 ml/h
                    Bolus dose 4 ml
                    Injection lock 20 min

Epinephrine addition in obstetrics
Epinephrine has both alpha-mimetic and beta-mimetic effects. Adding epinephrine causes a dose-dependent reduction in uterine activity and leads to a delay in birth. If there is inadvertent intravascular injection of a local anesthetic with epinephrine, adverse circulatory reactions can occur both in the mother (hypertonia, cardiac rhythm disturbances) and in the child (reduced placental perfusion due to vasoconstriction).
Any addition of epinephrine in obstetrics must therefore be strictly indicated.

Lumbar catheter epidural anesthesia in Caesarean section

When a Caesarean section is being carried out, the spread of the injected local anesthetic must reach segments T4 to T6. The higher the spread of the anesthesia, the greater the risk of severe hypotension.
Segments L5, S1 and S2 are not always adequately anesthetized and there is often a delay in anesthesia in this area.

Procedure

Preparation, materials, prerequisites
(See Chap. 33, pp. 233, 243)

Patient positioning
Left lateral decubitus for L2/3 or L3/4, or sitting (e. g. in obese patients or those with spinal deformities).

Puncture of the epidural space, test dose, incremental administration of local anesthetic

After identification of the epidural space and aspiration, a catheter is placed (see Chap. 33, section on continuous catheter epidural anesthesia, p. 243) and a test dose is administered.

After about five minutes incremental injection of a local anesthetic can be carried out in small increments of up to 5 ml each (several test doses), until adequate anesthesia reaches the desired segmental level of T4 to T6. If the catheter is already in position, there is the following choice: if there has been no injection within the previous 30 minutes, then after testing of the spread of the anesthesia about 12–15 ml 0.75 % ropivacaine or 0.5 % bupivacaine can be injected on an incremental basis. Alternatively, if an injection has been given shortly before, then initially only 5–10 ml 0.75 % ropivacaine or 0.5 % bupivacaine is injected.

In a protracted birth with a large total dose of local anesthetic and subsequent Caesarean section or marked fetal acidosis, 2–3 % chloroprocaine should be used, due to its fast onset of effect and short half-life in both mother and child.

Additional safety measures

▨ Supine positioning, with left lateral shift of the uterus until emergence of the child (slight Trendelenburg 10° if appropriate).
▨ Oxygen administration.
▨ Precise circulatory monitoring.
▨ Thorough checking of the spread of anesthesia shortly before the start of surgery.

Local anesthetics for Caesarean section

About 15–30 ml of local anesthetic is necessary for adequate anesthesia up to T4–6 (Table 35.1).

Adjuvant opioids

The addition of sufentanil or fentanyl to bupivacaine or lidocaine improves sensory analgesia substantially. The following dosages can be used:
▨ Sufentanil: 30–50 µg.
▨ Fentanyl: 50–100 µg.

Tab. 35.1 Local anesthetics for Caesarean section

Local anesthetic	Volume (ml)	Onset of effect (min)	Duration of effect (min)
0.75 % ropivacaine	15–20	10–20	180–300
0.5 % ropivacaine	25–30	10–15	120–150
0.5 % bupivacaine	15–30	15–20	120–180
1.5–2 % lidocaine	15–25	10–15	45–60
(with addition 1 : 400 000; 0,05 ml in 20 ml local anesthetic)			
2–3 % 2-chloroprocaine	15–25	ca. 10	45–60

Record and checklist

Obstetric catheter epidural anesthesia

Name: _____ Date: _____

Diagnosis: _____

Premedication: ☐ No ☐ Yes

Neurological abnormalities: ☐ No ☐ Yes _____

Purpose of block: ☐ *Vaginal delivery* ☐ *Caesarean section*

Needle: ☐ ____ *G Tuohy* ☐ *Other* ____

i. v. access and infusion: ☐ *Yes*

Monitoring: ☐ *ECG* ☐ *Pulse oximetry*

Ventilation facilities: ☐ *Yes (equipment checked)*

Emergency equipment *(drugs):* ☐ *Checked*

Patient: ☐ *Informed* ☐ *Consent*

Prerequisites met: ☐ *Adequate volume*

☐ *Fetal monitoring* ☐ *No oxytocin drip* ☐ *No amniotomy*

☐ *Monitoring of bladder function* ☐ *Cervix 5–6 cm (primipara)*

☐ *Cervix 3–4 cm (multipara)*

Position: ☐ *Left lateral* ☐ *Sitting*

Approach: ☐ *Median* ☐ *Paramedian*

Puncture level: ☐ *L3/4* ☐ *Other* _____

Puncture technique: ☐ *Loss of resistance* ☐ *Other* _____

Epidural space: ☐ *Identified*

Catheter: ☐ *Advanced 3–4 cm cranially*

Aspiration test: ☐ *Carried out*

Catheter end: ☐ *Positioned lower than the puncture site*

Bacterial filter: ☐

Test dose: _____ Epinephrine added: ☐ *Yes* ☐ *No*

Checking of motor and sensory function after 5 min: ☐ *Carried out*

Abnormalities: ☐ *No* ☐ *Yes* _____

Injection:

☐ Local anesthetic: _____ ml ____ %
   (incremental)

☐ Addition: _____ *µg/mg*

☐ Additional injection (incremental): _____ ml ____ %

Patient's remarks during injection:

☐ *None* ☐ *Pain* ☐ *Paresthesias* ☐ *Warmth*

Duration and area: _____

Objective anesthetic effect after 20 min:

☐ *Cold test* ☐ *Temperature measurement before* _____ °C *after* _____ °C

☐ *Sensory: L* _____ *T* _____ ☐ *Motor*

Complications:

☐ *None* ☐ *Radicular symptoms* ☐ *BP drop* ☐ *Vascular puncture* ☐ *Massive epidural anesthesia* ☐ *Subdural spread* ☐ *Drop in body temperature* ☐ *Bladder emptying disturbances* ☐ *Back pain* ☐ *Aortocaval compression syndrome* ☐ *Pain* ☐ *Vasovagal reactions* ☐ *Dural puncture* ☐ *Intravascular injection* ☐ *Total spinal anesthesia* ☐ *Respiratory disturbance* ☐ *Muscle tremor* ☐ *Postdural puncture headache* ☐ *Neurological complications*

Special notes:

_____

_____

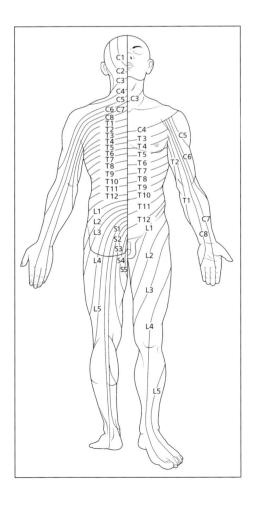

36 Lumbar epidural anesthesia in pediatric patients

Advantages and disadvantages

Advantages

- Better anatomic relationships and thus easier orientation and less time required for puncture.
- Better distribution of the injected local anesthetic than in adults.
- Highly effective anesthesia and analgesia with smaller amounts of local anesthetic.
- Easier advancing of the epidural catheter than in the adult.
- Due to immaturity of the sympathetic nervous system, circulatory problems are very rare, particularly in children younger than eight.
- Very fast recovery phase due to shallow basic general anesthesia and sparing of muscle relaxants.
- Quiet postoperative phase and sparing of opioids and thus fewer side effects such as nausea, vomiting or urinary retention.
- The need for subsequent postoperative intensive care is reduced.

Disadvantages

- Light general anesthesia is recommended, so that precise testing of the spread of anesthesia is not possible.

Distinctive features of pediatric anatomy
[35, 47]

The following anatomic characteristics must be noted before carrying out epidural puncture in children (Fig. 36.1):

- In the neonate, the spinal cord ends in the area of the L3 segment; at the end of the first year of life, it reaches the L1 segment.
- In the one-year-old child, the dural sac ends in the area of S2 and in the neonate it can even reach as far as the sacral foramina of S3 or S4.
- In infants, the iliac crest line crosses the midline in the area of L5 and at about L5/S1 in neonates.

- Lumbar lordosis has not yet developed in neonates and infants.
- The distance from the skin to the epidural space correlates with the child's age. According to Busoni, measured in millimeters in the L2/L3 segment it is equivalent to 10 mm + (age in years × 2) mm [35].

Characteristics of the pediatric epidural space
(See Chap. 40, p. 302)

Indications

Single-shot technique

- All surgical procedures in the region of dermatomes T5–S5 involving operating times of up to 90 minutes – e. g., perineal and perianal procedures orchidopexy (including undescended testis), hypospadias, inguinal hernia, repositioning of incarcerated hernia, umbilical hernia, superficial surgical procedures in the lower extremities, etc.

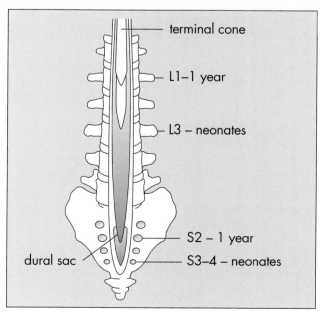

Fig. 36.1 Anatomic features

Continuous technique
- In combination with basic general anesthesia in more prolonged operations in the upper and lower abdomen, as well as urogenital and orthopedic procedures (dermatomes T5–S5) [27].

Advantages
- Shorter recovery time due to sparing of intraoperative drugs.
- Postoperative pain therapy.

Disadvantage
- The dosage is not as reliable as with caudal application.

Contraindications

(See Chap. 33, p. 232)

Procedure

Preparation and materials
These are the same as for epidural anesthesia in adults. Mild basic general anesthesia or more rarely sedation combined with local application of Emla cream is used for both the single-shot technique and for continuous epidural anesthesia.
- Strict asepsis:
  thorough, repeated and wide skin prep, drying and covering of the puncture site with a drape.
- Local anesthesia or application of Emla cream.
- Preparation of the drugs:
  - Syringe with 1 ml epinephrine-containing local anesthetic (test dose).
  - Syringe with the calculated amount of local anesthetic.
- In the *continuous* technique, the length of the puncture needle should be compared with the marking points on the catheter, for better identification of the depth of the catheter after it has been introduced. The ability of the catheter to pass through the puncture needle is tested at the same time.
- Skin incision with a hemostylet or large-lumen needle.

A **precordial stethoscope** is also required.
The use of a ready-supplied set is recommended.

Epidural puncture technique in pediatric patients:

Single-shot technique
- Up to four years of age: Tuohy needle with a metal stylet and 0.5 cm calibration marks, 22 G (0.73 × 50 mm) or 20 G (0.9 × 50 mm), e. g. Perican Paed, B. Braun Melsungen.
- Over four years of age: Tuohy needle with a plastic stylet and 0.5 cm calibration marks, 18 G (1.3 × 50 mm), e. g. Perican Paed, B. Braun Melsungen.

Continuous technique
- Up to four years of age: Tuohy needle with a metal stylet and 0.5 cm calibration marks, 20 G (0.9 × 50 mm), epidural catheter (0.6 mm–75 cm long) with central opening.
- Over four years of age: Tuohy needle with a plastic stylet and 0.5 cm calibration marks, 18 G (1.3 × 50 mm), epidural catheter (0.85 mm–100 cm long) with central opening (e. g. Perifix Paed, B. Braun Melsungen).

Single-shot technique

Patient positioning
Lateral decubitus, with legs bent.

Puncturing the epidural space

> Caution
> Epidural puncture must only be carried out after a preliminary incision with a large-diameter needle or hemostylet and a puncture needle with a stylet must always be used.

The puncture is carried out in the midline, usually between the spinous processes of L2/3 or L3/4 (Fig. 36.2). A Tuohy needle, with its bevel directed cranially, is advanced through the skin incision at an angle of 90° in neonates or 70° in infants, until it is lying firmly in the interspinous ligament (Fig. 36.3).
- Removal of the stylet and attachment of a smoothly moving syringe with saline (injection of a maximum of 0.5 ml in the neonate or 3 ml in older children).

> Caution
> Advancing the catheter further after leaving the interspinous ligament must be carried out gradually and gently, in the direction of the ligamentum flavum.

- Identification of the epidural space is carried out using the loss-of-resistance technique.
- Any fluid escaping from the end of the needle (CSF, blood) should be noted.
- Aspiration test.
- Test dose of 1 ml of an epinephrine-containing local anesthetic.
  During the subsequent waiting period: precise cardiovascular monitoring (plus precardial stethoscope) in order to recognize the development of tachycardia or arrhythmia. However, this test may lead to unreliable results in fully anesthetized children [28].
- Incremental injection of local anesthetic: after a negative result with the test dose, the calculated quantity of local anesthetic is administered on an incremental basis.

Checking the spread of anesthesia

In children who are not receiving light general anesthesia, the spread of the anesthesia should always be checked.

> **Caution**
> Since correct checking of the spread of anesthesia is not possible in fully anesthetized children, this method should only be used by highly experienced pediatric anesthetists.

A detailed examination of sensory and motor function is conducted postoperatively in recovery. The child should only be moved to the ward when he or she can move the legs freely.

Continuous lumbar epidural anesthesia

Comparison with continuous caudal anesthesia
Advantage:
Since the risk of contamination of the lumbar epidural catheter is lower (4 %) than that with a caudally placed catheter (22 %) [47], a lumbar epidural catheter is preferable when there is a need for postoperative pain therapy.
Disadvantage:
The dosage scheme is less reliable than with the caudal application.

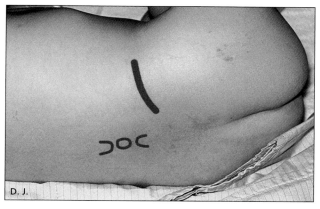

Fig. 36.2 The spinous processes of L3/4 or L2/3 are marked

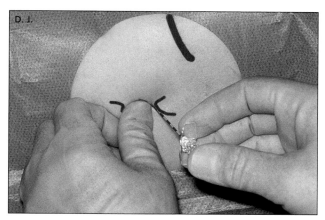

Fig. 36.3 Introduction of the Tuohy needle and identification of the epidural space

Puncture technique

A median puncture in the region of the L5/S1 segment has proved particularly favorable for placing a catheter in the lumbar area (modified Taylor access) [47].
Identification of the epidural space is carried out as described above. After the epidural space has been reached and loss of resistance has been confirmed at two levels, an aspiration test is carried out. Before the introduction of a catheter, it must be checked that the needle bevel is directed cranially.
The thumb and index finger of the left hand, the side of which rests on the patient's back, secure the epidural needle. Using the thumb and index finger of the right hand, the catheter is advanced cranially by a maximum of 2–3 cm (Fig. 36.4). A catheter must never be advanced against resistance – since this may be created by dura, a nerve or a blood vessel.

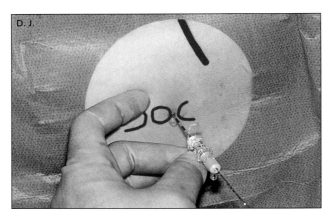

Fig. 36.4 Advancing the catheter

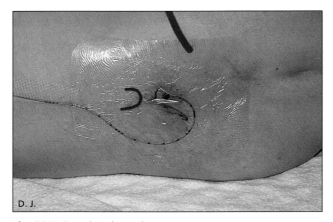

Fig. 36.5 Securing the catheter

> **Caution**
>
> If technical difficulties occur, the catheter and puncture needle are always removed simultaneously. A catheter must never be withdrawn through a positioned puncture needle.

After the catheter has been placed in the desired position, the puncture needle is very carefully withdrawn, with the thumb and index finger of the left hand simultaneously securing the catheter at the injection site. An adapter is attached to the end of the catheter. The patency of the catheter is tested by injecting 1 ml of saline.

After *aspiration*, the syringe is disconnected and the open end of the catheter is placed on a sterile drape below the level of the puncture site.

Any escaping fluid (CSF, blood) should be noted.

A bacterial filter is then placed and the catheter is secured (Fig. 36.5). An epinephrine-containing *test dose* is administered, followed by incremental injection of local anesthetic.

After a risk–benefit assessment, a catheter for postoperative pain therapy is usually left in place for 48–72 hours. After this period, the risk of infection and migration of the catheter increases.

Local anesthetic and dosage

Age-dependent dosages as proposed by Bromage [9] for lumbar epidural administration in adults also apply to pediatric patients. For testing, 2% lidocaine is used (see Chap. 33, p. 247). This schema is not suitable for children under the age of four.

Busoni used 2 % mepivacaine for testing and after statistical evaluation developed valuable diagrams that became very popular with anesthetists. However, in comparison with caudal epidural administration (where the local anesthetic only spreads cranially) (Fig. 36.6 A), these diagrams are less reliable for lumbar epidural administration (with both cranial and caudal spread) (Fig. 36.6 B) [35].

Another formula recommends 0.25 % bupivacaine: 0.75 ml/kg b. w. (children under eight years of age or under 25 kg) [35]. Yet another [48] is recommended for children under eight years of age: 0.7 ml/kg 1 % mepivacaine, 0.25 % bupivacaine or 0.2 % ropivacaine. In children over eight years of age, higher concentrations are used at a reduced dosage, based on height and weight as in adults.

> **Caution**
>
> The injection site should be as close as possible to the center of the area to be anesthetized.

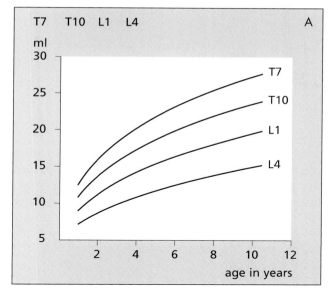 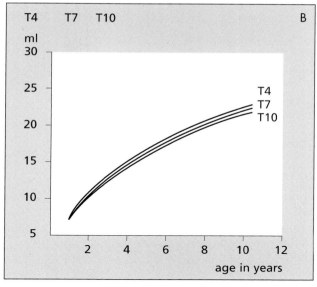

Fig. 36.6 A, B Diagram of the relation between dose, spread and age for various segmental levels in caudal **(A)** and lumbar **(B)** administration [adapted from Busoni, in Saint-Maurice C, Schulte-Steinberg O, Armitage E, eds., *Regional Anesthesia in Children* (Appleton & Lange/Mediglobe, 1990)]

Concentration of local anesthetic

Bupivacaine	0.25–0.5 %
Ropivacaine	0.2 %
Mepivacaine	1–1.5 % (2 %)
Lidocaine	1–1.5 % (2 %)

The concentration of the local anesthetic is based on the location and severity of the procedure. For more extensive abdominal procedures, slightly higher concentrations are required (2 % lidocaine, 0.5 % bupivacaine and 2 % mepivacaine with epinephrine added [35]).

Practical recommendations for postoperative pain therapy [47]

Local anesthetics
Initial dose: 0.25 % bupivacaine 2–2.5 mg/kg b. w.

Continuous epidural infusion with 0.125 % bupivacaine

Neonates and infants:	0.2 mg/kg/h
Small children:	0.3–0.4 mg/kg/h
Older children:	0.4–0.5 mg/kg/h

Opioids

Morphine	33 µg/kg/every 8–12 h
Fentanyl	0.5 µg/kg/h

Clonidine	2 µg/kg/24 h

Complications

(See Chap. 33, section on complications in adults, p. 249)

37 Epidural steroid injection

Introduction

Neuraxial techniques are recognized procedures in diagnostic and therapeutic pain treatment.

The first report in Europe describing the administration of steroids in the epidural space was published in 1952 [73]. Since 1961, authors in the United States and the United Kingdom in particular have regularly described lumbar [34, 36] and thoracic [31] epidural administration of methylprednisolone, and since 1986, cervical epidural steroid injections have increasingly been used in treatment-resistant cervical pain conditions [63, 74, 84].

The indications for epidural and intrathecal administration of methylprednisolone in anesthesia, orthopedics, neurology, neurosurgery, and rheumatology have included lumbosacral arachnoiditis, lumbar spine syndrome, multiple sclerosis, brachialgia, cluster headache, diabetic neuritis, post-herpetic neuralgia and causalgia, and Guillain-Barré syndrome.

The focus in neurology has been on intrathecal administration, and the success rates in arachnoiditis, lumbar spine syndrome, cluster headache, multiple sclerosis, and cervicobrachialgia have been estimated at 65 % (Cleveland Clinic, 1963: assessment of intrathecal hydrocortisone administration in over 1000 patients [79, 80, 81, 82]).

In 1970, a critical study by Goldstein et al. [37] for the first time pointed out the risks of intrathecal administration of methylprednisolone. Experimental studies on the neurotoxic effects of polyethylene glycol, the preservative used in the methylprednisolone preparation Depo-Medrol [55, 83] followed, using animal models. After reports from Australia describing increasing numbers of complications with intrathecal applications, but very rare complications with epidural applications, a reaction set in that led to the withdrawal of approval for Depo-Medrol for intrathecal – and consequently also epidural – applications.

This decision was criticized by numerous experienced specialists throughout the world, since epidural administration of methylprednisolone in carefully selected patients had established itself as an effective component of interdisciplinary pain therapy [1, 2, 6, 17, 19, 43, 88, 89, 98].

Even in large groups of patients – both Abram [1, 2] and Delaney et al. [26] reported more than 6000 applications – epidural administration of methylprednisolone was not associated with neurotoxic or meningeal reactions. In our own experience (more than 3000 epidural injections of Depo-Medrol, two-thirds of which were lumbar and one-third cervical), complications with the procedure were rare and confined to technical problems such as dural puncture.

According to the Australian and British Pain Societies, no evidence has been found that epidural steroid injections are injurious to the patient [39, 94]. "However … the Pain Societies of Great Britain and Australia now feel that a) there is good evidence that epidural steroids are helpful and b) no evidence that epidural steroids are harmful" if injected in the correct dose in the correct space (J.C.D. Wells, personal communication) [94]. When epidural steroid injection is carried out correctly by an experienced anesthetist, it is an important and useful component of the treatment of cervical and lumbar pain and is well tolerated by the patient.

Cervical epidural steroid injection

Anatomy

The narrowest sagittal diameter of the epidural space in the cervical region is 1–1.5 mm, but it may enlarge when the neck is flexed [10, 22, 57, 71]. The cervical spinous processes are not angled, and it is therefore advisable to use a median approach with the patient in a sitting position and with the neck flexed (see also Chap. 33, p. 231).

Indications

- Acute cervical pain, cervical radicular pain (when surgery is not indicated).
- Acute episodes of chronic cervical pain.
- Treatment-resistant cervicobrachial pain, genuine occipital neuralgia [63], post-herpetic neuralgia [63].
- After whiplash trauma [61].
- After cervical intervertebral disk surgery.
- Compressive lesions [74] and spinal stenoses [84].

Contraindications

(See Chap. 33, p. 232)

Relative
▨ Diabetes mellitus
When steroids are administered, regular checking of blood sugar levels must be carried out. The increased risk of infection must be taken into account.
▨ Neurological diseases
In individual cases, a strict risk-benefit assessment must be carried out. Epidural injections for surgical and therapeutic purposes have been safely carried out, and are continuing to be carried out safely, in thousands of patients – e. g., after intervertebral disk surgery with stable neurological deficits.

> **Caution**
> This block must only be carried out by highly experienced and skilled anesthetists with good anesthesiological training.

Procedure

Preparation and materials
▨ Availability and mastery of all anesthesiological facilities.
▨ Strict indication (risk-benefit assessment).
▨ The patient must be informed thoroughly.
▨ Check that the emergency equipment is complete and in working order; sterile precautions, anesthetic machine, intravenous access, BP monitoring, ECG monitoring, pulse oximetry.
▨ Maintain strict sepsis.

The use of a ready-supplied set for epidural anesthesia is recommended (e. g. from B. Braun Melsungen); disinfectant, endotracheal anesthesia set, emergency drugs.

Puncture needles
(See Chap. 33, p. 233, Fig. 33.3)
Tuohy needle:
The needle most widely used throughout the world is the 18-G Tuohy needle (there are also reports in the literature describing 17-G to 20-G Tuohy needles).

Weiss needle:
This needle (18–20 G) with wings and a blunt tip, is preferable with the "hanging drop" technique [75].

Spinal needle:
Spinal needles (3 ½, 20 G) are only used in connection with an epidurogram [94].

Patient positioning
Sitting (this increases the negative epidural pressure, particularly during inspiration), with the neck flexed (this relaxes the cervical muscles, and increases the size of the epidural space), if possible supported by an assistant (Fig. 37.1).
The patient must be informed about the importance of sitting still during the puncture procedure.

Skin prep
In all blocks.

Identifying the epidural space
The epidural space can be identified using either the loss-of-resistance technique (see below), with a subsequent epidurogram if appropriate [94], or using the "hanging drop" technique (see Chap. 33, p. 238, Fig. 33.11 A, B).

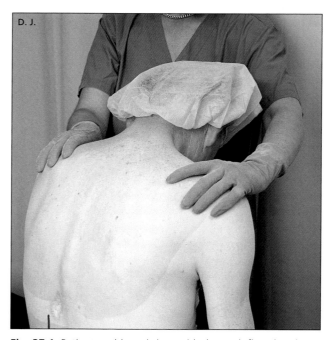

Fig. 37.1 Patient position: sitting, with the neck flexed and supported by an assistant

Injection technique

For puncture in the C7–T1 and T1–T4 regions, median approach is recommended.

Local infiltration

After thorough skin prep (strict asepsis), the puncture area is covered with a sterile drape, and local anesthesia with 1.5 ml 1 % mepivacaine is applied.

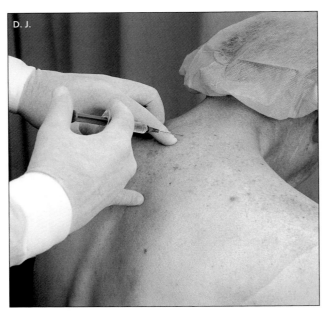

Fig. 37.2 Cutaneous, subcutaneous, and intraligamentous infiltration of the puncture area

Cutaneous, subcutaneous, and intraligamentous infiltration is carried out up to a depth of 2 cm (Fig. 37.2).

Reaching the ligamentum flavum

After palpation of the vertebra prominens (nuchal tubercle), the skin between the two spinous processes selected (C7–T1) is incised with a blade, to make it easier to introduce the Tuohy needle (Fig. 37.3).

The 18-G Tuohy needle, with its bevel directed cranially, is introduced in the midline. Depending on the flexion of the neck, the angle can be about 30° (Fig. 37.4). After about 1.5 cm, it reaches the interspinous ligament. A loss or resistance syringe filled with 10 ml isotonic saline, and with a small air bubble, is now attached to the needle.

Loss-of-resistance technique

(See Chap. 33, Fig. 33.10 A, B)

The needle is now advanced very slowly, millimeter by millimeter, with simultaneous pressure on the syringe plunger, using the right hand. The left hand is used to apply braking pressure.

As CSF pressure in the cervical region is very low and the elasticity of the ligamentum flavum is reduced in this area, aspiration must be carried out very frequently. When the epidural space is entered, the contents of the syringe can be easily injected. During the injection, brief paresthesias in the shoulder and arm region and as far as the fingertips are signs that the needle is positioned correctly.

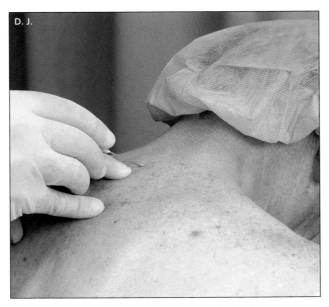

Fig. 37.3 Median approach: the skin is incised using a hemostylet

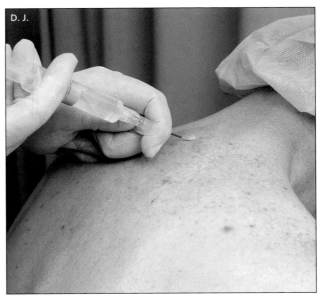

Fig. 37.4 Entering the epidural space using the loss-of-resistance technique. The 18-G Tuohy needle is advanced slowly. The angle is ca. 30°

Steroid injection into the epidural space
After this, slow injection of the solution of steroid, saline, and local anesthetic can be carried out without a prior test dose [75, 94], as the concentration of local anesthetic in the mixture is very low.
A false loss of resistance often occurs in the cervical region, with the epidural space not being reached. During the subsequent saline injection, the patient experiences severe local pain.

Effects of the block and onset
The analgesic and anti-inflammatory effects [49, 97] and resultant relaxation of the tensed neck muscles set in after one to six days.

Dosage
Local infiltration of the puncture site
1.5 ml local anesthetic, e. g. 1 % mepivacaine.

Identification of the epidural space
10 ml isotonic saline.

Injection solution
10 ml total volume: 1.5 ml (60 mg) soluble Volon A (triamcinolone acetonide), mixed with 2 ml 1 % mepivacaine and about 6.5 ml isotonic saline.
The mixture with saline and local anesthetic dilutes the steroid's preservative to an acceptable level [9]. The total volume guarantees adequate spread of the steroid. These are the reasons why the author prefers this particular injection mixture.

> **Caution**
> Immediately after the injection, transient fatigue (for about 20 minutes) and brief paresthesias in the shoulder, arm, and hand region are characteristic signs of a successful block.
> After the steroid injection, the patient remains lying down for about one hour (ECG, pulse oximetry, BP monitoring).
> After a further hour, the patient, who is not capable of driving, can be released if escorted. During the following 24–48 hours, pain may occur at the injection site.
> The risk of an epidural hematoma or abscess developing is extremely low, but it cannot be excluded. The patient must therefore be aware of the need to contact the hospital at the first sign of any complication.

Alternatives
4 ml total volume [75]: 2 ml (50 mg) intralesional Aristocort (triamcinolone diacetate) mixed with 2 ml 1 % lidocaine.
4 ml total volume [94]: 2 ml (80 mg) Kenalog (triamcinolone acetonide), mixed with 2 ml 0.25 % bupivacaine.

Block series
Patients who are completely free of pain after the first block, and those in whom the first block is not successful, do not receive a second injection [45].
A second or possible even a third block can only be carried out if there is evidence of improvement in the symptoms [7]. Steroid dosage should be reduced.
There is no justification for more than three injections at intervals of one to two weeks. If the symptoms deteriorate again, periodic single injections are possible after a careful risk-benefit assessment. It is best to wait at least three months prior to repeating steroids.

Complications
Dural puncture with postdural puncture headache
(See Chap. 29, p. 214)

Spinal cord injury
Neurological injuries may occur in all forms of neuraxial regional anesthesia. Spinal cord injury with paraplegia is caused by incorrect technique, but is extremely rare.
Prophylaxis requires extremely careful advancement of the needle, as well as frequent aspiration. It should be noted that CSF pressure is very low in the cervical region.

Bacterial meningitis
Strict asepsis is always necessary when carrying out this block. In septic diseases and infections in the area of the injection site, the block is contraindicated.

Epidural abscess
No connection has yet been identified between epidural steroid administration and the development of epidural abscesses. Numerous studies [1, 2, 11, 19, 38, 72, 87] report instead that there is evidence of a connection between prior septic disease and the development of abscesses after epidural anesthesia (see Chap. 33, p. 251).

Epidural hematoma
If the patient reports any symptoms of pain or fever, or radicular symptoms, these must be investigated without fail.

Constant contact with the patient is absolutely necessary, particularly after outpatient procedures. Immediate diagnostic investigation (myelography, CT, MRI) and immediate neurosurgical treatment within the first 12 hours are essential to reduce morbidity and mortality (see Chap. 33, p. 252).

During the preliminary examination to exclude contraindications, it should be clarified whether the patient is receiving any medication that might affect platelet function. Monotherapy with a platelet aggregation inhibitor does not lead to an increased risk of hemorrhage. By contrast, a combination of various drugs and treatment procedures must be taken into account. In connection with anatomic changes or technical difficulties, simultaneous administration of the following preparations can lead to incalculable risks:

Acetylsalicylic acid (ASA, aspirin) or mixed preparations containing ASA, nonsteroidal anti-inflammatory drugs, high-dose antibiotics, propranolol, furosemide, quinidine, heparin, heparinoids, thrombolytics, tricyclic antidepressants, phenothiazine, antilipemic drugs, chemotherapy drugs, dextrans, etc.

An epidural block with steroids should not take place within five days of the last intake of acetylsalicylic acid (ASA) and ASA-containing preparations. The last intake of nonsteroidal anti-inflammatory agents should be at least 24 hours previously. There is a lack of controlled studies here, and the topic is a controversial one.

Cushing's syndrome

In extremely rare cases, Cushing's syndrome may manifest as a result of an epidural block with steroids [30]. There is evidence of a reduced plasma cortisol level up to two weeks after the injection, even though the usual dosage of 40–80 mg per block is well below the maximum recommended corticosteroid dosage of 3 mg/kg b. w. per injection [91].

Cervical epidural steroid injection
Block no.

Record and checklist

Name: _____ Date: _____

Diagnosis: _____

Premedication: ☐ No ☐ Yes

Neurological abnormalities: ☐ No ☐ Yes _____

Purpose of block: ☐ *Diagnosis* ☐ *Pain treatment*

Needle: ☐ ___ *G Tuohy* ☐ *Other* ___

i. v. access and infusion: ☐

Monitoring: ☐ *ECG* ☐ *Pulse oximetry*

Ventilation facilities: ☐ *Yes (equipment checked)*

Emergency equipment *(drugs)*: ☐ *Checked*

Patient: ☐ *Informed* ☐ *Consent*

Position: ☐ *Sitting* ☐ *Lateral decubitus*

Approach: ☐ *Median* ☐ *Paramedian*

Puncture level: ☐ *C7 / Th 1*

Puncture technique: ☐ *Loss of resistance* ☐ *Other* _____

Test dose: ☐ *No* ☐ *Yes* _____ *ml* _____ *%*

Injection mixture: Steroid: _____ *mg*

NaCl 0,9%: _____ *ml*

Local anesthetic: _____ *ml* ____ *%*

Patient's remarks during injection:

☐ *None* ☐ *Pain* ☐ *Paresthesias* ☐ *Warmth*

Duration and area: _____

Objective anesthetic effect after 15 min:

☐ *Cold test* ☐ *Temperature measurement before* _____ *°C after* _____ *°C*

☐ *Sensory* ☐ *Motor*

Monitoring of block: ☐ *< 2 h* ☐ *> 2 h*

    Time of discharge: _____

    Abnormalities: _____

Complications:

☐ *None* ☐ *Vasovagal reactions* ☐ *Severe pain* ☐ *Fever*
☐ *Dural puncture* ☐ *Radicular symptoms* ☐ *Neurological complications*

Subjective effects of block: Duration: _____

☐ *None* ☐ *Increased pain*
☐ *Reduced pain* ☐ *No pain*

VISUAL ANALOG SCALE

|ııııııııı|ııııııııı|ııııııııı|ııııııııı|ııııııııı|ııııııııı|ııııııııı|ııııııııı|ııııııııı|ııııııııı|
0 10 20 30 40 50 60 70 80 90 100

Special notes:

_____

_____

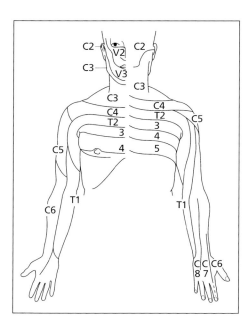

Lumbar epidural steroid injection

This method is not effective in:
Deforming spondylopathy, spondylochondrosis, deforming spondyloarthropathy, spondylolisthesis, spondylarthritis, scoliosis, functional back pain, chronic symptoms.

Indications

- Patients with a short history of pain.
- Unsuccessful discoidectomy (postlaminectomy syndrome).
- Irritative and compressive radiculopathies.
- Intervertebral disk prolapse (not requiring surgery).
- Spinal canal stenosis.
- Post-herpetic neuralgia in the lumbar area (best results within three months after the start of the disease).

Specific and relative contraindications

(See Chap. 33, p. 232, and section on cervical epidural steroid injection, p. 273)

> **Caution**
> This block must only be carried out by highly experienced and skilled anesthetists with good anesthesiological training.

Procedure

Preparation and materials
- Strict indication (risk-benefit assessment).
- The patient must be fully informed.
- Check that the emergency equipment is complete and in working order;
- Observe strict sepsis.
- Anesthetic machine, intravenous access, BP monitoring, ECG monitoring, pulse oximetry.

The use of a ready-supplied set for epidural anesthesia is recommended – e. g., from B. Braun Melsungen.

Puncture needles
- Tuohy needle, 17 G or 18 G (see Chap. 33, p. 233, Fig. 33.3.).
- Spinal needles (3 $^1/_2$, 20 G) are only used in connection with an epidurogram [94].

Patient positioning
Lateral decubitus with the patient lying on the painful side, or sitting (risk of collapse).

Skin prep, local anesthesia, skin incision, and identification of the epidural space
(See Chap. 33, p. 233)

After an intervertebral disk operation, the puncture is carried out about 1 cm above the scar. It can be carried out in the midline or paramedian.

Steroid injection into the epidural space
Injection of the steroid, mixed with a local anesthetic, must be carried out slowly.
After the injection, the patient remains in the lateral decubitus position for about 20 minutes.

Effects of the block and onset of effect
(See also the section on cervical epidural steroid injection, p. 275)

Immediately after the block, transient fatigue (for about 20 minutes), brief paresthesias, and a sensation of warmth in both legs are characteristic signs of a successful block. After an injection of steroid combined with local anesthetic, the patient remains recumbent for about one to two hours (20 minutes of this lying on the side), until the effect of the local anesthetic has declined.
Monitoring is obligatory during this period.
After a further hour, the patient, who should not drive, can be released if escorted. It should be checked and recorded beforehand that the effect of the local anesthetic is no longer present.
During the following 24–48 hours, pain may occur at the injection site. The risk of an epidural hematoma or abscess developing is extremely low, but it cannot be excluded. The patient must therefore be aware of the need to contact the hospital at the first sign of any complication.

Dosage

Injection solution

Test dose: 2 ml 1 % lidocaine.

Total volume 10 ml: 2 ml (50 mg) intralesional Aristocort (triamcinolone diacetate), mixed with 2 ml 0.9 % NaCl and 6 ml 1 % lidocaine [75].

Or:

Test dose: 2 ml 1 % lidocaine.

Total volume 10 ml: 2 ml (80 mg) soluble Volon A (triamcinolone acetonide), mixed with 8 ml local anesthetic consisting of equal halves of 1 % lidocaine and 0.25 % bupivacaine [94].

Block series

(See the section on cervical epidural steroid injection, p. 275)

Complications

(See Chap. 33, p. 275, and the section on cervical epidural steroid injection, p. 275)

Record and checklist

Lumbar epidural steroid injection

Block no.

Name: _____ Date: _____

Diagnosis: _____

Premedication: ☐ No ☐ Yes

Neurological abnormalities: ☐ No ☐ Yes _____

Purpose of block: ☐ Diagnosis ☐ Pain treatment

Needle: ☐ ____ G Tuohy ☐ Other ____

i. v. access and infusion: ☐

Monitoring: ☐ ECG ☐ Pulse oximetry

Ventilation facilities: ☐ Yes (equipment checked)

Emergency equipment (drugs): ☐ Checked

Patient: ☐ Informed ☐ Consent

Position: ☐ Sitting ☐ Lateral decubitus

Approach: ☐ Median ☐ Paramedian

Puncture level: ☐ L3/4 ☐ Other _____

Puncture technique: ☐ Loss of resistance ☐ Other _____

Test dose: ☐ Yes _____ ml _____ %

Injection mixture: Steroid: _____ mg

NaCl 0,9%: _____ ml

Local anesthetic: _____ ml _____ %

Patient's remarks during injection:

☐ None ☐ Pain ☐ Paresthesias ☐ Warmth

Duration and area: _____

Objective anesthetic effect after 15 min:

☐ Cold test ☐ Temperature measurement before _____°C after _____°C

☐ Sensory ☐ Motor

Monitoring of block: ☐ < 2 h ☐ > 2 h

Time of discharge: _____

Abnormalities: _____

Complications:

☐ None ☐ Vasovagal reactions ☐ Severe pain ☐ Fever

☐ Dural puncture ☐ Radicular symptoms ☐ Neurological complications

Subjective effects of block: Duration: _____

☐ None ☐ Increased pain

☐ Reduced pain ☐ No pain

VISUAL ANALOG SCALE

0 10 20 30 40 50 60 70 80 90 100

Special notes:

_____

_____

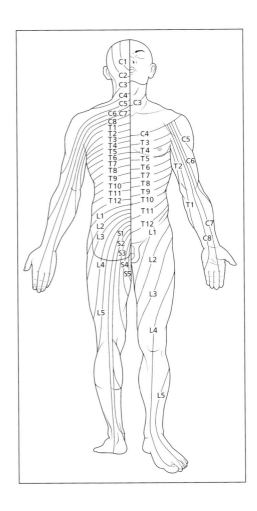

38 Combined spinal and epidural anesthesia (CSE)

Introduction

This combined technique was introduced in neuraxial regional anesthesia in order to exploit as many advantages of both procedures as possible and eliminate their disadvantages.

In CSE, the reliability, fast onset of effect, high success rate, excellent muscle relaxation and low toxicity of spinal anesthesia are combined with the advantages of epidural anesthesia: high flexibility, good controllability, ability to prolong the anesthesia as required and potential transition to postoperative pain treatment.

CSE allows better titration and a substantial reduction in the dose of local anesthetic, opioid, or combination of the two.

The advantages of this technique can be used particularly effectively in obstetrics, with results showing a substantial reduction in maternal hypotension during birth.

History

In 1937, the New York surgeon Soresi [85] reported that it was possible to inject procaine first epidurally and then subarachnoidally through the same needle.

In 1979, Curelaru [25] described the use of CSE in abdominal surgery, urology and orthopedics. After placement of an epidural catheter, a subarachnoid injection was carried out one or two segments below the puncture site.

In 1981, Brownridge [13] reported the use of CSE for Caesarean section. He used two different segments for puncture.

A modification of this technique with one-segment puncture ("needle through needle") was used in 1982 by Coates [20] and Mumtaz [60] in orthopedic surgery and in 1984 by Carrie [14] in obstetric surgery.

In 1988, Rawal [66] described the sequential (two-stage) CSE technique for Caesarean section.

Indications

Surgical procedures:
- General surgery.
- Outpatient surgery [92].
- Vascular surgery [93].
- Orthopedics [20, 44, 60, 95].
- Gynecology [16].
- Obstetrics [14, 66, 67, 68].
- Urology [25].
- Pediatric surgery [62].
- Postoperative pain therapy.

Contraindications

The contraindications are the same as those for spinal anesthesia (see Chap. 28, p. 200) and epidural anesthesia (see Chap. 33, p. 232).

Procedure

Preparation and materials
- Check that the emergency equipment is complete and in working order (intubation kit, emergency drugs); anesthetic machine.
- Set up the infusion and ensure adequate volume supplementation (500–1000 ml of a balanced electrolyte solution).
- Precise monitoring: ECG monitoring, BP control, pulse oximeter.
- Maintain strict asepsis.

The use of a prepacked set, e. g. Espocan from B. Braun Melsungen, is recommended (Fig. 38.1).

> **Caution**
> This procedure must only be carried out by an experienced anesthetist.

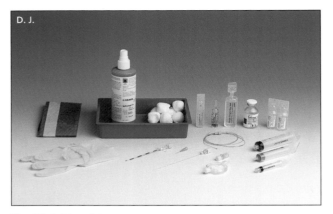

Fig. 38.1 Materials

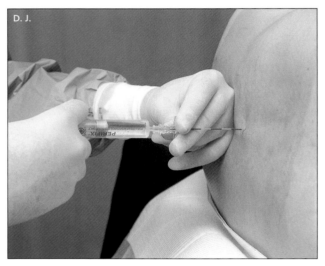

Fig. 38.2 Identifying the epidural space using the loss-of-resistance technique

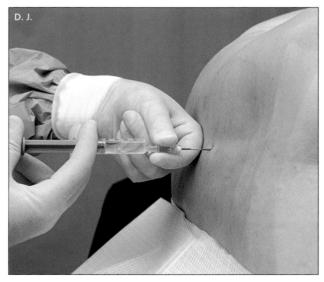

Fig. 38.3 Injecting a test dose

Patient positioning
The puncture is carried out below the L2 segment, with the patient either in the lateral decubitus position (preferable) or sitting.

Injection technique
"Needle through needle"
After locating and marking the puncture site (L2/3 or L3/4), thorough skin prep is carried out, followed by local anesthesia and the incision in skin using a hemostylet.
Puncture is carried out in the midline using an 18-G epidural Tuohy needle, with the tip directed cranially. Identification of the epidural space is carried out using the loss-of-resistance technique (Fig. 38.2).
After identification of the epidural space and injection of a test dose (Fig. 38.3), a thin 27-G pencil-point spinal needle is carefully advanced through the positioned epidural needle in the direction of the subarachnoid space, until dural perforation is confirmed by a dural click (Fig. 38.4 A).
The adapted form of the Tuohy needle tip, which has a central opening positioned in the needle axis ("back eye"), allows the needle to take a direct path, so that the spinal needle does not need to bend. The coating of the spinal needle with plastic expands its outer diameter, so that it fits the epidural needle precisely, maintains its central position as it is advanced and easily passes the axial opening ("back eye") (Fig. 38.4 B).
After careful aspiration of CSF, subarachnoid injection of a local anesthetic, opioid, or a combination of the two is carried out (Fig. 38.5). As this is done, the cone of the spinal needle should be secured with the thumb and index finger of the left hand, which rests on the patient's back. This is the critical phase of the puncture procedure.
The spinal needle is then withdrawn and the epidural catheter is introduced in a cranial direction up to a maximum of 3–4 cm (Fig. 38.6 A, B).
After aspiration, the open end of the catheter is laid on a sterile surface below the puncture site and any escaping fluid (CSF or blood) is noted (Fig. 38.7).
To test the patency of the catheter, 1–2 ml saline is then injected. The catheter is secured and a bacterial filter is attached (Fig. 38.8).

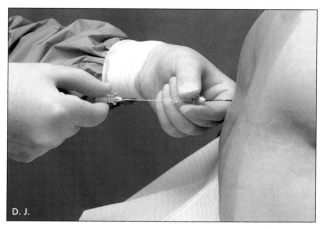

Fig. 38.4 A A 27-G pencil-point spinal needle is introduced through the positioned epidural needle

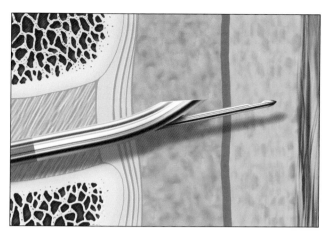

Fig. 38.4 B Identification of the subarachnoid space with the dural click

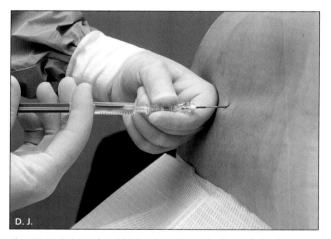

Fig. 38.5 Subarachnoid injection. The spinal needle is then withdrawn

Caution
- Repeated aspiration.
- As low a dose as possible.
- Always use incremental injections (several test doses).
- Maintain verbal contact.
- Check the spread of anesthesia immediately.
- Precise monitoring.

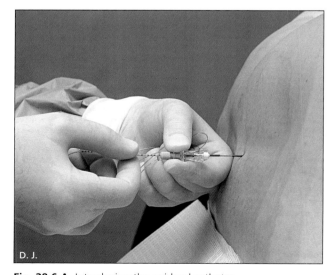

Fig. 38.6 A Introducing the epidural catheter

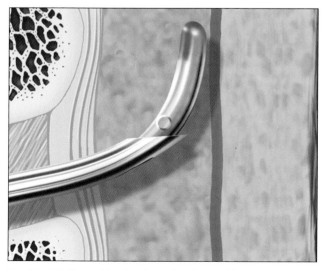

Fig. 38.6 B The epidural catheter is advanced by a maximum of 3–4 cm cranially

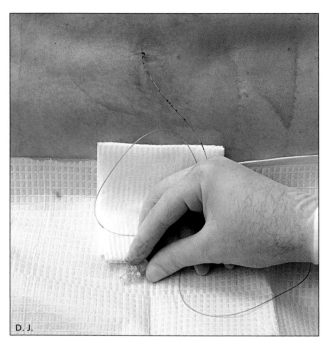

Fig. 38.7 The open end of the catheter is placed below the puncture site

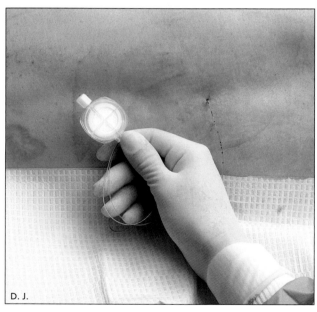

Fig. 38.8 The catheter is secured and a bacterial filter is attached

Problem situations
Specific problems during CSE occur in connection with the administration of a test dose to exclude subarachnoid positioning of the catheter.

As spinal anesthesia is in effect, it is not possible to test for incorrect intrathecal positioning of the catheter and incorrect positioning usually becomes evident through high or total spinal anesthesia. This technique should therefore only be carried out by experienced anesthetists.

Local anesthetics must only be injected in small incremental amounts (test doses), the spread of the anesthesia must be carefully checked and verbal contact with the patient must be maintained.

Two-segment technique
Puncture is carried out in the midline at the level of L2/3 or L3/4. An 18-G Tuohy needle is used. After identification of the epidural space, the epidural catheter is advanced cranially up to a maximum of 3–4 cm. A test dose is then administered. One or two segments lower, conventional spinal anesthesia is then carried out using a 27-G pencil-point needle. The remainder of the procedure is the same as in the "needle-through-needle" technique.

Dosages in the "needle-through-needle" and two-segment techniques [65, 66, 70]
Subarachnoid
- Opioid: 10 µg sufentanil + 1 ml 0.9 % saline.
- Local anesthetic: 0.5 % hyperbaric bupivacaine 1–1.5 ml (5–7.5 mg) ± 0.2 ml.
- Local anesthetic + opioid:
  0.5 % hyperbaric bupivacaine 1–2.5 mg + sufentanil 7.5–10 µg, or:
  0.5 % hyperbaric bupivacaine 1–2.5 mg + fentanyl 25 µg.

Epidural
- Top-up dose
  After the fixation period for the local anesthetic injected subarachnoidally (ca. 15 min):
  0.25–0.5 % bupivacaine, 1.5–2 ml per unblocked segment.

- Epidural infusion
  After bolus administration of 10 ml 0.0625–0.125 % bupivacaine + 10–20 µg sufentanil, or:
  10 ml 0.125–025 % bupivacaine + 50 µg fentanyl
  Continuous infusion of:
  0.031–0.0625 % bupivacaine + 0.2–0.3 µg/ml sufentanil at 6–10 ml/h, or:
  0.0625 % bupivacaine + 1–2 µg/ml fentanyl at 10 l/h.

Sequential (two-stage) CSE in Caesarean section
This technique has proved particularly useful for Caesarean section, reducing the frequency and severity of maternal hypotonia [69].

First stage: procedure in sitting position
- Identification of the epidural space (18-G Tuohy needle).
- Advancing the spinal needle (27-G pencil-point) until dural perforation is achieved (dural click and free CSF flow).
- Intrathecal administration of a local anesthetic and/or opioid. The aim is to reach the segmental level of S5–T9 with as low a concentration as possible (e. g. hyperbaric bupivacaine 1.5 ml ± 0.2 ml).
- Introduction of the epidural catheter.

Second stage: procedure in the supine position
(left lateral decubitus)
- 5–20-minute wait until full spread of the subarachnoid local anesthetic is achieved (fixation period).
- After subarachnoid spread of the local anesthetic, incremental epidural injection in small doses (top-up) is carried out through the epidural catheter. Ca. 1.5–2 ml 0.5 % bupivacaine is administered for each unblocked segment.

Advantages
The slow, incremental administration of the local anesthetic and/or opioid markedly reduces the risk of severe circulatory reactions during Caesarean section. The sympathetic block is less marked (lowest possible subarachnoid dosage and slow onset of epidural anesthesia). The body has time to activate compensatory mechanisms. This procedure is particularly suitable for high-risk patients.

Disadvantage
More time-consuming.
Invasive.

Dosage in Caesarean section [65]
Subarachnoid
- 0.5 % hyperbaric bupivacaine 1.5 ± 0.2 ml. Block target: S5–T8/9.

Epidural
- Top-up dose in left lateral decubitus position after the fixation period (ca. 15 min) of the local anesthetic injected subarachnoidally: 1.5–2 ml 0.5 % bupivacaine per unblocked segment.

Dosage in outpatient obstetrics [65]
Subarachnoid (single injection)
- 0.5 % hyperbaric bupivacaine 1–2.5 mg + 7.5–10 µg sufentanil, or:
  0.5 % hyperbaric bupivacaine 1–2.5 mg + 25 µg fentanyl.

Epidural top-up dose (continuous infusion 10 ml/h)
- Bupivacaine 1 mg + 0.075–1.0 µg/ml sufentanil, or
  Bupivacaine 1 mg + 2 µg fentanyl.

Complications
(See Chap. 29, p. 212 and Chap. 33, p. 249)

Record and checklist

Combined spinal and epidural anesthesia (CSE)

Name: _____ Date: _____

Diagnosis: _____

Premedication: ☐ No ☐ Yes

Neurological abnormalities: ☐ No ☐ Yes _____

Purpose of block: ☐ *Surgical* ☐ *Obstetric* ☐ *Postoperative*

Needle: Spinal: _____ *G Tip* _____

Epidural: *Tuohy* _____ *G* ☐ *Other*

i. v. access and infusion: ☐

Monitoring: ☐ *ECG* ☐ *Pulse oximetry*

Ventilation facilities: ☐ *Yes (equipment checked)*

Emergency equipment *(drugs):* ☐ *Checked*

Patient: ☐ *Informed* ☐ *Consent*

Position: ☐ *Lateral decubitus* ☐ *Sitting*

Approach: ☐ *Median* ☐ *Paramedian*

Puncture level: ☐ *L3/4* ☐ *L4/5* ☐ *Other* _____

Puncture technique: ☐ *"Needle through needle"* ☐ *Two-segment*

Epidural space: ☐ *Identified*

Test dose: _____ Epinephrine added: ☐ *Yes* ☐ *No*

Subarachnoid:

Puncture: ☐ *Carried out*

CSF aspiration: ☐ *Possible* ☐ *Not possible*

Local anesthetic: _____ *ml* _____ *%*

☐ Addition: _____ *µg/mg*

Epidural:

Epidural catheter: ☐ *Advanced 3–4 cm cranially*

Aspiration test: ☐ *Carried out*

Catheter attachment: ☐ *Positioned lower than the puncture site*

Bacterial filter: ☐

Local anesthetic: _____ *ml* _____ *%*

(incremental)

Abnormalities: ☐ *No* ☐ *Yes* _____

Patient's remarks during injection:

☐ *None* ☐ *Pain* ☐ *Paresthesias* ☐ *Warmth*

Duration and area: _____

Objective anesthetic effect after 20 min:

☐ *Cold test* ☐ *Temperature measurement before* _____ *°C after* _____ *°C*

☐ *Sensory: L* _____ *T* _____ ☐ *Motor*

Complications:

☐ *None* ☐ *Radicular symptoms* ☐ *BP drop* ☐ *Vascular puncture* ☐ *Massive epidural anesthesia* ☐ *Subdural spread* ☐ *Drop in body temperature* ☐ *Bladder emptying disturbances* ☐ *Back pain* ☐ *Pain* ☐ *Vasovagal reactions* ☐ *Inadvertent dural puncture* ☐ *Intravascular injection* ☐ *Total spinal anesthesia* ☐ *Respiratory disturbance* ☐ *Muscle tremor* ☐ *Postdural puncture headache* ☐ *Neurological complications*

Special notes:

_____

_____

	1. h			2. h		
	15	30	45	15	30	45
220						
200						
180						
160						
140						
120						
100						
80						
60						
40						
20						

mm Hg

O₂

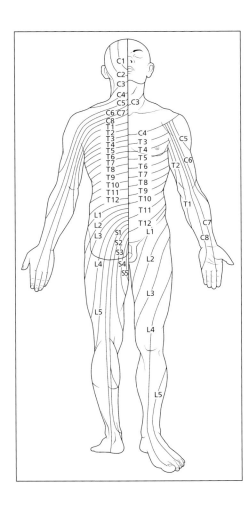

Epidural caudal anesthesia

39 Caudal anesthesia in adult patients

Epidural injection of a local anesthetic or a mixture of a local anesthetic and an opioid or steroid through a puncture needle positioned in the sacral canal or through a catheter.

Anatomy

(See also Chap. 27, section on the sacrum, p. 193)

The **sacral hiatus** is located in line with the median sacral crest. Its lateral boundary is formed by the sacral cornua and it is enclosed by the (superficial dorsal, deep dorsal and lateral) sacrococcygeal ligaments, which pass from the sacrum to the coccyx (Fig. 39.1). The hiatus represents the caudal entrance to the sacral canal.

The **sacral canal** has a diameter of 2–10 mm in an anteroposterior direction and its capacity varies from 12 ml to 65 ml (average 30–34 ml) [18] (Fig. 39.2). It encloses and protects the dura, arachnoid and subarachnoid space, which in most cases end at the level of the second sacral vertebra, as well as the sacral and coccygeal roots of the cauda equina, the sacral epidural venous plexus, lymphatic vessels and epidural fat.

The **dura** normally ends at the level of the second sacral foramen (1–1.5 cm medial and caudal to the dorsal cranial iliac spines), so that this connecting line externally marks the end of the dural sac (Fig. 39.3).

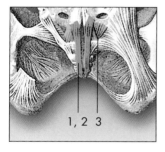

Fig. 39.1 Sacral hiatus, with the sacrococcygeal ligaments. (1) Superficial dorsal sacrococcygeal ligament, (2) deep dorsal sacrococcygeal ligament, (3) lateral sacrococcygeal ligament

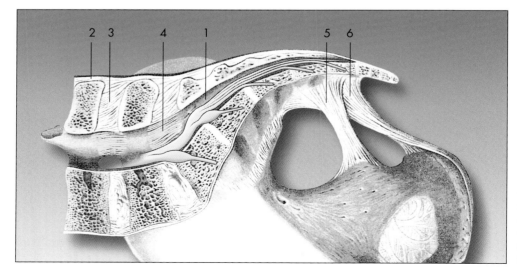

Fig. 39.2 Sacral canal. (1) Sacral canal, (2) supraspinous ligament, (3) interspinous ligament, (4) ligamentum flavum, (5) sacrospinous ligament, (6) sacrotuberal ligament

Anatomic variants are possible (e. g. S2 or S3), so that the distance from the dura to the hiatus can range from 1.6 cm to 7.5 cm (average 4.5 cm). This should be taken into account during puncture [15].

In children under one year of age, the dural sac may come up to the level of the fourth sacral vertebra and particular caution is therefore required during puncture in these cases.

The sacral canal is at its narrowest in the region of the hiatus and the surrounding area is very well vascularized. This block should only be carried out by experienced anesthetists or under their supervision.

Indications

Surgical
- Procedures and painful examinations in the perineal and perianal area (e. g. hemorrhoids or operations in the prostate, bladder or penis).
- Inguinal and femoral hernias.
- Procedures in the area of the coccyx.
- Superficial procedures in the lower extremities (e. g. skin transplants).

Gynecological
- Procedures and painful examinations (vulva, vagina, cervix, clitoris).

Obstetric
- Pain during the second stage of labor.

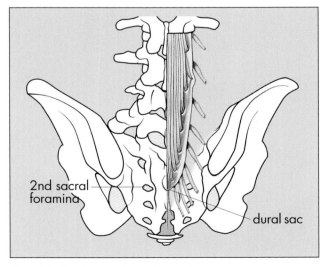

Fig. 39.3 Dural sac and sacral foramina

Diagnostic and therapeutic
- Various painful conditions in the area of the lumbar spine, pelvis, perineum, genitals, rectum and lower extremities.

Acute pain
- Postoperative and post-traumatic pain.
- Lumbar spine syndrome (only after excluding a surgical indication).
- Post-herpetic neuralgia.
- Vascular insufficiency.
- Ergotism.
- Frostbite.
- Hidradenitis suppurativa.

Chronic pain
- Lumbar radiculopathy.
- Spinal canal stenosis.
- Postlaminectomy syndrome.
- Diabetic polyneuropathy.
- Complex regional pain syndrome, types I and II (sympathetic reflex dystrophy and causalgia).
- Postamputation pain.
- Vasospastic diseases.
- Orchialgia.
- Proctalgia.

Tumor pain
- Genital and rectal, in the pelvis, in the perineum.
- Peripheral neuropathy (after radiotherapy or chemotherapy).

Contraindications

Specific
- Patient refusal or patients who are psychologically or psychiatrically unsuited.
- Coagulation disturbances, anticoagulant treatment.
- Sepsis.
- Local infections (skin diseases) at the puncture site.
- Immune deficiency.
- Severe decompensated hypovolemia, shock.
- Specific cardiovascular diseases of myocardial, ischemic or valvular origin, if the planned procedure requires higher sensory spread.
- Acute diseases of the brain and spinal cord.
- Increased intracranial pressure.
- A history of hypersensitivity to local anesthetics, without a prior intracutaneous test dose.

Relative
- Pilonidal cyst.
- Congenital anomalies of the dural sac and its contents.

Procedure

Preparation and materials
- Check that the emergency equipment is complete and in working order (intubation kit, emergency drugs); sterile precautions, intravenous access, anesthetic machine.
- Infusion of a balanced electrolyte solution (250–500 ml).
- Precise monitoring: ECG monitoring, BP control, pulse oximetry.
- Pillow for patient positioning.

The use of a pre-packed set is recommended (e. g. from B. Braun Melsungen) (Fig. 39.4).

Puncture needles
Single-shot technique
- Plastic indwelling catheter needle with stylet, e. g. Contiplex-A plastic indwelling catheter needle 1.3 × 45 mm, 30° bevel.
- Special caudal needle with stylet, e. g. Tuohy: Perican 0.90 × 50 mm 20 G, Perican 1.30 × 50 mm 20 G, Perican 1.30 × 50 mm 18 G × 2″ or Epican, special 32° tip at 0.9 × 50 mm.

Continuous technique
- Tuohy or Crawford or plastic indwelling catheter needle (e. g. Epican, B. Braun Melsungen).

> **Caution**
> Current information and standards show that only needles with a stylet should be used, particularly for caudal anesthesia in children.

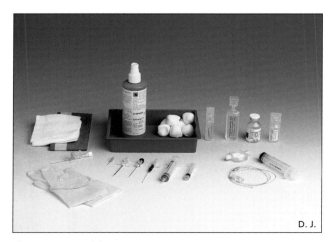

Fig. 39.4 Materials

Single-shot technique

Patient positioning
The puncture is most often carried out with the patient in the prone position, with a pillow under the pelvis and legs spread, so that the heels are turned out and the toes rotated inward. This allows optimal relaxation of the gluteal musculature (Fig. 39.5 A). In addition, particularly in obese patients, the gluteal cleft is separated by attaching a broad band of sticky plaster between the skin of the buttocks and the operating table (Fig. 39.5 B).
This procedure can also be carried out in the lateral decubitus position (particularly in children and in pregnant patients) or in the knee-elbow position (pregnant patients).

Location, skin prep, local anesthesia, skin incision
Locating and marking the sacral cornua
The sacral cornua or sacral hiatus and sacrococcygeal ligaments are palpated with the thumb and index finger (Fig. 39.6 A).

> **Caution**
> The thumb and index finger remain in place on the sacral cornua during the entire puncture procedure.

Palpation of the dorsal cranial iliac spines
A triangle is drawn to the sacral cornua (sacral hiatus). About 1–1.5 cm caudal and medial to the dorsal cranial iliac spines lies the second sacral foramen, the connecting line of which indicates the level of the dural sac in most patients. This line must not be reached when the puncture needle is being advanced (Fig. 39.6 B).
A swab is placed in the gluteal sulcus to protect the anal and perineal area from disinfectant (Fig. 39.5 B).

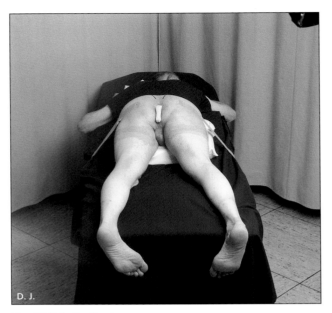

Fig. 39.5 A Positioning

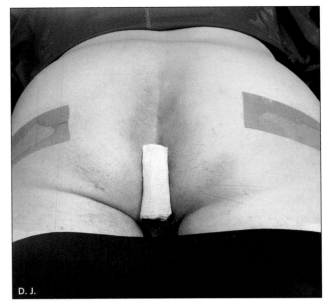

Fig. 39.5 B Attachment of a broad sticky plaster. Placement of a swab in the gluteal cleft

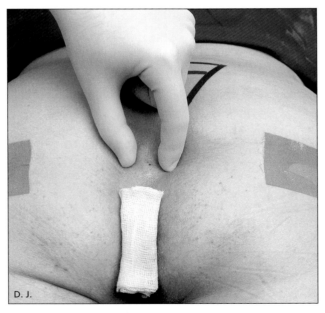

Fig. 39.6 A Palpation of the sacral cornua

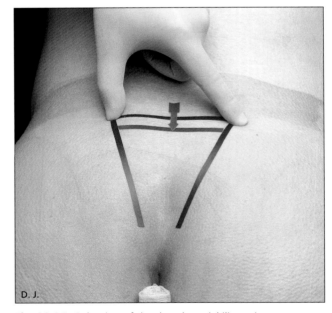

Fig. 39.6 B Palpation of the dorsal cranial iliac spines

Strict asepsis
Thorough, repeated wide skin prep, drying and covering of the puncture site with a sterile drape.

Local anesthesia
Local anesthesia with 1 % mepivacaine is applied in the subcutaneous tissue over and around the sacral hiatus. The periosteum around the sacral hiatus is particularly sensitive and should also be carefully injected.
The needle, which simultaneously identifies the path to the sacral hiatus, is introduced at an angle of 70° to the skin surface of the back of the sacrum (Fig. 39.7)

Preparing the drugs
A syringe with 3–4 ml of an epinephrine-containing local anesthetic (test dose).
A syringe with the calculated amount of local anesthetic.

Skin incision
Using a hemostylet or large-diameter needle (Fig. 39.8).

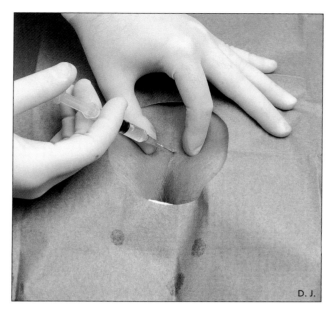

Fig. 39.7 Local anesthesia

Puncture of the caudal epidural space
Puncture
The puncture needle is introduced at an angle of 70° in the direction of the sacral hiatus until bone contact is made (Fig. 39.9 A).
The needle is now slightly withdrawn and the anesthetist slowly reduces the angle of the needle (Fig. 39.9 B) as far as about 20° in male patients or about 35° in women until perforation of the sacrococcygeal ligament is carried out and the needle can be advanced without resistance parallel to the posterior wall of the sacral canal to a depth of 3 cm [15] (Fig. 39.9 C).

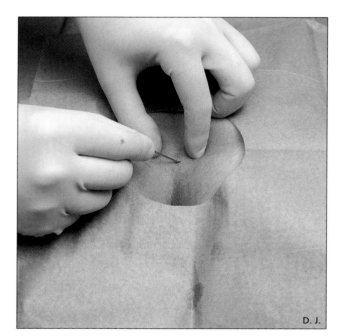

Fig. 39.8 Skin incision

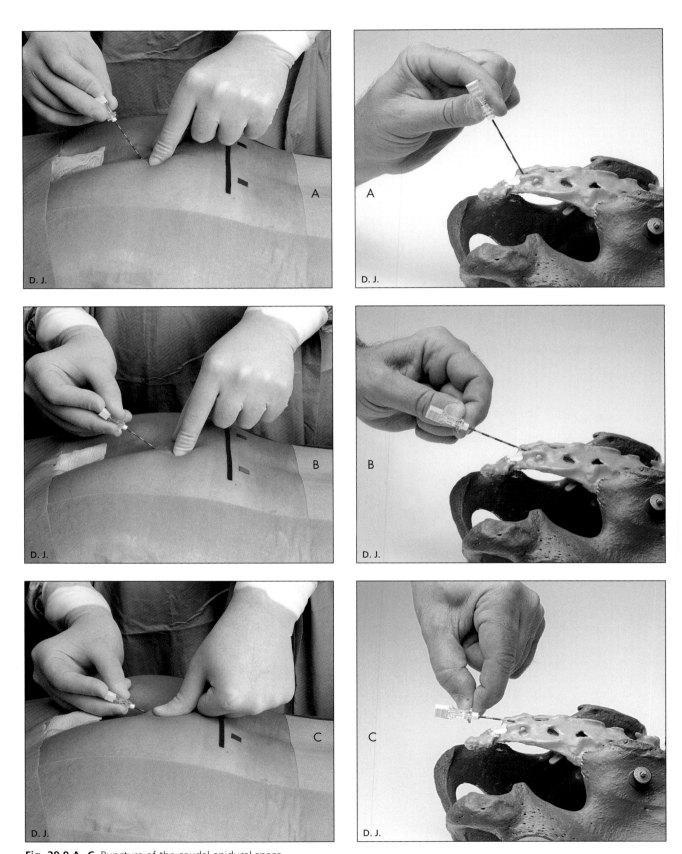

Fig. 39.9 A–C Puncture of the caudal epidural space.
A Puncture angle of 70°. **B** Lowering maneuver. **C** Introducing the needle into the sacral canal

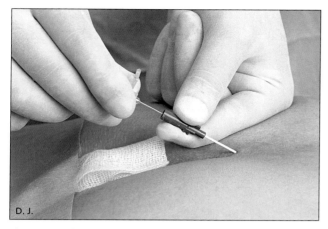

Fig. 39.10 Plastic indwelling catheter needle

When plastic indwelling catheter needles are used, the stylet is withdrawn slightly after the sacral canal has been entered and the plastic part is advanced 2–3 cm (Fig. 39.10).

Checking the position of the needle tip in the dural sac (second sacral foramen)
The stylet is withdrawn and the distance of the needle in the sacral canal checked. This is easily done by placing the stylet on the skin overlying the sacrum (Fig. 39.11 A, B).

Checking for escaping fluid (CSF or blood) (Fig. 39.12)

Aspiration test (Fig. 39.13)

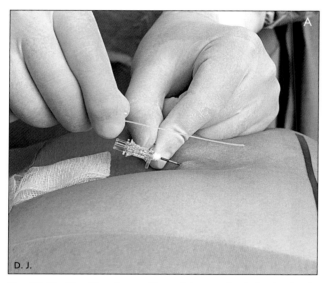

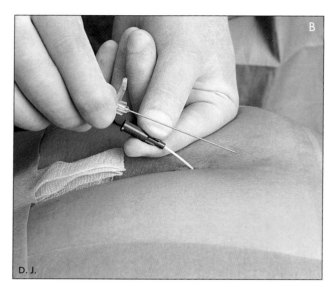

Fig. 39.11 Checking the position of the needle tip in the dural sac (second sacral foramen)

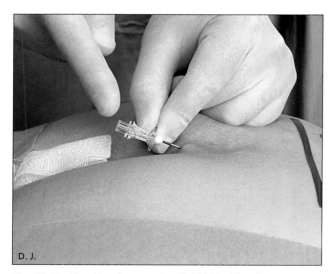

Fig. 39.12 Checking for escaping fluid (CSF, blood)

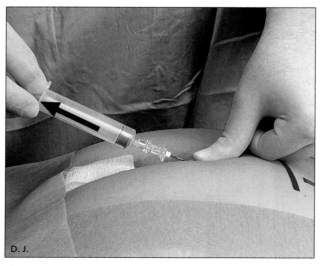

Fig. 39.13 Aspiration test

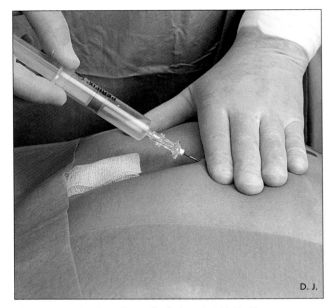

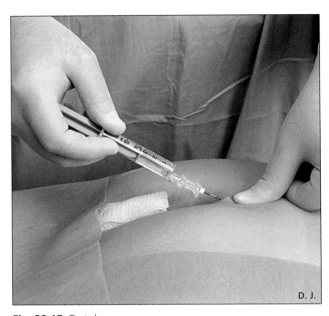

Fig. 39.14 Injection of 5 cm³ of air or 0.9 % NaCl

Fig. 39.15 Test dose

Injection of 5 cm³ of air or 0.9 % NaCl
If no blood or CSF escapes, a rapid injection of 5 cm³ of air or 0.9 % NaCl is carried out (Fig. 39.14).
The patient is then informed that he or she will feel pressure paresthesias in the legs (a sign of correct needle positioning). The anesthetist palpates the surface of the sacrum with the free hand (crepitation, swelling), to exclude the possibility that the catheter is positioned outside the canal.
If pain occurs during this injection, the needle is not correctly positioned.

Test dose
3–4 ml of an epinephrine-containing local anesthetic (Fig. 39.15).
During injection, the tissue over the sacrum should be observed for swelling.

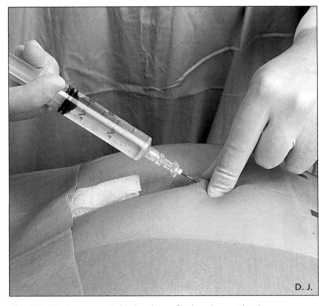

Fig. 39.16 Incremental injection of a local anesthetic

Waiting period
During the five-minute wait, precise cardiovascular monitoring is carried out. Verbal contact must be maintained with the patient constantly.
Five minutes after administration of the test dose, the lower extremities, abdomen and chest are tested for numbness, in order to exclude the possibility of inadvertent subarachnoid injection. Extensive spread suggests dural puncture.

Incremental injection of a local anesthetic
If there is no effect or only a minimal effect, in the form of hypoesthesia in the perineal and perianal area or over the coccyx and if the patient's sensory function is unchanged and the circulation is stable, then the injection of local anesthetic can be carried out (Fig. 39.16).

Problem situations

Aspiration of blood
- Steel needle or plastic indwelling catheter needle: Reinsert the stylet, then advance by 0.5–1 cm and wait for 2–3 minutes.
- Steel needle without a stylet: Advance by about 0.5–1 cm, inject 1 ml 0.9 % NaCl and wait for 2–3 minutes.

If blood is aspirated again, the puncture procedure must be interrupted.

Aspiration of CSF
The puncture procedure must be interrupted.

Failure rate
Owing to the highly variable anatomy in the sacral canal, a failure rate of 5–10 % must be anticipated [15]. Experience shows that the sacral hiatus cannot be identified in about 0.5–1 % of patients.

> **Caution**
> - The puncture needle must remain in the midline during the puncture procedure.
> - The thumb and index finger remain in position on the sacral cornua during the location and puncture process.
> - During the injection of the local anesthetic, the sacral area should be carefully observed for any swelling.
> - The local anesthetic should always be injected on an incremental basis.

Continuous caudal anesthesia

Puncture needles
As for the single-shot technique.

Catheter
Atraumatic epidural catheters with a central opening are used.

Before the puncture procedure
The length of the puncture needle must be compared with the calibration marks on the catheter to improve assessment of the depth of the catheter after introduction (Fig. 39.17). At the same time, the ability of the catheter to pass the puncture needle can be tested. Preparation, puncture and introduction of the needle into the sacral canal are the same as in the single-shot technique.

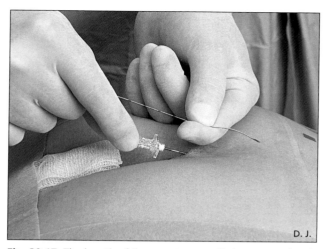

Fig. 39.17 The length of the puncture needle is compared with the calibration marks on the catheter

Further steps
After aspiration at two different levels, the catheter is advanced through the positioned needle to a depth of 3–4 cm.

> **Caution**
> - If there is any obstruction, the catheter must never be advanced using force, since the obstruction may be caused by the dura, a nerve or a blood vessel.
> - A catheter must never be withdrawn through the positioned puncture needle (risk of shearing).

Removing the puncture needle
After the catheter has been positioned as required, the puncture needle is carefully withdrawn, with the catheter being simultaneously secured with the thumb and index finger of the left hand at the injection site (Fig. 39.18 A, B).

Checking the patency of the catheter
An adapter is attached to the end of the catheter (Fig. 39.19 A) and 1 ml of saline is injected (Fig. 39.19 B).

> **Caution**
> Pain during the injection suggests that the catheter is positioned intraneurally. The injection must be interrupted and the position of the catheter must be corrected by withdrawing it minimally.

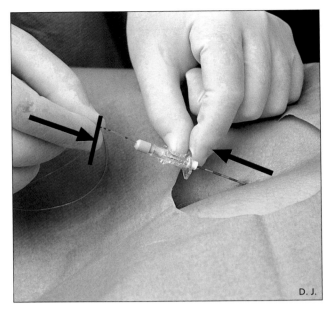

Fig. 39.18 A Withdrawing the puncture needle

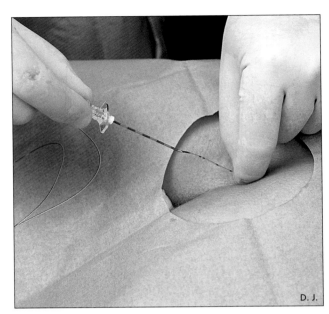

Fig. 39.18 B Securing the catheter with the thumb and index finger

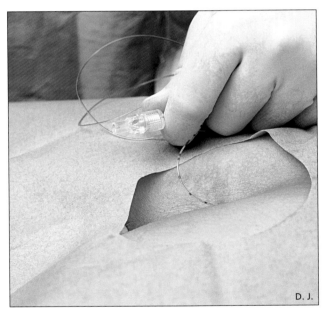

Fig. 39.19 A Attaching the adapter

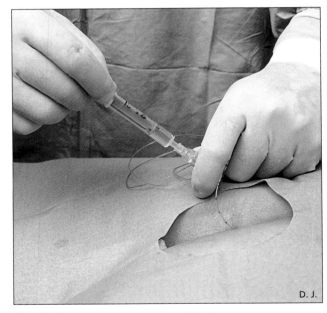

Fig. 39.19 B Injection of 1 ml 0.9 % NaCl

Aspiration test (Fig. 39.20)

Observe the open end of the catheter carefully
The syringe is disconnected and the open end of the catheter is placed on the sterile drape lower than the puncture site. Any escaping fluid (CSF or blood) is noted (Fig. 39.21).

Test dose
3–4 ml of an epinephrine-containing local anesthetic (Fig. 39.22).

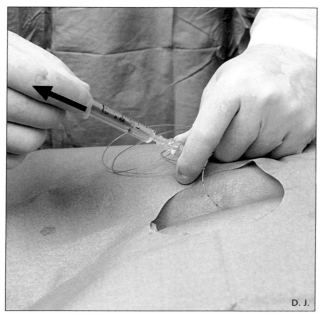

Fig. 39.20 Aspiration test

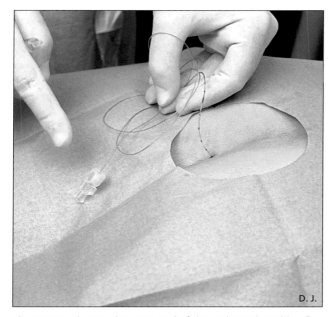

Fig. 39.21 Observe the open end of the catheter (CSF, blood) carefully

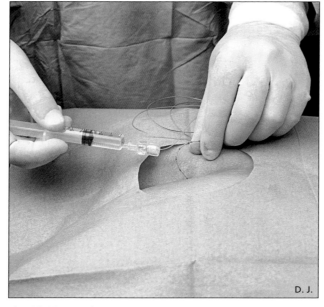

Fig. 39.22 Test dose

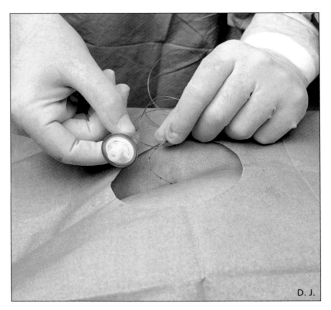

Fig. 39.23 Attaching a bacterial filter

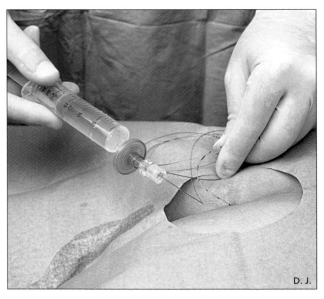

Fig. 39.24 Incremental injection of a local anesthetic

Waiting period
Wait for five minutes. During this time, precise cardio-vascular monitoring is carried out. Verbal contact must be maintained with the patient constantly.
Five minutes after administration of the test dose, the lower extremities, abdomen and chest are tested for possible numbness, to exclude the possibility of inadvertent subarachnoid injection.

Incremental injection of a local anesthetic
After placement of a bacterial filter (Fig. 39.23), sterile attachment of the catheter and repeated aspiration, the incremental injection of local anesthetic is carried out (Fig. 39.24).

Dosages

The same principles apply here as in lumbar epidural anesthesia. Due to the wide variations in the capacity of the sacral canal in the adult, it is difficult to give precise details of the volume of local anesthetic to be injected.
The concentration of local anesthetic determines the intensity of the block. Usually, 20–35 ml of local anesthetic is administered (2–3 ml per segment in the adult). A delay in the onset of effect must be anticipated. The time to onset of effect is shortened and the motor block is intensified when epinephrine is added.

Anesthetic spread (segment)	Local anesthetic (ml)
S5–L2	15–20
S5–T10	25–30

In pregnant patients and obese patients, the dose should be reduced by about 30 %.

Local anesthetics
Surgical procedures

Ropivacaine	0.75–1 %
Bupivacaine	0.375–0.5 %
Prilocaine	2 % (contraindicated in obstetrics)
Mepivacaine	1.5–2 %
Lidocaine	1.5–2 %

Diagnostic and therapeutic blocks
(no addition of epinephrine!)

Block	**Sensory**	**Sympathetic**
Ropivacaine	0.375–0.5 %	0.2 %
Bupivacaine	0.25 %	0.125 %
Prilocaine	1 %	0.5 %
Mepivacaine	1 %	0.5 %
Lidocaine	1 %	0.5 %

Pain therapy
Combination of local anesthetic and corticosteroids
- 15 ml 0.2 % ropivacaine or 15–20 ml 0.125 % bupivacaine mixed with 40–80 mg triamcinolone acetonide (soluble Volon A) (see Chap. 37, p. 279).
- In outpatient procedures, 0.5 % prilocaine or 0.5 % mepivacaine or 0.5 % lidocaine can be used as an alternative.

Opioids
Bolus injections
In combination with a local anesthetic:

Sufentanil:	30–50 µg
Fentanyl:	50 µg
Morphine:	2–5 µg

Continuous administration
(See Chap. 33, p. 249)

Complications (Fig. 39.25)

- Complications due to incorrect technique
  Intraosseous injection into the richly vascularized vertebral bodies, as the spongiosa is easily injured by the puncture needle.
  Puncture needle lying on the sacrum: crepitations or subcutaneous swelling may be noticed after injection of air, saline or local anesthetic.
  Subperiosteal positioning: this becomes evident through resistance during the injection and the associated pain.
  Needle positioned ventral to the sacrum: the needle is located between the sacrum and the coccyx. Advancing it further could lead to perforation of the rectum or in obstetric anesthesia to injury to the head of the fetus.
  Prophylaxis: strict observation of the midline.
- Infections: in about 0.2 % of patients. Strict asepsis is the best form of prophylaxis.
- Intravascular injection (see Chap. 4, pp. 42, 43).
- Intrathecal injection, with high or total spinal anesthesia (see Chap. 33, p. 250).
  Prophylaxis: in adults, the puncture needle should not be advanced further than 3.5 cm and in children not more than 1 cm.
  Check the position of the needle tip in relation to the dural sac. Particular care is required in children (the end of the dural sac is often at S3–4).
  Test dose, incremental injection of the local anesthetic, verbal contact with the patient, circulatory monitoring, testing the anesthetic spread.

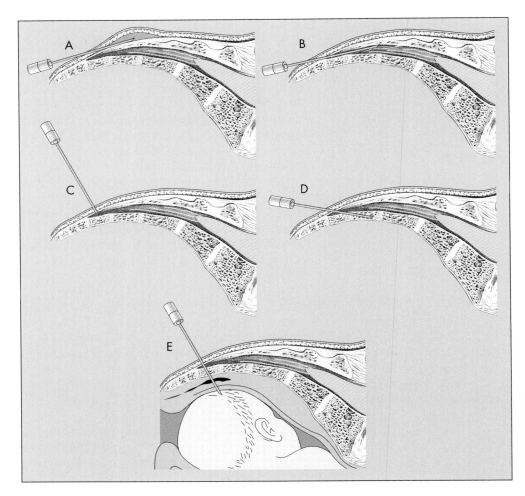

Fig. 39.25 A–E Complications due to incorrect technique. **A** Outside the sacral canal, **B** subperiosteal, **C** into the sacrococcygeal ligament, **D** spongiosa, **E** through the sacrum

- Massive epidural anesthesia
  When attempting to reach segment T10, unpredictable spread of the anesthesia caused by the local anesthetic must be anticipated.
- Hypotension, bradycardia, nausea, vomiting.
- Bladder emptying difficulties.
- Postdural puncture headache (see Chap. 29, p. 214).
- Breaking of the needle, or catheter shearing
  Check the puncture needle before the block and do not advance it over its full length. A catheter must never be withdrawn through the positioned needle.

- Neurological complications
  These arise very rarely and are usually caused by trauma to the lumbosacral plexus – e. g., by the child's head during delivery or by instruments. The complications include paresthesias, peroneal nerve paralysis or coccygodynia. These complications are not causally connected to the caudal anesthesia.
- Cauda equina syndrome (see Chap. 29, p. 218, Chap. 30, p. 223).
- Epidural abscess (see Chap. 33, p. 251).
- Epidural hematoma (see Chap. 33, p. 252).

Caudal anesthesia

Name: _____ Date: _____

Diagnosis: _____

Premedication: ☐ No ☐ Yes

Neurological abnormalities: ☐ No ☐ Yes _____

Purpose of block: ☐ *Surgical* ☐ *Therapeutic* ☐ *Diagnostic*

Needle: ☐ ____ *G* ☐ *With stylet* ☐ *Without stylet*

i. v. access and infusion: ☐

Monitoring: ☐ *ECG* ☐ *Pulse oximetry*

Ventilation facilities: ☐ *Yes (equipment checked)*

Emergency equipment *(drugs)*: ☐ *Checked*

Patient: ☐ *Informed* ☐ *Consent*

Position: ☐ *Prone* ☐ *Lateral decubitus*

Epidural space: ☐ *Identified*

Checking position of needle tip relative to dural sac (2nd sacral foramen): ☐ *Carried out*

Aspiration test: ☐ *Carried out*

Injection: *(5 cm³ air or 0.9% NaCl):* ☐ *Carried out*

Test dose: _____ Epinephrine added: ☐ *Yes* ☐ *No*

Motor and sensory function checked after 5 min: ☐ *Carried out*

Abnormalities: ☐ *No* ☐ *Yes* _____

Injection:

Local anesthetic: _____ *ml* ____ %
(incremental)

☐ Addition: _____ *µg/mg*

Patient's remarks during injection:

☐ *None* ☐ *Pain* ☐ *Paresthesias* ☐ *Warmth*

Duration and area: _____

Objective anesthetic effect after 20 min:

☐ *Cold test* ☐ *Temperature measurement before* ____ °C *after* ____ °C

☐ *Sensory: L* _____ *T* _____

☐ *Motor*

Complications:

☐ *None*   ☐ *Pain*
☐ *Radicular symptoms*   ☐ *Vasovagal reactions*
☐ *BP drop*   ☐ *Dural puncture*
☐ *Vascular puncture*   ☐ *Intravascular injection*
☐ *Massive epidural anesthesia* ☐ *Total spinal anesthesia*
☐ *Bladder emptying disturbances* ☐ *Respiratory disturbances*
☐ *Coccygodynia*   ☐ *Postdural puncture headache*
☐ *Neurological complications*

Special notes:

_____

_____

Record and checklist

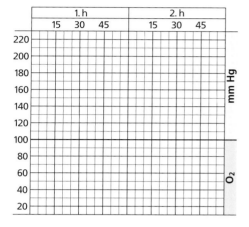

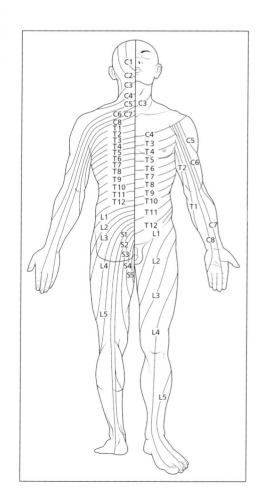

40 Caudal anesthesia in pediatric patients

In pediatric patients, caudal approach is the easiest and safest route to the epidural space.

Advantages and disadvantages

Advantages [5, 9]
- Better anatomic relationships and thus easier orientation and shorter time required for puncture.
- Perforation of the sacrococcygeal ligament is more clearly palpable.
- Better distribution of the injected anesthetic than in the adult.
- Very effective anesthesia and analgesia with small amounts of local anesthetic.
- An 18-G epidural catheter can be used in children of almost any age group.
- It is easier to advance the epidural catheter than in the adult.
- Higher positioning of the catheter is possible, particularly in neonates and infants.
- The immaturity of the sympathetic nervous system means that circulatory problems are extremely rare, particularly up to the age of eight.
- There is a very rapid recovery phase due to the shallow supplementary light general anesthesia and avoidance of muscle relaxants.
- There is a quiet postoperative phase and thus reduced opioids and therefore fewer side effects such as nausea, vomiting or urinary retention.
- The need for subsequent postoperative intensive-care treatment is reduced.

Disadvantages
- Mild light general anesthesia is needed on principle, so that precise testing of the spread of anesthesia is not possible [5]. When Emla cream is used in combination with sedation, this problem can sometimes be overcome.
- The risk of contamination with caudal epidural catheters is higher than with lumbar epidural catheters.

Characteristics of the epidural space in children [5]

In children under one year of age, the dural sac reaches to the third or even to the fourth sacral foramen.
The gelatin-like epidural fatty tissue is more permeable and allows the injected local anesthetic to spread much better than in the adult. When advancing the epidural catheter, hardly any resistance is produced. In neonates and infants up to 6 kg in body weight in particular, it is possible to reach almost any height due to the relatively wide epidural space, which is almost empty and runs parallel to the dura.
In older children, obstruction occurs more often when advancing the catheter, particularly in the area from L2 to L5.

Indications

Single-shot technique
- All surgical procedures below the T10 dermatome with an operating time of up to 90 minutes, e. g. perineal and perianal procedures, orchidopexy (not undescended testis), hypospadias, inguinal hernia, repositioning of incarcerated hernias.
- Superficial surgical procedures in the lower extremities, e. g. skin transplantations, etc.

Contraindications

These correspond to those in caudal anesthesia in the adult (see Chap. 39, p. 288).

Procedure

Mild light general anesthesia or more rarely sedation in combination with local application of Emla cream, is used both with the single-shot technique and in continuous caudal anesthesia.

Preparation
▨ Location and marking of the sacral cornua.
▨ Palpation of the dorsal cranial iliac spines.
▨ Strict asepsis (thorough skin prep).
▨ Local anesthesia or application of Emla cream.
▨ Preparation of the drugs:
   Syringe with 1 ml epinephrine-containing local anesthetic (test dose).
   Syringe with the calculated quantity of local anesthetic.
▨ Skin incision using a hemostylet or large-diameter needle.

Preparation and materials
These correspond to those for caudal anesthesia in the adult (see p. 289); a **precordial stethoscope** is also needed.

Caudal puncture needles
A wide variety of needle types are used all over the world for caudal puncture in pediatric patients: normal steel needles, Tuohy or Crawford needles, plastic indwelling catheter needles and in children weighing less than 4 kg, 23-G butterfly needles as well [11].
There are no standardized criteria for assessing these, so that the choice is a matter of personal preference and experience on the part of the anesthetist concerned.
Based on numerous publications, the following summary can be given: the use of puncture needles without a stylet can lead to dangerous transport of free skin particles with epidermal cells into the spinal canal, with later development of epidermoid tumors (malformation tumors) [3, 10, 12, 17].
For this reason, the following recommendation has been made: caudal puncture in children should only be carried out after a preliminary skin incision using a large-diameter needle or hemostylet and a puncture needle with a stylet should always be used [4].
The use of a ready-supplied epidural set is recommended (e. g. Epican Paed, B. Braun Melsungen).

Pediatric caudal needles:
▨ Size: 0.53 × 30 mm, 25 G, with 32° short bevel and steel stylet.
▨ Or 0.73 × 35 mm, 22 G, also with 32° short bevel and steel stylet.
▨ Or 0.90 × 50 mm, 20 G, also with 32° short bevel and steel stylet.

Single-shot technique

Patient positioning
Lateral decubitus, with the legs bent (Fig. 40.1).

Puncture of the caudal epidural space

> **Caution**
> In children younger than one year, the dural sac reaches as far as the third or even fourth sacral foramen.

The puncture needle is introduced in a cranial direction at an angle of 60–70°, towards the sacral dorsum (Fig. 40.2). After the very clear sensation of the sacrococcygeal ligament, the needle reaches the sacral canal ("sudden give"). The needle position is not altered any further.
The thumb and index finger remain on the sacral cornua throughout the whole of the location and puncture procedure.
Then:
▨ Withdraw the stylet.
▨ Check the end of the needle for escaping fluid (CSF, blood).
▨ Carry out aspiration in two different planes.
▨ Inject a test dose of 1 ml of an epinephrine-containing local anesthetic.

During the subsequent waiting period:
Precise cardiovascular monitoring is carried out, along with the precordial stethoscope, to recognize the development of tachycardia or arrhythmia.
However, this test can lead to unreliable results in fully anesthetized children [8].

Incremental injection of local anesthetic
After a negative result with the test dose, the calculated quantity of local anesthetic is injected on an incremental basis (Fig. 40.3).
As this is done, the index and middle finger are laid on the surface of the sacrum, so that subcutaneous injection can be recognized quickly.

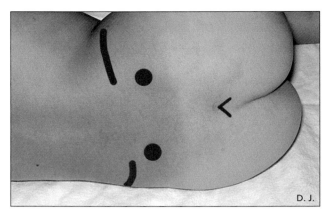

Fig. 40.1 Lateral decubitus position, with the legs bent

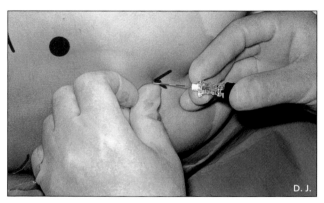

Fig. 40.2 Introducing the needle

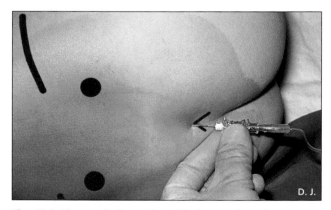

Fig. 40.3 The needle is positioned in the sacral canal. Incremental injection of a local anesthetic

Checking the spread of anesthesia

The spread of anesthesia should always be checked in children who have not received light general anesthesia.

As correct testing of the anesthetic spread is not possible in fully anesthetized children, this method is reserved only for highly experienced anesthetists.

Postoperatively, a detailed examination of sensory and motor function is carried out. The child should be moved to the normal ward only if he or she is able to move the legs freely.

Continuous caudal anesthesia

Indications

In combination with light general anesthesia in longer-lasting operations in the upper and lower abdominal areas, in the urogenital area and in the area of the lower extremities.

Contraindications

(See Chap. 39, p. 288)

Disadvantage

Due to the risk of infection (proximity to the anogenital region), the catheter should be withdrawn immediately after the end of the operation.

Preparation, materials, patient positioning

(See Chap. 39, pp. 289, 295)

Puncture of the caudal epidural space

- Skin incision using a hemostylet or large-diameter needle.
- The plastic indwelling catheter needle (or Tuohy) is advanced at an angle of 60–70° in the direction of the sacrococcygeal ligament. After perforation of the ligament, the needle is advanced 1 cm into the sacral canal, the stylet is removed and the plastic part is advanced a further 0.5 cm.
- After palpation of the iliac crests through the drapes, the catheter should be measured to allow the desired dermatome to be located.
- The catheter is now advanced to the desired dermatome. In neonates, infants and small children, the catheter meets hardly any resistance, so that it is easy to advance it to the upper lumbar or thoracic segments.

Caution
A catheter must never be advanced against resistance, which might be caused by the dura, a nerve or a blood vessel.

Checking the catheter position
- Removal of the plastic indwelling catheter needle.
- Checking the patency of the catheter:
  An adapter is attached to the end of the catheter and 1 ml saline is injected.
- Aspiration in two different planes.
- The open end of the catheter should be carefully observed.
  The syringe is disconnected, the open end of the catheter is placed on the sterile drape below the level of the puncture and any escaping fluid (CSF or blood) is noted.

Test dose of an epinephrine-containing local anesthetic
During the waiting period: precise circulatory monitoring (ECG, pulse oximetry, precordial stethoscope).

Placement of a bacterial filter, sterile attachment of the catheter

Administration of local anesthetics
- Injection of one-quarter of the calculated dose of local anesthetic.
- When there is no resistance to the injection, the remaining dose can be administered at a speed of 0.7 ml/s.
  Larger amounts of the local anesthetic are needed if the injection is carried out more slowly [5].

Dosages

The following parameters are particularly important for the dosage of local anesthetics in neonates, infants and small children:
- Better penetration of the local anesthetic solution takes place due to the incomplete myelinization of the nerves in infants and due to the small diameter of the nerves in small children. This means that lower doses are required!
- Muscle relaxation, particularly in extensive abdominal or orthopedic procedures, can be produced by adding epinephrine.
- The "threshold block" is much more extensive, reaching as far as five dermatomes.

- Surprisingly low plasma concentrations are found in children after administration of the maximum dose of a local anesthetic.
- In comparison with adults, the dosage of local anesthetic is more reliable and precise and is based on the tried and tested parameters of age, weight and height.

The following guidelines may be helpful for the dosage of local anesthetic:

Schulte-Steinberg schema [16]
The age of the child is used according to the following formula:
0.1 ml per segment to be blocked × age in years
The pin-prick test is taken into account here and thin C fibers are blocked.

Busoni and Andreucetti schema [5, 6, 7]
For clinical applications, particularly in longer, more extensive surgical procedures, the **age and weight** of the child are used as the parameters, with 1 % mepivacaine being tested. Testing of the analgesia is carried out by pinching (thicker A-delta fibers) and pin-pricks (thin C fibers). The anesthesia lies about four to six dermatomes lower ("threshold block").
In neonates and infants, weight is a reliable parameter; in small children, age has proved to be a better parameter for assessing the required dosage. Experienced anesthetists have found Busoni's diagrams (Fig. 40.4) particularly useful.

Armitage schema [1, 2]
This schema is easy to use and has also proved itself with less experienced anesthetists.
The following dosage is recommended:
Lumbosacral block: 0.50 ml/kg b. w.
Thoracolumbar block: 1.00 ml/kg b. w.
Mid-thoracic block: 1.25 ml/kg b. w.

Local anesthetics
The most frequently used local anesthetics are:
Bupivacaine: 0.25–0.375 %
Ropivacaine: 0.2 %
Mepivacaine: 1 %
Lidocaine: 1 %

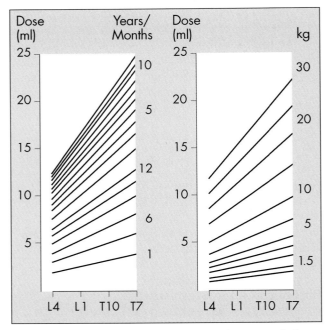

Fig. 40.4 Diagram of the relation between dose, spread of analgesia, age and body weight for various segmental levels [adapted from Busoni, in: Saint-Maurice C, Schulte-Steinberg O, Armitage E (eds.), *Regional Anesthesia in Children* (Appleton & Lange/Mediglobe, 1990]

After the volume has been calculated, the maximum dose for the body weight should be calculated and the local anesthetic should be diluted accordingly.

If the calculated quantity of local anesthetic is less than 20 ml, administration of 0.25 % bupivacaine, for example, is recommended. If the calculated quantity is over 20 ml, dilution in saline should be carried out until a concentration of 0.19 % bupivacaine is reached [9].

Complications

(See Chap. 39, section on complications, p. 299)

41 Adjuncts to local anesthesia in neuraxial blocks

Opioids, vasopressors, clonidine (an alpha-2-adrenoceptor antagonist), ketamine and – in subarachnoid administration in particular – glucose, can be used as adjuncts to a neuraxially administered local anesthetic.

Glucose

In the hyperbaric spinal anesthesia technique, glucose is mixed at concentrations of 5–10 % with a local anesthetic in order to produce a higher density than that of the CSF (see Chap. 28, p. 208, Table 28.1).

Vasopressors

Vasopressors that can be used to prolong the duration of effect of a local anesthetic are:

▨ Phenylephrine (Neosynephrine)
0.5–5 mg (0.05–0.5 ml in a 1 % solution), with which the duration of effect of the local anesthetic is extended by 30–100 % [31].

▨ Epinephrine (adrenaline)
0.2–0.5 mg (0.2–0.5 ml, 1 : 1000 in solution), with which the duration of effect of the local anesthetic can be extended by 40–50 % [31].

Advantages and disadvantages of phenylephrine/epinephrine
The addition of a vasopressor leads to slower vascular resorption of the local anesthetic. This slows down contact with neural tissue, while at the same time reducing the systemic toxicity.

Reservations regarding the possible association of added vasopressors with spinal cord ischemia, with subsequent neurological complications, have not been confirmed clinically [10, 23].

The causes of neurological injury are rather multifactorial, and include the technique, equipment and injected drugs. In addition, the patient's individual situation and possible distinctive anatomic features play a role. However, this topic continues to be a controversial one [31].

Opioids [13, 27, 28, 42]

Neuraxial administration of an opioid – as a single agent, or in combination with a low-dose local anesthetic – produces very good analgesia during surgery and in the postoperative period.

Central or systemic side effects are only caused very rarely.

The receptors specific for opioids are located alongside areas in the brain and particularly in the gelatinous substance of the spinal cord. Their concentration there is at its most dense.

In comparison with a local anesthetic, an opioid injected in the vicinity of the spinal cord has a selective effect – i. e., it produces a pure analgesia, without sensory or motor block and with only a slight sympathetic block.

In comparison with systemic administration, opioids are strongly potent in effect and have marked segmental limitation, a long duration of effect and a low tendency to produce side effects.

The following characteristics of opioids are important for optimal effectiveness:

▨ **High affinity with the receptor** and thus **high analgesic potency.**

▨ **High lipophilia,** causing acceleration of their passage through the dura and CSF to the spinal cord. At the same time, however, there is a high elimination speed, which is reflected in a short duration of effect. Agents such as sufentanil or fentanyl, for example, remain in the CSF for only a very short time and are quickly absorbed by the lipid-rich structures of the spinal cord. They are characterized by a short gradient of effect, but also by a short duration of effect.

▨ **Low hydrophilia** and thus a short period of persistence in the CSF.
The strongly hydrophilic opioids – the main representative being morphine – remain in the CSF for a longer period, so that a larger proportion is transported to the brain before binding with opioid receptors can take place.

The consequences of this are slow systemic resorption, a slower gradient of effect, a long duration of effect, a low elimination rate and the risk of cranial diffusion. Due to the physiological slow circulation of CSF, the patient is at risk of **respiratory depression** even after several hours. This applies particularly to hydrophilic substances, so that after morphine administration, depending on the dosage, respiratory depression can be expected even after 18–24 hours.

- **Long receptor binding and thus a long duration of effect** (e. g. buprenorphine).
- **Low tendency for tolerance to develop.**

Pharmacokinetic data for the most frequently used opioids

Administration of an opioid can be carried out subarachnoidally or epidurally. It is mainly pure opioid agonists that are used.

Strongly lipophilic opioids
- Sufentanil
  High lipophilia, high receptor affinity, 1000 times more effective than morphine – drug of the future in neuraxial applications.
  Suitable for acute pain therapy.
  Epidural:
  Dosage 30–50 µg, onset of effect after 10 min, duration of effect 4–5 h.
  Subarachnoid:
  Dosage 7.5–10 µg, onset of effect after 2–10 min, duration of effect 1–3 h.
- Fentanyl
  Strongly lipophilic and 75 times more effective than morphine. Suitable for acute pain therapy.
  Epidural:
  Dosage 50–100 µg, onset of effect after 5–10 min, duration of effect 2–3 h.
  Subarachnoid:
  Dosage 25–50 µg, onset of effect after 2–10 min, duration of effect 30–120 min.

Strongly hydrophilic opioids
- Morphine
  Epidural:
  Dosage 2–5 mg, onset of effect after 30–60 min, duration of effect 8–22 h.
  Subarachnoid:
  Dosage 0.2–0.5 mg, onset of effect after 10–20 min, duration of effect 8–24 h.

Combinations

In some clinical situations, the effect of opioids alone is not adequate. A combination of opioids and local anesthetics leads to an additive or multiplied analgesic effect, characterized by faster onset of effect, longer duration of effect and reduced motor block. The blocking of pain takes place at various sites: at the neural axon and via the opioid receptors in the spinal cord.

The use of such combinations is becoming more and more routine.

Types of application [27]

Epidural bolus injection
The lowest possible volume should be selected, with volumes of 5–10 ml being normally preferred.

Epidural infusion
A bolus dose of 10 ml bupivacaine (0.0625–0.125 %) in combination with 1–2 µg/ml sufentanil is followed by infusion of a mixture of bupivacaine (0.031 %) and sufentanil (0.2–0.3 µg/ml) at a speed of 6–10 ml/h. These low dosages are used in obstetrics in particular.

Patient-controlled epidural anesthesia (PCEA)
This mode of application leads to a significant reduction in the total dose, by up to 30 %.
A bolus dose of 10–30 µg sufentanil is followed by a baseline infusion rate of 5 µg/h. The maximum single dose is 5 µg, with a 10–20-minute injection lock.

Factors influencing epidural infusion

Important factors that influence the opioid/local anesthetic dosage in epidural infusions are:
- Location and type of surgery.
- Pain type (obstetric, post-traumatic).
- Opioid type and its initial dosage.
- Injection volume.
- Concentration of the local anesthetic.
- Patient characteristics (age, obesity, concomitant diseases).
- Intraoperative blood loss.
- Pharmacokinetics of the injected opioid.
- Position of the catheter tip in the epidural space.

Complications and side effects [13, 28]

Respiratory depression

This is the most feared complication, particularly after subarachnoid administration.

The cause is either overdosage, or systemic resorption of the opioid. Respiratory depression occurs relatively shortly after administration, or may be delayed by slow rostral diffusion to the respiratory center. Delayed respiratory depression is particularly seen after morphine administration, since its marked hydrophilia leads to larger amounts remaining in the slowly circulating CSF and spreading towards the respiratory center. Slowly circulating CSF takes 6–10 hours to pass from the lumbar subarachnoid space to the fourth ventricle.

Low levels of respiratory depression are possible even after the administration of lipophilic opioids [16, 34]. Monitoring of respiration when applying both hydrophilic and lipophilic opioids is therefore strongly recommended. Despite the binding of lipophilic opioids to the receptors in the spinal cord, the analgesic effect of these agents is mainly systemic, rather than spinal. Thus, the same quality of analgesia can thus be achieved independently of the catheter position (lumbar or thoracic, after a thoracotomy: see Chap. 34, p. 257).

The following measures are regarded as effective forms of prophylaxis to reduce the risk of respiratory depression:

- Careful monitoring of respiration and circulation.
- Use of lipophilic opioids.
- Individual dose adjustment and dose reduction by titration.
- Low volumes.
- Dose reduction in older patients, pregnant patients and obese patients.
- If the patient becomes somnolent, it is a warning signal.
- Particular caution should be used when there is intraoperative blood loss and a drop in blood pressure.
- Lumbar application and epidural infusion are preferable.
- Possible catheter dislocation should be carefully observed.
- Avoid the use of intravenous supplementation (opioids or sedatives).

Therapy

Naloxone	0.1–0.2 mg i. v. as a bolus, or as infusion 5–10 µg/h
Nalbuphine	5–10 mg i. v.

Pruritus

This is a harmless side effect, which can be observed in a large proportion of patients (40 %) after administration of an initial dose. In most cases, it resolves spontaneously after 10–20 minutes without any treatment being needed.

In resistant cases, treatment with nalbuphine, 5–10 mg i. v., or naloxone is recommended.

Alternatively, propofol (10–20 mg) and antihistamines can be used.

Urinary retention

This is often observed after spinal administration of opioids.

Treatment: carbachol (Doryl) i. m., or catheterization.

Nausea/vomiting

These side effects are often seen after the administration of pethidine.

Treatment: metoclopramide 10–20 mg i. v., nalbuphine 5–10 mg i. v. or propofol 10–20 mg i. v. A last alternative is naloxone 0.2–0.4 mg.

Drop in blood pressure

Occurs in 11.5 % of cases [13].

Bradycardia

Occurs in 1.6 % of cases [13].

Muscle relaxation

Occurs in 7 % of cases [13].

Clonidine

Clonidine, a derivative of imidazoline, binds to alpha-2-adrenoceptors.

The alpha-2-receptors are mainly found in the intermediomedial nucleus (preganglionic sympathetic cells of origin for T4–L2/3), in the intermediolateral nucleus (preganglionic parasympathetic cells of origin for the sacral spinal cord) and in the gelatinous substance of the dorsal horn.

The receptor density in the sacral cord is 50 % greater than in the thoracic and lumbar spinal cord [29, 30].

The high lipid solubility with low plasma protein binding (20 %) of clonidine allows it to pass the blood-brain barrier more quickly.

Its analgesic effect is segmental. Maximum CSF levels are observed 30 minutes after epidural administration of clonidine and these are about 100 times higher than the simultaneous plasma levels.

The elimination half-life in CSF is about 80 minutes and in plasma 12 ± 7 hours. The elimination is mainly renal.

Hemodynamic side effects

As clonidine is a potent hypotensive drug, bradycardia, hypotension, or sedation can be expected after epidural or subarachnoid application. Administration of clonidine in patients with cardiac insufficiency or hypovolemia is therefore contraindicated.

Neurotoxic injury in the form of ischemia due to vasoconstriction has not as yet been observed after epidural or subarachnoid administration of clonidine.

Combination with local anesthetics or opioids

Clonidine has a very good additive effect when combined with local anesthetics or opioids.

Subarachnoid administration

Subarachnoid administration of clonidine (150 µg) combined with a local anesthetic leads to a prolonged duration of effect and prolonged motor block in spinal anesthesia, due to its very good additive effect.

The dosage required for adequate effect in subarachnoid injection is about one-third of the epidural dose.

In subarachnoid combination with a local anesthetic, clonidine does not lead to more severe circulatory depression in comparison with pure spinal anesthesia with a local anesthetic.

Long-term subarachnoid administration of clonidine in pain therapy has been reported [18].

Epidural administration

The combination of clonidine with a local anesthetic or an opioid leads to a significant improvement in the quality and duration of analgesia. This has been reported in particular in orthopedics [12], obstetrics [21], pediatric anesthesia [17] and in long-term pain therapy [20].

Dosage recommendations for clinical application

If opioids and alpha-2-agonists are being used in neuraxial analgesia procedures, it can be assumed that antinociception undergoes an additive effect, if not a synergistic one. This is associated with a doubling of the duration of effect and has been reported for combinations of clonidine with morphine, fentanyl and sufentanil.

Suggested dosages

- Subarachnoid:
  Clonidine 150 µg in combination with a local anesthetic.
- Epidural:
  Clonidine 2–4 µg/kg b. w. + morphine 30–50 µg/kg b. w. [29].
  Clonidine 4 µg/kg b. w. + fentanyl 2 µg/kg b. w. + 0.25 % bupivacaine ad 50 ml, infusion at 0.05 ml/kg/h [29].
  Clonidine 150 µg + fentanyl 100 µg [29].
  Clonidine 150 µg + sufentanil 10 µg [29].
  Clonidine 2–4 µg/kg b. w. + sufentanil 0.2–0.3 µg/ml + 0.125 % bupivacaine ad 50 ml, infusion at 6–10 ml/h [29].

Ketamine

Ketamine was synthesized in 1963 and is structurally related to the addictive hallucinogen phencyclidine (PCP, "angel dust"). It is used as an analgesic, narcotic and for intubation in status asthmaticus. It has a firmly established place in anesthesia, intensive-care medicine and in emergency medicine.

Its importance as a low-dose co-analgesic drug in neuraxial applications is growing. In particular, intravenous or epidural administration of the stereoisomer S-(+)-ketamine is likely to become more important. In comparison with the racemate form, it has double the analgesic and anesthetic potency, an equally fast onset of effect, shorter recovery times and a wider range of therapeutic application [2, 3, 4].

Mechanism of effect [2, 3, 4]

Ketamine is a nonspecific N-methyl-D-aspartate (NMDA) receptor antagonist. The most important binding site for the analgesic effect of ketamine is the NMDA-sensitive glutamate receptor channel. The NMDA receptors belong to the excitatory amino acid system (EAA) of the central nervous system. Glutamate is the most important excitatory neurotransmitter in the central nervous system of vertebrates. PCP receptor agonists such as ketamine inhibit the effect of glutamate at the NMDA receptor channels noncompetitively and thus prevent calcium transport into the cells. The analgesic effect of ketamine is mainly produced by this process.

The local anesthetic effect of ketamine, by contrast, is based on sodium ion channel inhibition, with raised concentrations being found at the site of application.

At low dosages, the local anesthetic effect (in the spinal cord) is very low. Ketamine is also thought to have a neuroprotective effect in the context of NMDA receptor antagonism [3].

There is an affinity with other receptors, but the significance of these in mediating the effect has not yet been fully clarified:

Opioid receptors, nicotinic (nACh) and muscarinic (mACh) acetylcholine receptors, dopamine receptors (indirectly), serotonin receptors (indirectly), adrenoceptors (indirectly), ion channel block (voltage-operated channels, particularly Na^+, K^+, Ca^{++}), GABA receptor A binding (modulation of the chloride channel).

Neuraxial application of ketamine

The use of ketamine in combination with an opioid or local anesthetic (rarely as a monoanalgesic) has proved its value in the following areas:

- Postoperative pain therapy.
- Various chronic pain syndromes that are treatment-resistant.
- Carcinoma pain.

A combination of subanalgesic doses of ketamine and morphine synergistically enhances the effect of morphine and interaction with various receptors. This leads to the following advantages:

- Very good analgesia, comparable with that of high-dose morphine administration [40].
- A substantial reduction in the rate of adverse side effects, particularly respiratory depression, resulting from the reduced dosage of morphine.
- Prophylaxis against developing opioid tolerance.

In cases of morphine tolerance, ketamine is a good way of potentiating the effect through an additional attack at the NMDA receptor.

Subarachnoid application

Subarachnoid administration of ketamine as a co-analgesic (rarely as a single agent) is **not recommended**, due to the **neurotoxicity** of the preservative benzethonium chloride that is contained in ketamine preparations. Ketamine may only be used exceptionally and in the form of a preservative-free solution for subarachnoid applications [14, 15, 37, 40].

Carcinoma pain

Treatment-resistant carcinoma pain is the principal indication for the subarachnoid administration of ketamine as a co-analgesic with morphine [41], or as an addition to clonidine and a local anesthetic [24] in the form of a continuous infusion.

The potentiating effect of ketamine leads to a substantial reduction in the morphine dosage and thus a reduction in the risk of adverse side effects.

Anesthesiology

The use of ketamine as a single agent in anesthesiology has not as yet proved successful. The reasons for this are the high dosages required (0.7–0.95 mg/kg), the short duration of effect and its dose-dependent central sympathomimetic side effects [15].

Epidural application

The first publications reporting the epidural use of ketamine date from 1982.

The administration of ketamine as a co-analgesic, usually with morphine (more rarely as a single drug) leads to a very good postoperative analgesia, particularly when administered preemptively.

The nociceptors are blocked to an extent such that a subsequent pain stimulus does not lead to increased sensitivity in its effects on the nerve cell. Pain-related central adaptation processes, which increase postoperative pain, are thereby prevented.

Ketamine should be used without a preservative substance and at a concentration of 0.1–0.3 % [15, 37, 40].

Surgical indications

- Gynecological procedures [1, 19].
- Upper abdominal procedures via a thoracic catheter [9].
- General surgery [8].
- Cholecystectomy [25].
- Orthopedic endoprostheses [37, 38].
- Pediatric surgery (orchidopexy) via caudal administration [11, 32].

The epidural dosage of ketamine is 20–50 mg [14].

Indications in pain therapy

- Post-herpetic neuralgia [39].
- Complex regional pain syndrome (CRPS), types I and II [22, 35].
  A dosage of 7.5–10 mg in combination with 0.75–1 mg morphine and 0.1 % bupivacaine is recommended here.
  For continuous epidural infusion, a dosage of 25 μg/kg/h is recommended [35].
- Phantom pain [26].
- Carcinoma pain.

Specific contraindications

- Poorly adjusted or untreated arterial hypertension.
- Preeclampsia and eclampsia.
- Manifest hyperthyroidism.

Relative contraindications

- Unstable angina pectoris.
- Myocardial infarction within the previous six months.
- Raised intracranial pressure without adequate ventilation.
- Glaucoma and perforating eye injuries.

Interactions

Combined application with thyroid hormones leads to severe hypertension and tachycardia.

References

Chapter 1: Regional nerve blocks in clinical practice

1. Basler, H.-D., Ernst, A., Flöter, Th., Gerbershagen, H.-U., Hankemeier, U., Jungck, D., Müller-Schwefe, G., Zimmermann, M.: Gemeinsame Richtlinien der Deutschen Gesellschaft zum Studium des Schmerzes e. V. (DGSS) und des SCHMERZtherapeutischen Kolloquiums e. V. (StK) für die Zusatzweiterbildung zum Algesiologen DGSS / STK. SCHMERZtherapeutisches Kolloquium **11** (1995) 3–5
2. Bonica, J. J., Buckley, P. F.: Regional analgesia with local anesthetics. In: Bonica, J. J. (ed.): Management of Pain. (2nd ed.) Lea & Febiger, Philadelphia – London (1990)
3. Borchard, U., Niesel, H. C.: Grundlagen der Pharmakologie der Lokalanästhetika. In: Niesel, H. C. (Hrsg.): Regionalanästhesie, Lokalanästhesie, Regionale Schmerztherapie. Georg Thieme Verlag, Stuttgart – New York (1994)
4. Campbell, J. N., Raja, S. N., Cohen, R. H., Manning, D. C., Khan, A. A., Meyer, R. A.: Peripheral neural mechanisms of nociception. In: Wall, P. D., Melzack, R. (eds.): Textbook of Pain. (2nd ed.) Churchill Livingstone, Edinburgh (1989)
5. Devor, M.: Central changes mediating neuropathic pain. In: Dubner, R., Gebhart, G. F., Bond, M. R. (eds.): Proceedings of the Vth World Congress on Pain. Pain Research and Clinical Management. Elsevier, Amsterdam (1988)
6. Hildebrandt, A. G. (Bundesgesundheitsamt): Bekanntmachung über die Zulassung und Registrierung von Arzneimitteln. Abwehr von Arzneimittelrisiken, Stufe II – Lidocain- und Etidocain-haltige Arzneimittel (Ausgenommen sind Lidocain-haltige Arzneimittel, die zur anti-arrhythmischen Therapie angewendet werden). Bundesanzeiger Nr. **149**, Jahrgang 45 (1993) 7494
7. Tryba, M.: Lokalanästhetika. In: Zenz, M., Jurna, I. (Hrsg.): Lehrbuch der Schmerztherapie. Grundlagen, Theorie und Praxis für Aus- und Weiterbildung. Wissenschaftliche Verlagsgesellschaft, Stuttgart (1993)
8. Weninger, E.: Pharmakodynamik der Lokalanästhetika. Anästhesiologie & Intensivmedizin **5** (37) (1996) 249–267
9. Zimmermann, M.: Physiologie von Nozizeption und Schmerz. In: Zimmermann, M., Handwerker, H. O. (Hrsg.): Schmerz-Konzepte und ärztliches Handeln. Springer-Verlag, Berlin (1984)

Chapter 2: Occipital nerves

1. Bonica, J. J.: Block of cranial nerves. In: Bonica, J. J. (ed.): The management of Pain. (2nd ed.) Lea & Febiger, Philadelphia (1990)
2. Murphy, T. M.: Somatic blockade of head and neck. In: Cousins, M. J., Bridenbaugh, P. O. (eds.): Neural Blockade. (2nd ed.) Lippincott, Philadelphia (1988)
3. Netter, F. H.: Anatomie. In: Firbas, W. (Hrsg.): Farbatlanten der Medizin (Band 7). Bewegungsapparat I: Anatomie, Embryologie, Physiologie und Stoffwechselkrankheiten. Georg Thieme Verlag, Stuttgart – New York (1992)
4. Steenks, M. H., deWijer, A.: Kiefergelenksfehlfunktionen aus physiotherapeutischer und zahnmedizinischer Sicht. Quintessenz, Berlin (1991)
5. Tilscher, H., Eder, M.: Infiltrationstherapie. Hippokrates, Stuttgart (1994)
6. Travell, J. G., Simons, D. G.: Myofascial Pain and Dysfunction. The Trigger Point Manual. Williams & Wilkins, Baltimore – London (1983)

Chapter 3: Trigeminal nerve

1. Amster, L. J.: Sphenopalatine ganglion block for the relief of painful vascular and muscular spasm with special reference to lumbosacral pain. NY State J. Med. **48** (1948) 2475–2480
2. Auberger, H. G., Niesel, H. C.: Gesichtsschädel: Proximale Leitungsanästhesie im Bereich des N. trigeminus. In: Auberger, H. G., Niesel, H. C. (Hrsg.): Praktische Lokalanästhesie. (4. Auflage) Georg Thieme Verlag, Stuttgart – New York (1982)
3. Berger, J. J., Pyles, S. T., Saga-Rumley, S. A.: Does topical anesthesia of the sphenopalatine ganglion with cocaine or lidocaine relieve low back pain? Anesth. Analg. **65** (1986) 700–702
4. Bonica, J. J.: Block of cranial nerves. In: Bonica, J. J. (ed.): The management of Pain. (2nd ed.) Lea & Febiger, Philadelphia (1990)

5. Byrd, H., Byrd, W.: Sphenopalatine phenomena: Present status of knowledge. Arch. Intern. Med. **46** (1930) 1026–1038

6. Devogel, J. C.: Cluster headache and sphenopalatine block. Acta Anesth. Belg. **32** (1981) 101–107

7. Jenkner, F. L.: Nervenblockaden auf pharmakologischem und auf elektrischem Weg. Springer, Wien (1980)

8. Lebovits, A. H., Alfred, H., Lefkowitz, M.: Sphenopalatine ganglion block: Clinical use in the pain management clinic. Clin. J. Pain **6** (1990) 131–136

9. Moore, D. C.: Regional Block. (4th ed.) Charles Thomas, Springfield (1976)

10. Murphy, T. M.: Somatic Blockade of Head and Neck. In: Cousins, M. J., Bridenbaugh, P. O. (eds.): Neural Blockade. (2nd ed.) Lippincott, Philadelphia (1988)

11. Netter, F. H.: Nervengeflechte und periphere Nerven. In: Krämer, G. (Hrsg.): Farbatlanten der Medizin. (Band 5). Nervensystem I: Neuroanatomie und Physiologie. Georg Thieme Verlag, Stuttgart – New York (1987)

12. Prasanna, A., Murthy, P. S. N.: Sphenopalatine ganglion block and pain of cancer. J. of Pain **8** (3) (1993) 125

13. Petren, T.: Anatomie des Nervus trigeminus. In: Eriksson, E. (Hrsg.): Atlas der Lokalanästhesie. (2. Auflage) Springer-Verlag, Berlin – Heidelberg – New York (1980)

14. Reder, M., Hymanson, A. S., Reder, M.: Sphenopalatine ganglion block in treatment of acute and chronic pain. In: Hendle, N. H., Long, D. M., Wise, T. N. (eds.): Diagnosis and treatment of chronic pain. John Wright, Boston (1982)

15. Rosen, S., Shelesnyak, M. C., Zacharias, L. R.: Nasogenital relationship II. Pseudopregnancy following extirpation of sphenopalatine ganglion in rat. Endocrinology **27** (1940) 463–468

16. Ruskin, A. P.: Sphenopalatine (nasal) ganglion: Remote effects including "psychosomatic" symptoms, rage reaction, pain and spasm. Arch. Phys. Med. Rehabil. **60** (1979) 353–358

17. Ruskin, S. L.: The neurologic aspects of nasal sinus infections. Headaches and systemic disturbances of nasal ganglion origin. Arch. Otolaryng. **4** (10) (1929) 337–382

18. Saade, E., Paige, G. B.: Patient administrated sphenopalatine ganglion block. Reg. Anesthesia **21** (1) (1996) 68–70

19. Sluder, G.: Injection of the nasal ganglion and comparison of methods. In: Nasal Neurology, Headaches and Eye disorders. CV Mosby, St. Louis (1918)

20. Waldman, S. D.: Sphenopalatine ganglion block – 80 years later. Reg. Anesthesia **18** (1993) 274–276

21. Zacharias, L. R.: Further studies in naso-genital relationship: Anatomical studies of perihypophyseal region in rat. J. Comp. Neurol. **74** (1941) 421–445

Chapter 4: Cervicothoracic ganglion (stellate ganglion)

1. Abram, S. E., Boas, R. A.: Sympathetic and visceral nerve blocks. In: Benumof, L. J. (ed.): Clinical procedures in anesthesia and intensive care. Lippincott, Philadelphia (1992)

2. Bonica, J. J.: Cervicothoracic sympathetic block. In: Bonica, J. J. (ed.): Management of Pain. (2nd ed.) Lea & Febiger, Philadelphia – London (1990)

3. Carron, H., Litwiller, R.: Stellate ganglion block. Anesth. Analg. **54** (1975) 567–570

4. Colding, A.: The effect of regional sympathetic blocks in the treatment of herpes zoster. Acta Anesth. Scand. **13** (1969) 133–141

5. Dan, K., Higa, K., Noda, B.: Nerve block for herpetic pain. In: Fields, H. L. et al. (eds.): Advances in Pain Research and Therapy (Vol. 9.) Raven Press, New York (1985)

6. Davies, R. M.: Stellate ganglion block: A new approach. Anesthesia **7** (1952) 151–153

7. Dukes, R. R., Leroy, A. A.: Transient locked-in syndrome after vascular injection during stellate ganglion block. Reg. Anesthesia **18** (1993) 378–380

8. Fine, P. G., Ashburn, M. A.: Effect of stellate ganglion block with fentanyl on postherpetic neuralgia with a sympathetic component. Anesth. Analg. **67** (1988) 897–899

9. Floyd Jr., J. B.: Traumatic cerebral edema relieved by stellate ganglion anesthesia. South Med. J. **80** (1987) 1328

10. Ganz, H., Klein, H.: Verläufe und Spätergebnisse beim Hörsturz. HNO **16** (11) (1968) 334–339

11. Goto, F., Fujita, T., Kitani, Y., Kano, M.: Hyperbaric oxygen and stellate ganglion blocks for idiopathic sudden hearing loss. Acta Otorinolaring. **88** (1979) 335–342

12. Hardy, P. A. J., Wells, J. C. D.: Extent of sympathetic blockade after stellate ganglion block with bupivacaine. Pain **36** (1989) 193–196

13. Haug, O., Draper, W. L., Haug, S. A.: Stellate ganglion blocks for idiopathic sensorineural hearing loss. Arch. Otorinolaring. **102** (1) (1976) 5–8

14. Hickey, R.: Lokalanästhetikumstoxizität. In: Ramamurthy, S., Rogers, J. N. (Hrsg.): Schmerztherapeutische Entscheidungen. Ullstein Mosby, Berlin – Wiesbaden (1995)

15. Jankovic, D.: Die Effektivität der Ganglion stellatum Blockade bei Kopf- und Gesichtsschmerzen. Speyerer-Tage: Zeitgemäße Diagnostik und Therapie von Kopf-, Gesichts- und Schulterschmerzen, Speyer (1993)

16. Katz, J., Renck, H.: Stellatumblockade. In: Katz, J., Renck, H. (Hrsg.): Thorakoabdominale Nervenblockaden. Edition Medizin, Weinheim (1988)

17. Lang, J.: Klinische Anatomie der Halswirbelsäule. Thieme, Stuttgart – New York (1991)

18. Lang, J.: Einige Befunde zur Anatomie des Halssympathikus. Med. Orth. Tech. **112** (1992) 194–200

19. Löfström, B. J., Cousins, M. J.: Sympathetic neural blockade of upper and lower extremity. In: Cousins, M. J., Bridenbaugh, P. O. (eds.): Neural Blockade. (2nd ed.) Lippincott, Philadelphia (1988)

20. Malmquist, R. N., Bengtsson, M., Sörensen, J.: Efficacy of stellate ganglion block: A clinical study with bupivacaine. Reg. Anesthesia **17** (1992) 340–347

21. Matsuoka, H., Tokutomi, Y., Muteki, T., Yokoyama, M. M.: Influence of stellate ganglion block on the immune system. Masui Jap. J. Anesthesiology **34** (7) (1985) 917–923

22. Mays, K. S., North, W. C., Schnapp, M.: Stellate ganglion blocks with morphine in sympathetic type pain. J. Neurol. Neurosurg. Psychiat. **44** (1981) 189–190

23. Milligan, N. S., Nash, T. P.: Treatment of postherpetic neuralgia. A review of 77 consecutive cases. Pain **23** (1985) 381–386

24. Miyazaki, H., Tashiro, M., Kakiuchi, Y.: The effect of drug therapy and stellate ganglion block with or without oxygen inhalation on sudden hearing loss. Masui Jap. J. Anesthesiology **40** (8) (1991) 1251–1255

25. Moore, D. C.: Anterior (paratracheal) approach for block of the stellate ganglion. In: Moore, D. C. (ed.): Regional Block. (4th ed.) Charles Thomas, Springfield (1976)

26. Nabil, M. K. A.: Does sympathetic ganglionic block prevent postherpetic neuralgia? Reg. Anesthesia **20** (3) (1995) 227–233

27. Naveira, F. A., Morales, A.: Treatment of persistent cough after stellate ganglion block. Reg. Anesthesia **18** (1993) 312–314

28. Netter, F. H.: Autonomes Nervensystem. Autonome Innervation von Kopf und Hals. In: Krämer, G. (Hrsg.): Farbatlanten der Medizin (Band 5). Nervensystem I: Neuroanatomie und Physiologie. Georg Thieme Verlag, Stuttgart-New York (1987)

29. Olson, E. R., Ivy, H. B.: Stellate block for trigeminal zoster. J. Clin. Neuro-Ophth. 1 (1) (1981) 53–55

30. Scott, D. B.: Stellate ganglion block. In: Scott, D. B. (ed.): Techniques of Regional Anesthesia. Mediglobe, Singapore (1989)

31. Stannard, C. F., Glynn, C. J., Smith, S. P.: Dural puncture during attempted stellate ganglion block. Anesthesia **15** (1990) 952–954

32. Tenicella, R., Lovasik, D., Eaglstein, W.: Treatment of herpes zoster with sympathetic blocks. Clin. J. Pain **1** (1985) 63–67

33. Thompson, G. E., Brown, D. L.: Stellate block. In: Nunn, J. F., Utting, J. E., Brown Jr., B. R. (eds.): General Anesthesia. (5th ed.) Butterworths, London (1989)

34. Umeda, S., Hasihida, T., Kakita, T.: Clinical application of stellate ganglion morphine infiltration for chronic pain relief. Masui Jap. J. Anesthesiology **31** (1982) 1403–1406

35. Waldman, S. D., Waldman, K.: Reflex sympathetic dystrophy of the face and neck: Report of six patients treated with stellate ganglion block. Reg. Anesthesia **12** (1987) 15–17

36. Winnie, A. P., Hartwell, P. W.: Relationship between time of treatment of acute herpes zoster with sympathetic blockade and prevention of postherpetic neuralgia: Clinical support for a new theory of the mechanism by which sympathetic blockade provides therapeutic benefit. Reg. Anesthesia **18** (1993) 277–282

Chapter 5: Superior cervical ganglion

1. Gross, D.: Therapeutische Lokalanästhesie des Halsgrenzstranges. In: Gross, D. (Hrsg.): Therapeutische Lokalanästhesie. Hippokrates, Stuttgart (1972)

2. Harder, H. J.: Die Behandlung der Migraine Blanche und Ophthalmique mit Blockaden des Ganglion cervicale superius. Regional-Anaesthesie **4** (1981) 1–9

3. Jenkner, F. L.: Blockade des Ganglion cervicale superius. In: Jenkner, F. L. (Hrsg.): Nervenblockaden auf pharmakologischem und auf elektrischem Weg. Springer, Wien (1980)

4. Lang, J.: Klinische Anatomie der Halswirbelsäule. Thieme, Stuttgart – New York (1991)

5. Lang, J.: Einige Befunde zur Anatomie des Halssympathikus. Med. Orth. Techn. **112** (1992) 194–200

6. Matsuoka, H., Tokutomi, Y., Muteki, T., Yokojama, M. M.: Influence of stellate ganglion block on the immune system. Masui, Jap. J. Anesthesiology **34** (7) (1985) 917–923

7. Netter, F. H.: Nervengeflechte und periphere Nerven. In: Krämer, G. (Hrsg.): Farbatlanten der Medizin (Band 5). Nervensystem I: Neuroanatomie und Physiologie. Georg Thieme Verlag, Stuttgart – New York (1987)

Chapter 6: Deep (and superficial) cervical plexus

1. Castresana, E. J., Shaker, I. J:, Castresana, M. R.: Incidence of shunting during carotid endarterectomy: Regional versus general anesthesia. Reg. Anesthesia **22** (2, Suppl.) (1997)

2. Davies, M. J., Silbert, B. S., Scott, D. A., Cook, R. J., Mooney, P. H., Blyth, C.: Superficial and deep cervical plexus block for carotid artery surgery: A prospective study of 1000 blocks. Reg. Anesthesia **22** (5) (1997) 442–446
3. Moore, D. C.: Block of the cervical plexus. In: Moore, D. C. (ed.): Regional Block. (4th ed.) Charles Thomas, Springfield (1976)
4. Murphy, T. M.: Somatic blockade of head and neck. In: Cousins, M. J., Bridenbaugh, D. L. (eds.): Neural Blockade. (2nd ed.) Lippincott, Philadelphia (1988)

Chapter 7: Brachial plexus

1. Allesio, J. G., Rosenblum, M., Shea, K., Freitas, D.: A retrospective comparison of interscalene block and general anesthesia for ambulatory surgery and shoulder arthroscopy. Reg. Anesthesia **20** (1) (1995) 62–68
2. Barutell, C., Vidal, F., Raich, M., Montero, A.: A neurological complication following interscalene brachial plexus block. Anesthesia **35** (1980) 365–367
3. Blanchard, J., Ramamurthy, S.: Brachial plexus. In: Benumof, L. J. (ed.): Clinical procedures in anesthesia and intensive care. Lippincott, Philadelphia (1992)
4. Bridenbaugh, D. L.: The upper extremity: Somatic blockade. In: Cousins, M. J., Bridenbaugh, D. L. (eds.): Neural Blockade. (2nd ed.) Lippincott, Philadelphia (1988)
5. Büttner, J., Kemmer, A., Argo, A., Klose, R., Forst, R.: Axilläre Blockade des Plexus brachialis. Reg. Anaesth. **11** (1988) 7
6. Cockings, E., Moore, P. L., Lewis, R. C.: Transarterial brachial plexus blockade using high doses of 1,5% mepivacaine. Reg. Anesthesia **12** (1987) 159–164
7. Cooper, K., Kelley, M. N., Carrithers, J.: Perceptions of side effects following axillary block used for outpatient surgery. Reg. Anesthesia **20** (3) (1995) 212–216
8. De Jong, R. H.: Axillary block of the brachial plexus. Anesthesiology **22** (1961) 215–225
9. De Jong, R. H.: Modified axillary block. Anesthesiology **26** (1965) 615
10. De Jong, R. H., Wagman, I. H.: Physiological mechanisms of peripheral nerve block by local anesthetics. Anesthesiology **24** (1963) 684–727
11. Durrani, Z., Winnie, A. P.: Brainstem toxicity with reversible locked-in syndrome after interscalene brachial plexus block. Anesth. Analg. **72** (1991) 249–252
12. Fletcher, D., Kuhlman, G., Samii, K.: Addition of fentanyl to 1,5% lidocaine does not increase the success of axillary plexus block. Reg. Anesthesia **19** (3) (1994) 183–188

13. Gentili, M. E., Le foulon-Gourves, M., Mamelle, J. C.: Acute respiratory failure following interscalene block: Complications of combined general and regional anesthesia. Reg. Anesthesia **19** (4) (1994) 292–293
14. Greene Jr., E. R.: Intravascular injection of local anesthetics after veni puncture of axillary vein during attempted brachial plexus block. Anesth. Analg. **65** (1986) 421
15. Groh, G. I., Gainor, J. B., Jeffries, J. T., Brown, M.: Pseudoaneurysm of the axillary artery with median-nerve deficit after axillary block anesthesia. Bone Joint Surg. **72** (1990) 1407–1408
16. Haasio, J., Tuominen, M. K., Rosenberg, P. H.: Continuous interscalene brachial plexus block during and after shoulder surgery. Ann. Chir. Gynaecol. **79** (1990) 103–107
17. Hickey, R., Rogers, J., Hoffman, J., Ramamurthy, S.: Comparison of the clinical efficacy of three perivascular techniques for axillary brachial plexus block. Reg. Anesthesia **18** (1993) 335–338
18. Hirschel, G.: Anästhesierung des Plexus brachialis bei Operationen an der oberen Extremität. Münchn. med. Wschr. **58** (1911) 1555–1556
19. Jankovic, D.: Blockadetechniken des Plexus brachialis. Eine prospektive klinische Studie über 430 Blockaden. Inauguraldissertation. Mainz (1981)
20. Kardash, K., Schools, A., Concepcion, M.: Effects of brachial plexus fentanyl on supraclavicular block. Reg. Anesthesia **20** (4) (1995) 311–315
21. Kulenkampff, D.: Die Anästhesierung des Plexus brachialis. Dtsch. med. Wschr. **38** (1912) 1878–1880
22. Kumar, A., Battit, G. E., Froese, A. B., Long, M. C.: Bilateral cervical and thoracic epidural blockade complicating interscalene brachial plexus block: Report of two cases. Anesthesiology **35** (1971) 650–652
23. Lanz, E., Theiss, D., Jankovic, D.: The extent of blockade following various techniques of brachial plexus block. Anesth. Analg. **62** (1983) 55–58
24. Lennon, R. L., Stinson Jr., L. W.: Continuous axillary brachial plexus catheters. In: Morrey, B. F. (ed.): The Elbow and its Disorders. (2nd ed.) W. B. Saunders, Philadelphia (1993)
25. Löfström, B., Wennberg, A., Widen, L.: Late disturbances in nerve function after block with local anesthetic agents. Acta Anesth. Scand. **10** (1966) 111–122
26. Mehler, D., Otten, B.: Ein neuer Katheterset zur kontinuierlichen axillären Plexusanaesthesie. Regional-Anaesthesie **6** (1983) 43–46
27. Moore, D. C.: Supraclavicular (axillar) approach for block of the Brachial plexus. In: Moore, D. C. (ed.): Regional Block. (4th ed.) Charles Thomas, Springfield (1976)

28. Neil, R. S.: Postoperative analgesia following brachial plexus block. Br. J. Anaesth. **50** (1978) 379–382

29. Netter, F. H.: Nervengeflechte und periphere Nerven. In: Krämer, G. (Hrsg.): Farbatlanten der Medizin (Band 5). Nervensystem I: Neuroanatomie und Physiologie. Georg Thieme Verlag, Stuttgart – New York (1987)

30. Ott, B., Neuberger, L., Frey, H. P.: Obliteration of the axillary artery after axillary block. Anesthesia **44** (1989) 773–774

31. Pere, P.: The effect of continuous interscalene brachial plexus block with 0,125% bupivacaine plus fentanyl on diaphragmatic motility and ventilatory function. Reg. Anesthesia **18** (1993) 93–97

32. Poeck, K.: Therapie der peripheren Nervenschädigungen. In: Poeck, K. (Hrsg.): Neurologie. (9. Aufl.) Springer, Berlin – Heidelberg – New York (1994)

33. Postel, J., März, P.: Elektrische Nervenlokalisation und Kathetertechnik. Ein sicheres Verfahren zur Plexus brachialis Anaesthesie. Regional-Anaesthesie 7 (1984) 104–108

34. Raj, P. P., Montgomery, S. J., Nettles, D., Jenkins, M. T.: Infraclavicular brachial plexus block – A new approach. Anesth. Analg. **52** (1973) 897–904

35. Ross, S., Scarborough, C. D.: Total spinal anesthesia following brachial plexus block. Anesthesiology **39** (1973) 458

36. Sada, T., Kobayashi, T., Murakami, S.: Continuous axillary brachial plexus block. Can. Anaesth. Soc. J. **30** (1983) 201

37. Selander, D.: Catheter technique in axillary plexus block. Acta Anesth. Scand. **21** (1977) 324–329

38. Selander, D., Dhuner, K. G., Lundborg, G.: Peripheral nerve injury due to injection needles used for regional anesthesia. Acta Anesth. Scand. **21** (1977) 182–188

39. Selander, D., Brattsand, R., Lundborg, G., Nordborg, C., Olsson, Y.: Local anesthetics: Importance of mode of application, concentration and adrenaline for the appearance of nerve lesions. Acta Anesth. Scand. **23** (1979) 127–136

40. Selander, D., Edshage, S., Wolff, T.: Paraesthesiae or no paraesthesiae? Acta Anesth. Scand. **23** (1979) 27–33

41. Siler, J. N., Liff, P. I., Davis, J. F.: A new complication of interscalene brachial plexus block. Anesthesiology **38** (6) (1973) 590–591

42. Stan, T. C., Krantz, M. A., Solomon, D. L.: The incidence of neurovascular complications following axillary brachial plexus block using a transarterial approach. Reg. Anesthesia **20** (6) (1995) 486–492

43. Stark, P., Watermann, W. F.: Die Anwendung des Nervenstimulators zur Nervenblockade. Regional-Anaesthesie **1** (1978) 16–19

44. Stinson Jr., L. W., Lennon, R. L., Adams, R. A., Morrey, B. F.: The technique and efficacy of axillary catheter analgesia as an adjunct to distraction elbow arthroplasty: A prospective study. J. Shoulder Elbow Surg. **2** (1993) 182–189

45. Tetzlaff, J. E., Yoon, H. J., Brems, J.: Interscalene brachial plexus block for shoulder surgery. Reg. Anesthesia **19** (5) (1994) 339–343

46. Tetzlaff, J. E., Yoon, H. J., Dilger, J., Brems, J.: Subdural anesthesia as a complication of an interscalene brachial plexus block. Reg. Anesthesia **19** (5) (1994) 357–359

47. Theiss, D., Robbel, G., Theiss, M., Gerbershagen, H. U.: Experimentelle Bestimmung einer optimalen Elektrodenanordnung zur elektrischen Nervenlokalisation. Anaesthesist **26** (1977) 411–417

48. Travell, J. G., Simons, D. G.: Myofascial Pain and Dysfunction. The Trigger Point Manual. (Vol. 1) Williams & Wilkins, Baltimore (1983)

49. Urban, M. K., Urquhart, B.: Evaluation of brachial plexus anesthesia for upper extremity surgery. Reg. Anesthesia **19** (3) (1994) 175–182

50. Viel, E. J., Eledjam, J. J., de la Coussage, J. E., D'Athis, F.: Brachial plexus block with opioids for postoperative pain relief: Comparison between buprenorphine and morphine. Reg. Anesthesia **14** (1989) 274–278

51. Wall, J. J.: Axillary nerve blocks. Am. Fam. Physician **11** (1975) 135–142

52. Winchell, S. W., Wolf. R.: The incidence of neuropathy following upper extremity nerve blocks. Reg. Anesthesia **10** (1985) 12–15

53. Winnie, A. P.: An "immobile needle" for nerve blocks. Anesthesiology **31** (1969) 577–578

54. Winnie, A. P.: Interscalene brachial plexus block. Anesth. Analg. **49** (1970) 455–466

55. Winnie, A. P.: Regional Anesthesia. Surg. Clin. North America **54** (1975) 861–881

56. Winnie, A. P.: Does the transarterial technique of axillary block provide a higher success rate and a lower complication rate than a paresthesia technique? Reg. Anesthesia **20** (6) (1995) 482–485

57. Winnie, A. P., Collins, V. J.: The subclavian perivascular technique of brachial plexus anesthesia. Anesthesiology **25** (1964) 353–363

58. Winnie, A. P., Radonjic, R., Akkineni, S. R., Durrani, Z.: Factors influencing distribution of local anesthetics injected into the brachial plexus sheath. Anesth. Analg. **58** (1979) 225–234

59. Zipkin, M., Backus, W. W., Scott, B.: False aneurysm of the axillary artery following brachial plexus block. J. Clin. Anesth. **3** (1991) 143–145

Chapter 8: Suprascapular nerve
Chapter 9: Subscapular nerve blocks

1. Bonica, J. J., Buckley, P. F.: Regional analgesia with local anesthetics. In: Bonica, J. J. (ed.): Management of Pain. (2nd ed.) Lea & Febiger, Philadelphia-London (1990)
2. Mercadante, S., Sapio, M., Villari, P.: Suprascapular nerve block by catheter for breakthrough shoulder cancer pain. Reg. Anesthesia **20** (4) (1995) 343–346
3. Moore, D. C.: Block of the suprascapular nerve. In: Moore, D. C. (ed.): Regional Block. (4th ed.) Charles Thomas, Springfield (1976)
4. Mumenthaler, M.: Der Schulter-Arm-Schmerz. Huber, Bern – Stuttgart – Wien (1980)
5. Netter, F. H.: Nervengeflechte und periphere Nerven. In: Krämer, G. (Hrsg.): Farbatlanten der Medizin (Band 5). Nervensystem I: Neuroanatomie und Physiologie. Georg Thieme Verlag, Stuttgart – New York (1987)
6. Travell, J. G., Simons, D. G.: Myofascial Pain and Dysfunction. The Trigger Point Manual. (Vol. 1) Williams & Wilkins, Baltimore (1983)

Chapter 10: Peripheral nerve blocks in the elbow region
Chapter 11: Peripheral nerve blocks in the wrist region

1. Bridenbaugh, D. L.: The upper extremity: Somatic blockade. In: Cousins, M. J., Bridenbaugh, D. L. (eds.): Neural-Blockade. (2nd ed.) Lippincott, Philadelphia (1988) 405–416
2. Brown, D. L.: Distal upper extremity blocks. In: Atlas of Regional Anesthesia. W. B. Saunders (1992) 48–54
3. Covic, D.: Blockaden peripherer Nerven im Ellenbogenbereich. Blockade peripherer Nerven im Handwurzelbereich. In: Hoerster, W., Kreuscher, H., Niesel, H. C, Zenz, M. (Red.): Regionalanaesthesie. Gustav Fischer Verlag, Stuttgart (1989) 86–101
4. Löfström,B.: Blockade der peripheren Nerven des Armes in der Ellenbeuge. Blockade der peripheren Nerven des Armes in der Handwurzelgegend. In: Eriksson, E. (Hrsg.): Atlas der Lokalanaesthesie. (2. Auflage) Springer (1980) 86–92
5. Netter, F. H.: Nervengeflechte und periphere Nerven. In: Krämer, G. (Hrsg.): Farbatlanten der Medizin (Band 5). Nervensystem I: Neuroanatomie und Physiologie. Georg Thieme Verlag, Stuttgart – New York (1987)

Chapter 12: Intravenous sympathetic block with guanethidine (Ismelin®)

1. Hannington-Kiff, J.: Intravenous regional sympathetic block with guanethidine. Lancet I, (1974) 1010–1020
2. Hannington-Kiff, J.: Antisympathetic drugs in limbs. In: Wall, P. D., Melzack, R. (eds.): Textbook of Pain. Churchill Livingstone, London (1984)
3. Wahren, K. L., Gordh, T., Torebjörk, E.: Effects of regional intravenous guanethidine in patients with neuralgia in the hand, a follow up study over a decade. Pain **62** (1995) 379–385

Chapter 13: Thoracic spinal nerve blocks
Chapter 14: Lumbar paravertebral somatic nerve block
Chapter 15: Lumber sympathetic block
Chapter 16: Iliolumbosacral ligaments
Chapter 17: Celiac plexus block

1. Brown, D. L.: Intercostal Block. In: Brown, D. L.(ed.): Atlas of Regional Anesthesia. W. B. Saunders Company (1992) 211–217
2. Buy, J. N., Moss, A. A., Singler, R. C.: CT guided celiac plexus and splanchnic nerve neurolysis. J. Comput. Ass. Tomogr. **6** (1982) 315
3. Galizia, E. J., Lahiri, S. K.: Paraplegia following coeliac plexus block with phenol. Br. J. Anaesth. **46** (1974) 539
4. Gerbershagen, H. U., Panhans, C., Waisbrod, H., Schreiner, K.: Diagnostische Lokalanaesthesie zur Differenzierung des Kreuzschmerzursprungs. Teil I, Kreuzschmerz bei ilio-lumbo-sakraler Bänderinsuffizienz. Rohrer GmbH, Bielefeld (1986)
5. Hegedues, V.: Relief of pancreatic pain by radiography-guided block. Am. J. Roentgenol. **133** (1979) 1101
6. Jenkner, F. L.: Blockade der Interkostalnerven; Blockade der thorakalen Spinalnerven (paravertebral). In: Jenkner, F. L.: Nervenblockaden auf pharmakologischen und auf elektrischem Weg. Springer Verlag, Wien (1980)
7. Katz, J., Renck, H.: Thorakale paravertebrale Blockade (S. 130); Interkostale Nervenblockade (S. 132–134). In: Katz, J., Renck, H. (Hrsg.): Thorakoabdominale Nervenblockaden. Edition Medizin, Weinheim (1988)
8. Kirvelä, O., Antila, H.: Thoracic paravertebral block in chronic postoperative pain. Reg. Anesth. **17** (1992) 348–350

9. Klein, S. M., Greengrass, R. A., Weltz, C., Warner, D. S.: Paravertebral somatic nerve block for outpatient inguinal herniorrhaphy: An expanded case report of 22 patients. Reg. Anesth. and Pain Med. **23** (3) (1998) 306–310

10. Moore, D. C.: Intercostal Nerve Block; Paravertebral thoracic somatic Nerve Block. In: Moore, D. C. (ed.): Regional Block. (4th ed.) Charles Thomas, Springfield (1976) 163–166, 200–204

11. Netter, F. H.: Nervengeflechte und periphere Nerven. In: Krämer, G. (Hrsg.): Farbatlanten der Medizin (Band 5). Nervensystem I: Neuroanatomie und Physiologie. Georg Thieme Verlag, Stuttgart – New York (1987)

12. Sayed, I., Elias, M.: Acute chemical pericarditis following celiac plexus block. Middle East J. Anesthesiol. **14** (3) (1997) 201–205

13. Thompson, G. E., Moore, D. C.: Celiac plexus, intercostal and minor peripheral blockade. In: Cousins, M.J., Bridenbaugh, D.L. (eds.): Neural Blockade. (2nd ed.) Lippincott, Philadelphia (1988)

14. Wassef, M. R., Randazzo, T., Ward, W.: The paravertebral nerve root block for inguinal herniorrhaphy – A comparison with the field block approach. Reg. Anesth. and Pain Med. **23** (5) (1998) 451–456

15. Wong, G. Y., Brown, D. L.: Transient paraplegia following alcohol celiac plexus block. Reg. Anesth. **20** (4) (1995) 352–355

1. Berkowitz, A., Rosenberg, H.: Femoral block with mepivacaine for muscle biopsy in malignant hyperthermia patients. Anesthesiology **62** (1985) 651–652

2. Bridenbaugh, P. O.: The lower extremity: Somatic blockade. In: Cousins, M. J., Bridenbaugh, D. L. (eds.): Neural Blockade in Clinical Anesthesia and Management of Pain. (2nd ed.) Lippincott, Philadelphia (1988) 417–441

3. Chayen, D., Nathan, H., Clayen, M.: The psoas compartment block. Anesthesiology **45** (1976) 95–99

4. Elmas, C., Atanassoff, P.: Combined inguinal paravascular (3 in 1) and sciatic nerve blocks for lower limb surgery. Reg. Anesth. **18** (1993) 88–92

5. Frerk, C. M.: Palsy after femoral nerve block. Anaesthesia **43** (1988) 167–168

6. Hirst, G. C., Lang, S. A., Dust, W. N., Cassidy, D., Yip, R.W.: Femoral nerve block. Single injection versus continuous infusion for total knee arthroplasty. Reg. Anesth. **21** (4) (1996) 292–297

7. Hoerster, W.: Blockaden peripherer Nerven im Bereich des Kniegelenkes; Blockaden im Bereich des Fußgelenkes (Fußblock). In: Hoerster, W., Kreuscher, H., Niesel, H. C., Zenz, M. (Red.): Regionalanaesthesie. Gustav Fischer Verlag, Stuttgart (1989) 124–139

8. Kofoed, H.: Peripheral nerve blocks at the knee and ancle in operations for common foot disorders. Clin. Orthop. **168** (1982) 97–101

9. Lynch, J.: Prolonged motor weakness after femoral nerve block with bupivacaine 0,5%. Anaesthesia **45** (1990) 421

10. McCutcheon, R.: Regional anesthesia for the foot. Can. Anaesth. Soc. J. **12** (1995) 465

11. Misra, U., Pridie, A. K., McClymont, C., Bower, S.: Plasma concentrations of bupivacaine following combined sciatic and femoral 3 in 1 nerve blocks in open knee surgery. Br. J. Anaesth. **66** (1991) 310– 313

12. Moore, D. C.: Regional Block. (4th ed.) Charles Thomas, Springfield (1976)

13. Ringrase, N. H., Cross, M. J.: Femoral nerve block in knee joint surgery. Am. J. Sports Med. **12** (1984) 398–402

14. Rooks, M., Fleming, L. L.: Evaluation of acute knee injuries with sciatic femoral nerve blocks. Clin Orthop. **179** (1983) 185–188

15. Rorie, D. K., Beyer, D. E., Nelson, D. O.: Assessment of block of the sciatic nerve in popliteal fossa. Anesth. Analg. **59** (1980) 371–376

16. Singelyn, F. J., Gouverneur, J. M.: The continuous "3-in-1" block as postoperative pain treatment after hip, femoral shaft or knee surgery: A large scale study of efficacy and side effects. Anesthesiology **81** (1994) 1064

17. Smith, B. E., Fischer, A. B. J., Scott, P. U.: Continuous sciatic nerve block. Anaesthesia **39** (1984) 155–157

18. Winnie, A. P., Ramamurthy, S., Durani, Z.: The inguinal paravascular technic of lumbar plexus anesthesia: The "3-in-1" block. Anesth. Analg. **52** (1973) 989–996

Chapter 27: **Neuraxial anatomy**
Chapter 28: **Spinal anesthesia**
Chapter 29: **Complications of spinal anesthesia**
Chapter 30: **Continuous spinal anesthesia (CSA)**
Chapter 31: **Continuous spinal anesthesia (CSA) in obstetrics**
Chapter 32: **Chemical intraspinal neurolysis with phenol in glycerine**

1. Abboud, T. K., Raya, J., Noueihed, R., Daniel, J.: Intrathecal morphine for relief of labor pain in parturient with severe pulmonary hypertension. Anesthesiology **59** (1983) 477–479

2. Abouleish, E., de la Vega, S., Blendinger, I., Tio, T.: Long-term follow up of epidural blood patch. Anaesth. Analg. **54** (1975) 459–463

3. Arkoosh, V.: Continuous spinal analgesia and anesthesia in obstetrics. Reg. Anesth. **18** (1993) 402–405

4. Armstrong, L. A., Littlewood, D. G., Chambers, W. A.: Spinal anesthesia with tetracaine – the effect of added vasoconstrictors. Anaesth. Analg. **62** (1983) 793

5. Atulkumar, M. K., Foster, P. A.: Adrenocorticotropic hormone infusion as a novel treatment for postdural puncture headache. Reg. Anesth. **22** (5) (1997) 432–434

6. Bannister, R.: Brain's clinical neurology. (6th ed.) Oxford University Press (1985) 52

7. Barash, P. G., Cullen, B. F., Stoelting, R. K. In: Barash, P. G., Cullen, B. F., Stoelting, R. K. (eds.): Clinical Anesthesia. Lippincott Comp, Philadelphia (1989) 778–780

8. Baxter, A.: Continuous spinal anesthesia: The Canadian perspective. Reg. Anesth. **18** (1993) 414–418

9. Beards, S. C., Jackson, A., Griffiths, A. G., Horsman, E. L.: Magnetic resonance imaging of extradural blood patches: Appearances from 30 min to 18 h. Br. J. Anaesth. **71** (1993) 182–188

10. Bergmann, H.: Komplikationen, Fehler und Gefahren der Spinalanaesthesie. In: Nolte, H., Meyer, J. (Hrsg.): Die rückenmarksnahen Anaesthesien. Georg Thieme Verlag, Stuttgart (1972) 45

11. Bevacqua, B.: Continuous spinal anesthesia: Operative indication and clinical experience. Reg. Anesth. **18** (1993) 394–401

12. Bolton, V. E., Leicht, C. H., Scanlon, T. S.: Postpartum seizure after epidural blood patch and intravenous caffeine sodium benzoate. Anesthesiology **70** (1989) 146–149

13. Bridenbaugh, P. O., Greene, N.: Spinal (subarachnoid) Neural Blockade. In: Cousins, M. J., Bridenbaugh, P. O. (eds.): Neural Blockade. (2nd ed.) Lippincott, Philadelphia (1988)

14. Brizgys, R. V., Shnider, S. M: Hyperbaric intrathecal morphine analgesia during labor in a patient with Wolff-Parkinson-White syndrome. Obstet. Gynecol. **64** (3) (1984) 44–46

15. Caldwell, C., Nielsen, C., Baltz, T., Taylor, P.: Comparison of high dose epinephrine and phenylephrine in spinal anesthesia with tetracaine. Anesthesiology **62** (1995) 804

16. Camann, W. R., Murray, R. S., Mushlin, P. S., Lambert, D. H.: Effects of oral caffeine on postdural puncture headache: a double-blind, placebo-controlled trial. Anesth. Analg. **70** (1990) 181–184

17. Carp, H., Singh, P. J., Vahera, R., Jayaram, A.: Effects of the serotonin-receptor agonist sumatriptan on postdural puncture headache: Report of six cases. Anesth. Analg. **79** (1994) 180–182

18. Carrie, L. E. S.: Postdural puncture headache and extradural blood patch. Br. J. Anaesth. **71** (1993) 179

19. Cass, W., Edelist, G.: Postspinal headache. JAMA **227** (1974) 786–787

20. Chambers, W. A., Littlewood, D. G., Logan, M. R., Scott, D. B.: Effect of added epinephrine on spinal anesthesia with lidocaine. Anesth. Analg. **60** (1981) 417

21. Chambers, W. A., Littlewood, D. G., Scott, D. B.: Spinal anesthesia with bupivacaine: Effect of added vasoconstrictors. Anesth. Analg. **61** (1982) 49

22. Chibber, A. K., Lustik, S. J.: Unexpected neurologic deficit following spinal anesthesia. Reg. Anesth. **21** (4) (1996) 355–357

23. Clayton, K. C.: The incidence of Horner's syndrome during lumbar extradural for elective caesarean section and provision of analgesia during labour. Anaesthesia **38** (1983) 583–585

24. Collier, B. B: Treatment for dural puncture headache. Br. J. Anaesth. **72** (1994) 366

25. Concepcion, M., Maddi, R., Francis, D.: Vasoconstrictors in spinal anesthesia. A comparison of epinephrine and phenylephrine. Anesth. Analg. **63** (1984) 134

26. Craft, J. B., Epstein, B. S., Coakley, C. S.: Prophylaxis of dural-puncture headache with epidural saline. Anesth. Analg. **52** (1973) 228–231

27. Dahlgren, N., Törnebrandt, K.: Neurological complications after anaesthesia. A follow-up of 18000 spinal and epidural anaesthetics performed over three years. Acta. Anaesth. Scand. **39** (1995) 872–880

28. Day, C. J., Schutt, L. E.: Auditory, ocular and facial complications of central neural block. A review of possible mechanisms. Reg. Anesth. **21** (3) (1996) 197–201

29. Di Giovanni, A. J., Dunbar, B. S.: Epidural injections of autologous blood for postlumbar-puncture headache. Anesth. Analg. **49** (1970) 268–271

30. Drasner, K.: Cauda equina syndrome and continuous spinal anesthesia (Letter). Anesthesiology **78** (1993) 215–216
31. Drasner, K.: Models for local anesthetic toxicity from continuous spinal anesthesia. Reg. Anesth. **18** (1993) 424–438
32. Dripps, R. D., Vandam, L. D.: Long-term follow-up of patients who received 10098 spinal anesthetics. I. Failure to discover major neurological sequelae. JAMA **156** (1954) 1486
33. Dunteman, E., Turner, S. W., Swarm, R.: Pseudo-spinal headache. Reg. Anesth. **21** (4) (1996) 358–360
34. Ford, C. D., Ford, D. C., Koenigsberg, M. D.: A simple treatment of post-lumbar-puncture headache. J. Emerg. Med. **7** (1989) 29–31
35. Freye, E.: Peridurale Analgesie mit Opioiden. In: Freye, E. (Hrsg): Opioide in der Medizin. Wirkung und Einsatzgebiete zentraler Analgetika. Springer (1995)
36. Gazmuri, R. R., Ricke, C. A., Dagnino, J. A.: Trigeminal nerve block as a complication of epidural anesthesia. Reg. Anesth. **17** (1992) 50–51
37. Gerbershagen, H. U., Baar, H. A., Kreuscher, H.: Langzeitnervenblockaden zur Behandlung schwerer Schmerzzustände. Die intrathekale Injektion von Neurolytika. Anaesthesist **21**, Springer (1972) 112–121
38. Giering, H., Glözner, F. L., Pock, H. G.: Persistierendes Querschnittsyndrom nach Spinalanaesthesie. Anaest. Intensivmed. **10** (38) (1997) 505–508
39. Gogarten, W., Van Aken, H., Wulff, H., Klose, R., Vandermeulen, E., Harenberg, J.: Rückenmarksnahe Regionalanaesthesien und Thromboembolieprophylaxe/Antikoagulation. Empfehlung der Deutschen Gesellschaft für Anaesthesiologie und Intensivmedizin. Anaesth. Intensivmed. **12** (38) (1997) 623–628
40. Gonsales-Carrasco, J., Nogues, S., Aguilar, J. L., Vidal-Lopez, F., Llubia, C.: Pneumocephalus after accidental dural puncture during epidural anesthesia. Reg. Anesth. **18** (1993) 193–195
41. Harrington, T. M.: An alternative treatment for spinal headache. J. Fam. Pract. **15** (1982) 172–177
42. Hawkins, J. L.: Wet tap during labor – now what? Am. Soc. Reg. Anesth. 12th Annual Meeting, Syllabue (1995) 259–270
43. Heavner, J. R., De Jong, R. H.: Lidocaine blocking concentration for B and C nerve fibers. Anaesthesiology **40** (1974) 228–233
44. Hönig, O., Winter, H., Baum, K. R., Schöder, P., Winter, P.: Sectio caesarea in Katheter-Spinalanästhesie bei einer kardiopulmonalen Hochrisikopatientin. Anaesthesist **47**, Springer Verlag (1998) 685–689
45. Hurey, R.: Continuous spinal anesthesia: A historical perspective. Reg. Anesth. **18** (1993) 390–393
46. Jaradeh, S.: Cauda equina syndrome: A neurologist's perspective. Reg. Anesth. **18** (1993) 473–480
47. Jarvis, A. P., Greenawalt, J. W., Fagraeus, L.: Intravenous caffeine for postdural puncture headache. Anesth. Analg. **65** (1986) 316–317
48. Kalichman, M.: Physiologic mechanisms by which local anesthetics may cause injury to nerve and spinal cord. Reg. Anesth. **18** (1993) 448–452
49. Kubina, P., Gupta, A., Oscarsson, A., Axelsson, K., Bengstsson, M.: Two cases of cauda equina syndrome following spinal-epidural anesthesia. Reg. Anesth. **22** (5) (1997) 447–450
50. Larsen, R.: Spinalanaesthesie. In: Larsen, R. (Hrsg): Anaesthesie. (4. Auflage) Urban & Schwarzenberg (1985)
51. Lehmann, L. J., Hacobian, A., De Sio, M.: Successful use of epidural blood patch for postdural puncture headache following lumbar sympathetic block. Reg. Anesth. **21** (4) (1996) 347–349
52. Leicht, C. H., Evans, D. E., Durkan, W. J., Noltner, S.: Sufentanil versus fentanyl intrathecally for labor analgesia. Anesth Analg **72** (1991) 159
53. Le Polain, B., De Kock, M., Scoltes, J. L., Vanleirde, M.: Clonidine combined with sufentanil and bupivacaine with adrenaline for obstetric analgesia. Br. J. Anaesth. **71** (1993) 657–660
54. Levinson, G.: Spinal Anesthesia. In: Benumof, J.: Clinical procedures in anesthesia and intensive care. Lippincott, Philadelphia (1992) 645–661
55. Lowe, D. M., Mc Cullough, A. M.: 7th nerve palsy after extradural blood patch. Br. J. Anaesth. **65** (1990) 721–722
56. Lund, P. C.: Principles and practise of spinal anesthesia. IL Charles Thomas, Springfield (1971)
57. Maher, R., Mehta, M.: Spinal (intrathecal) and extradural analgesia. In: Lipton, S. (ed.): Persistant pain. Modern methods of treatment. (Vol. 1) Academic Press, London (1977)
58. Möllmann, M., Auf der Landwehr, U.: Post-operative Analgesia following continuous Spinal Anesthesia (CSA). B. Braun Satellite Symposium: Continuous Regional post-operative Analgesia: Breaking up some taboos. 17 ESRA Congress Geneva, (Sept. 1998)
59. Möllmann, M.: St. Franziskus Hospital Münster. Persönliche Mitteilung (1998)
60. Netter, F. H.: Knöcherne Bedeckung des Gehirns und des Rückenmarks; Makroskopische Anatomie des Gehirns und des Rückenmarks. In: Krämer, G. (Hrsg.): Farbatlanten der Medizin (Band 5). Nervensystem I. Neuroanatomie und Physiologie. Thieme Verlag, Stuttgart – New York (1987)

61. Norris, M. C., Leighton, B. L.: Some useful information for obstetrical anesthesia. In: Physician Education Program in Regional Anesthesia. (Volume 2) Becton & Dickinson, (1994)

62. Paech, M. J.: Unexplained neurologic deficit after uneventful combined spinal and epidural anesthesia for ceasarean delivery. Reg. Anesth. **22** (5) (1997) 479–482

63. Palmer, C. M.: Early respiratory depression following intrathecal fentanyl-morphine combination. Anesthesiology **74** (1991) 1153–1155

64. Perez, M., Olmos, M., Garrido, J.: Facial nerve paralysis after epidural blood patch. Reg. Anesth. **18** 1(1993) 96–198

65. Poeck, K.: Die wichtigsten neurologischen Syndrome. In: Poeck, K. (Hrsg.): Neurologie. (9. Aufl.) Springer Verlag, Berlin – Heidelberg – New York (1994)

66. Ravindran, R. S., Bond, V. K., Tasch, M. D., Gupta, C. D., Leurssen, T. G.: Prolonged neural blockade following regional anesthesia with 2-chloroprocaine. Anesth. Analg. **59** (1980) 447–454

67. Rawal, N.: Klinischer Einsatz der rückenmarksnahen Opioidanalgesie. Teil 1. Der Schmerz **10**, Springer Verlag (1996) 176–189

68. Rawal, N.: Klinischer Einsatz der rückenmarksnahen Opioidanalgesie. Teil 2. Der Schmerz **10**, Springer Verlag (1996) 226–236

69. Ray, B. S., Hindey, J. C., Geohegan, W. A.: Preservations of the distribution of the sympathetic nerves to the pupil and upper extremity as determined by stimulation of the anterior nerve roots in man. Ann. Surg. **118** (1943) 647–655

70. Renck, H.: Neurological complications of central nerve blocks. Acta. Anaesth. Scand. **39** (1995) 859–868

71. Rigler, M. L., Drasner, K., Krejcie, T. C., Yelich, S. J., Scholnick, F. T., De Fontes, J., Bohner, D.: Cauda equina syndrome after continuous spinal anesthesia. Anesth. Analg. **72** (1991) 275–281

72. Sechzer, P. H., Abel, L.: Post-spinal anesthesia headache treated with caffeine: evaluation with demand method. Part I. Curr. Ther. Res. **24** (1978) 307–312

73. Sechzer, P. H.: Post-spinal anesthesia headache treated with caffeine, part II: intracranial vascular distention, a key factor. Curr. Ther. Res. **26** (1979) 440–448

74. Shigematsu, T., Wang, H., Nagano, M.: Trigeminal nerve palsy after lumbar epidural anesthesia. Anaesth. Analg. **64** (1985) 653

75. Spencer, H.: Postdural puncture headaches: what matters in technique. Reg. Anesth. and Pain Med. **23** (4) (1998) 374–379

76. Spivey, D. L.: Epinephrine does not prolong lidocaine spinal anesthesia in term parturients. Anaesth. Analg. **64** (1985) 468

77. Sprung, J., Haddox, J. D., Maitra-D'Cruze, A. M.: Horner's syndrome and trigeminal nerve palsy following epidural anesthesia for obstetrics. Can. J. Anesth. **38** (1991) 767–771

78. Stevens, D. S., Peeters-Asdourian, C.: Treatment of postdural puncture headache with epidural dextran patch. Reg. Anesth. **18** (1993) 324–325

79. Tetzlaff, J., O'Hara, J., Bell, G., Grimm, K., Yoon, H.: Influence of baricity on the outcome of spinal anesthesia with bupivacaine for lumbar spine surgery. Reg. Anesth. **20** (6) (1995) 533–537

80. Thomas, P. K.: Other cranial nerves. In: D. J., Ledingham, J. G. G., Warell, D. A. (eds.): Weatherall, Oxford Textbook of Medicine 21. (2nd ed.) Oxford University Press, Oxford (1988) 92

81. Usubiaga, J. E.: Neurological complications following epidural anesthesia. Int. Anaesth. Clin. **13** (1975) 33–96

82. Zenz, M., Donner, B.: Regionale Opioidanalgesie. In: Niesel, H. C. (Hrsg.): Regionalanaesthesie, Lokalanaesthesie, Regionale Schmerztherapie. Thieme Verlag (1994)

83. Zoys, T. N.: An overview of postdural puncture headaches and their treatment. In: ASRA Supplement of the American Society of Regional Anesthesia (1996)

Chapter 33: Lumbar epidural anesthesia
Chapter 34: Thoracic epidural anesthesia
Chapter 35: Epidural anesthesia in obstetrics
Chapter 36: Lumbar epidural anesthesia
**   in pediatric patients**
Chapter 37: Epidural steroid injection
Chapter 38: Combined spinal and epidural
**   anesthesia (CSE)**

1. Abram, S. E.: Perceived dangers from intraspinal steroid injections. Arch. Neurol. **46** (1989) 719–720

2. Abram, S. E., O'Connor, T.: Complications associated with epidural steroid injections. Reg. Anesth. **21** (2) (1996) 149–162

3. Bachmann-Mennenga, B.: Epidurale Analgesie in der Geburtshilfe. In: Van Aken, H. (Hrsg.): Regionalanaesthesiologische Aspekte, Band 10. Ein neues Lokalanaesthetikum – Naropin. Arcis Verlag, (1997)

4. Badner, N. H., Sandler, A. N., Koren, G.: Lumbar epidural fentanyl infusions for post-thoracotomy patients: analgesic, respiratory, and pharmacokinetic effects. J. Cardiothorac. Anesth. **4** (1990) 543

5. Baker, A. S., Ojemann, R. G., Schwarz, M. N., Richardson, E. P.: Spinal epidural abscess. N. Engl. J. Med. **293** (1975) 463–468

6. Benzon, H. R.: Epidural injections for low back pain and lumbosacral radiculopathy. Pain **24** (1986) 277–295

7. Bogduk, N.: Back pain: Zygapophysial blocks and epidural steroids. In: Cousins, M. J., Bridenbaugh, P. O. (eds.): Neural Blockade. (2nd ed.) Lippincott, Philadelphia (1988) 935–954

8. Brodsky, J. B., Kretzschmar, M., Mark, J. B. D.: Caudal epidural morphine for post-thoracotomy pain. Anesth. Analg. **67** (1988) 409

9. Bromage, P. R.: Diagnostic and therapeutic applications. In: Bromage, P. R. (ed.): Epidural Block. Saunders, Philadelphia (1978) 601–643

10. Bromage, P. R.: Anatomy. In: Bromage, P. R. (ed.): Epidural Block. Saunders, Philadelphia (1978) 8–67

11. Bromage, P. R.: Spinal extradural abscess: Pursuit of vigilance. Br. J. Anesth. **70** (1993) 471–473

12. Bromage, P., Benumof, J.: Paraplegia following intracord injection during attempted epidural anesthesia under general anesthesia. Reg. Anesth. and Pain Med. **23** (1) (1998) 104–107

13. Brownridge, P.: Epidural and subarachnoid analgesia for elective caesarean section. Anaesthesia **36** (1981) 70

14. Carrie, L. E. S., O'Sullivan, G: Subarachnoid bupivacaine 0,5% for caesarean section. Eur. J. Anaesth. **1** (1984) 275–283

15. Castagnera, L., Maurette, P., Pointillart, V., Vital, J., Erny, P., Senegas, J.: Long-term results of cervical epidural steroid injection with and without morphine in chronic cervical radicular pain. Pain **58** (1994) 239–243

16. Cherng, Y. G., Wang, Y. P., Liu, C. C., Shi, J. J., Huang, S. C.: Combined spinal and epidural anesthesia for abdominal hysterectomy in a patients with myotonic dystrophy. Reg. Anesth. **19** (1994) 69–72

17. Cherry, D. A.: Epidural depotcorticosteroids. Med. J. Austr. **2** (1983) 420

18. Chestnut, D. H., Owen, C. L., Brown, C. K., Vandewalker, G. E., Weiner, C. P.: Does labor affect the variability of maternal heart rate during induction of epidural anesthesia? Anesthesiology **68** (1988) 622

19. Cicala, R. S., Turner, R., Morgan, B. S. et al.: Methylprednisolone acetate does not cause inflammatory changes in the epidural space. Anesth. Analg. **72** (1990) 556–558

20. Coates, M.: Combined subarachnoid and epidural techniques. A single space technique for surgery of the hip and lower limb. Anaesthesia **37** (1982) 89

21. Coda, B., Bausch, S., Haas, M., Chavkin, C.: The hypothesis that antagonism of fentanyl analgesia by 2-chloroprocaine is mediated by direct action on opioid receptors. Reg. Anesth. **22** (1) (1997) 43–52

22. Cousins, M. J., Bromage, P. R.: Epidural Neural Blockade. In: Cousins, M. J., Bridenbaugh, P. O. (eds.): Neural Blockade. (2nd ed.) Lippincott, Philadelphia (1988) 253–274

23. Cousins, M. J., Bromage, P. R.: Epidural Neural Blockade. In: Cousins, M. J., Bridenbaugh, P. O. (eds.): Neural Blockade. (2nd ed.) Lippincott, Philadelphia (1988) 341

24. Covino, B. G., Scott, B. D.: Epidurale Anästhesie und Analgesie. Lehrbuch und Atlas. Edition Medizin, Weinheim (1987)

25. Curelaru, I.: Long duration subarachnoid anaesthesia with continuous epidural block. Prakt. Anästh. **14** (1979) 71–78

26. Delaney, T. J., Rowlingson, J. C., Carron, H., Butler, A.: Epidural steroid effects on nerves and meninges. Anesth. Analg. **58** (1980) 610–614

27. Delleur, M. M.: Continuous lumbar epidural block. In: Saint-Maurize, C., Schulte-Steinberg, O., Armitage, E. (eds.): Regional Anaesthesia in Children. Appleton & Lange, Mediglobe (1990) 106–109

28. Desparmet, J., Mateo, J., Ecoffey, C., Mazoit, X.: Efficacy of an epidural test dose in children anesthetized with halothane. Anesthesiology **72** (1990) 249

29. Eddleston, J. M., Holland, J. J., Griffin, R. P., Corbett, A., Horsman, E. L., Reynolds, F.: A double-blind comparison of 0,25% ropivacaine and 0,25% bupivacaine for extradural analgesia in labour. Br. J. Anaesth. **76** (1996) 66–71

30. Edmonds, C. L., Vance, L. M., Hughes, M.: Morbidity from paraspinal depot corticosteroid injections for analgesia: Cushing's syndrome and adrenalin suppression. Anesth. Analg. **72** (1991) 820–822

31. Forrest, J.: The response to epidural steroids in chronic dorsal root pain. Can. Anesth. Soc. J. **27** (1980) 40–46

32. Fromme, G. A., Steidl, L. J., Danielson, D. R.: Comparison of lumbal and thoracic epidural morphine for relief of postthoracotomy pain. Anesth. Analg. **64** (1985) 454

33. Gambling, D. R., Yu P. Cole, McMorland, G. H., Palmer, L.: A comparative study of patient controlled epidural analgesia (PCEA) and continuous infusion epidural analgesia (CIEA) during labour. Can. J. Anaesth. **35** (1988) 249–254

34. Gardner, W. J., Goebert, H. W., Sehgal, A. D.: Intraspinal corticosteroids in the treatment of sciatica. Trans. Am. Neurol. Assoc. **86** (1961) 214–215

35. Giaufre, E.: Single shot lumbar epidural block. In: Saint-Maurize, C., Schulte Steinberg, O., Armitage, E. (eds.): Regional Anaesthesia in Children. Appleton & Lange, Mediglobe (1990) 98–105

36. Goebert, H. W., Jallo, S. J., Gardner, W. J., Asmuth, C. E.: Painful radiculopathy treated with epidural

injections of procaine and hydrocortisone acetate. Results in 113 patients. Anesth. Analg. **140** (1961) 130–134

37. Goldstein, N. P., McKenzie, B. F., McGuckin, W. F., Mattox, V. R.: Experimental intrathecal administration of methylprednisolone acetate in multiple sclerosis. Trans. Am. Neurol. assoc. **95** (1970) 243–244

38. Goucke, C. R., Graziotti, P.: Extradural abscess following local anaesthetic and steroid injection for chronic low back pain. Br. J. Anaesth. **65** (1990) 427–429

39. Gronow, D. W., Mendelson, G.: Epidural injection of depot corticosteroids. Position Statement. Med. J. Austr. **157** (1992) 417–420

40. Guinard, J. P., Mulroy, M. F., Carpenter, R. L., Knopes, K. D.: Test doses optimal epinephrine content with and without acute beta-adrenergic blockade. Anesthesiology **73** (1990) 386

41. Guinard, J. P., Mulroy, M. F., Carpenter, R. L.: Aging reduces the reliability of epidural epinephrine test doses. Reg. Anesth. **20** (1995) 193

42. Harik, S. I., Raichle, M. E., Reis, D. J.: Spontaneously remitting spinal epidural hematoma in a patient on anticoagulants. N. Engl. J. Med. **284** (1971) 1355

43. Haynes, G., Melinda, K. B., Davis, S., Mahaffey, J. E.: Use of methylprednisolone in epidural analgesia. Arch. Neurol. **46** (1989) 1167–1168

44. Holmström, B., Laugaland, K., Rawal, N., Hallberg, S.: Combined spinal epidural block versus spinal and epidural block for orthopedic surgery. Can. J. Anaesth. **40** (1993) 601–606

45. Hopwood, M. B., Abram, S. E.: Factors associated with failure of lumbar epidural steroids. Reg. Anesth. **18** (1993) 238–243

46. Hurford, W. E., Dutton, R. P., Alfille, P. H., Clement, D., Wilson, R. S.: Comparison of thoracic and lumbar epidural infusions of bupivacaine and fentanyl for post-thoracotomy analgesia. J. Cardiothorac. Vasc. Anesth. **7** (1993) 521

47. Ivani, G.: Continuous epidural techniques for postoperative pain relief in paediatric use. B. Braun Satellite Symposium: Continuous Regional postoperative Analgesia: Breaking up some taboos. 17. ESRA Congress Geneva (Sept. 1998)

48. Ivani, G. (Head dept. of Anaesth. & Intensive Care, Regina Margherita Children's Hospital, Turin, Italy). Persönliche Mitteilung (1998)

49. Johansson, A., Hao, J., Sjolund, B.: Local corticosteroid application blocks transmission in normal nociceptive C-fibers. Acta Anesth. Scand. **34** (1990) 335–338

50. Katz, J., Renck, H.: Thorakoabdominale Nervenblokkaden. Lehrbuch und Atlas. Edition Medizin, Weinheim (1988)

51. Krane, E., Dalens, B. J., Murat, I., Murell, D.: The safety of epidurals placed during general anesthesia. Editorial. Reg. Anesth. and Pain Med. **23** (5) (1998) 433–438

52. Kumar, C.: Combined subarachnoid and epidural block for caesarean section. Can. J. Anaesth. **34** (1987) 329–330

53. Leighton, B. L., Norris, M. C., Sosis, M., Epstein, R., Chayen, B., Larijani, G. E.: Limitations of epinephrine as a marker of intravascular injection in laboring women. Anesthesiology **66** (1987) 688–691

54. Liu, S. L., Carpenter, R. L.: Hemodynamic responses to intravascular injection of epinephrine containing epidural test doses in adults during general anesthesia. Anesthesiology **84** (1996) 81

55. McKinnon, S. E., Hudson, A. R., Gentili, F.: Peripheral nerve injury with steroid agents. Plast. Reconstr. Surg. **69** (1982) 482–489

56. Melendez, J. A., Cirella, V. N., Delphin, E. S.: Lumbar epidural fentanyl analgesia after thoracic surgery. J. Cardiothorac. Anesth. **3** (1989) 150

57. Mense, S., Kaske, A. (Institut für Anatomie und Zellbiologie, Ruprecht-Karls-Universität Heidelberg). Persönliche Mitteilung (1995)

58. Moore, D. C., Batra, M. S.: The components of an effective test dose prior to epidural block. Anesthesiology **55** (1981) 693

59. Mulroy, M. F.: The epinephrine test dose for epidural anesthesia – Is it necessary? In: ASRA Supplement of the American Society of Regional Anesthesia (1996)

60. Mumtaz, M. H., Daz, M., Kuz, M.: Combined subarachnoid and epidural techniques. Anaesthesia **37** (1982) 30

61. Nelson, D. A.: Intraspinal therapy using methylprednisolone acetate – 23 years of clinical controversy. Spine **18** (2) (1993) 278–286

62. Peutrell, J., Hughes, D. G.: Combined spinal and epidural anaesthesia for inguinal hernia repair in babies. Pediatric Anaesth. **4** (1994) 221–227

63. Purkis, I. E.: Cervical epidural steroids. The Pain Clinic **1** (1986) 3–7

64. Rao, A. K., Carvalho, A. C. A.: Aquired qualitative platelat defects. In: Colman, R. W., Hirsh, J., Marder, V. J., Salzman, E. W. (eds.): Hemostasis and Thrombosis. (3rd ed.) Lippincott, Philadelphia (1994)

65. Rawal, N.: The combined spinal-epidural technique. Permanyer, S. L. Publications, (1997)

66. Rawal, N.: Single segment combined spinal-epidural block for caesarean section. Can. Anaesth. Soc. J. **33** (1986) 254–255

67. Rawal, N.: Combined spinal-epidural anesthesia. In: Van Zundert, A., Ostheimer, G. W. (eds.): Pain relief and anaesthesia in obstetrics. Churchill Livingstone, New York (1996) 413–426

68. Rawal, N., Schollin, J., Wesström, G.: Epidural versus combined spinal-epidural block for caesarean section. Acta Anaest. Scand. **32** (1998) 61–66

69. Rawal, N., Van Zundert, A., Holmström, B., Crowhurst, J.: Combined spinal-epidural technique. Reg. Anesth. **22** (5) (1997) 406–423

70. Rawal, N.: Klinischer Einsatz der rückenmarknahen Opioidanalgesie. Teil 1. Der Schmerz **10** (1996) 176–189

71. Reisner, L. S., Ellis, J.: Epidural and caudal puncture. In: Benumof, L. J. (ed.): Clinical procedures in anesthesia and intensive care. Lippincott, Philadelphia (1992) 663–679

72. Reisner, L. S., Ellis, J.: Epidural and caudal puncture. In: Benumof, L. J. (ed.): Clinical procedures in anesthesia and intensive care. Lippincott, Philadelphia (1992) 691

73. Robecci, A., Capra, R.: L'idrocortisone (composto F): Prime esperience cliniche in campo reumatologico. Minerva Med. **43** (1952) 1259–1263

74. Rowlingson, J. C., Kirchenbaum, L. P.: Epidural analgesic techniques in the management of cervical pain. Anesth. Analg. **65** (1986) 938–942

75. Rowlingson, J. C. (Health Sciences Center, University of Virginia). Persönliche Mitteilung (1995)

76. Saberski, L. R., Kondamuri, S., Osinubi, O. Y. O.: Identification of the epidural space: Is loss of resistance to air safe technique? A review of the complications related to the use of air. Reg. Anesth. **22** (1) (1997) 3–15

77. Schneider, M. C., Alon, E.: Die geburtshilfliche Epiduralanalgesie. Anaesthesist 45 Springer Verlag, (1996) 393–409

78. Scott, D. B.: Identification of the epidural space: Loss of resistance to air or saline? Editorial. Reg. Anesth. **22** (1) (1997) 1–2

79. Seghal, A. D., Gardner, W. J.: Corticosteroids administrated intradurally for relief of sciatica. Cleveland Clin. Quart. **27** (1960) 198–201

80. Seghal, A. D., Gardner, W. J., Dohn, D. F.: Pantopaque arachnoiditis treatment with subarachnoid injection of corticosteroids. Cleveland Clin. J. Med. **29** (1962) 177–178

81. Seghal, A. D., Gardner, W. J.: Place of intrathecal methylprednisolone acetate in neurological disorders. Trans Am. Neurol. Assoc. **88** (1963) 275–276

82. Seghal, A. D., Tweed, D. E., Gardner, W. J., Foote, M. K.: Laboratory studies after intrathecal corticosteroids: Determination of corticosteroids in plasma and cerebrospinal fluid. Arch. Neurol. **9** (1963) 64–68

83. Selby, R.: Complications from Depo-Medrol. Surg. Neurol. **19** (1983) 393–394

84. Shulman, M.: Treatment of neck pain with cervical epidural steroid injection. Reg. Anesth. **11** (1986) 92

85. Soresi, A.: Episubdural anesthesia. Anesth. Analg. **16** (1937) 306–310

86. Sreerama, V., Ivan, L. P., Dennery, J. M., Richard, M. T.: Neurosurgical complications of anticoagulant therapy. Can. Med. Assoc. J. **108** (1973) 305

87. Strong, W. E.: Epidural abscess associated with epidural catheterisation: A rare event? Anesthesiology **74** (1991) 943–946

88. Strong, W. E., Wesley, R., Winnie, A. P.: Epidural steroids are safe and effective when given appropriately. Arch. Neurol. **48** (1991) 1012

89. Sugar, O.: Steroid injections. Surg. Neurol. **19** (1983) 91

90. Tanaka, M., Yamamoto, S., Ashimura, H., Iwai, M., Matsumiya, N.: Efficacy of an epidural test dose in adult patients anesthetized with isoflurane: lidocaine containing 15 mcg epinephrine reliably increases arterial blood pressure, but not heart rate. Anesth. Analg. **80** (1995) 310

91. Tuel, S., Meythaler, M., Cross, L.: Cushing's syndrome from epidural methylprednisolone. Pain **40** (1990) 81–84

92. Urmey, W. F., Stanton, J., Peterson, M., Sharrock, N. E.: Combined spinal epidural anesthesia for outpatient surgery. Dose-response characteristic of intrathecal isobaric lidocaine using a 27-gauge Whitacre needle. Anesthesiology **83** (1995) 528–534

93. Vercauteren, M. P., Geernaert, K., Vandeput, D. M., Adriansen, H.: Combined continuous spinal-epidural anaesthesia with a single interspace, double catheter technique. Anaesthesia **48** (1993) 1002–1004

94. Wells, J. C. D. (Director Pain Relief Center, Walton Hospital, Liverpool). Persönliche Mitteilung (1995)

95. Wilhelm, S., Standl, T.: CSA vs. CSE bei Patienten in der Unfallchirurgie. Anaesthesist **46** (1997) 938–942

96. Williams, K. N., Jackowski, A., Evans, P. J. D.: Epidural hematoma requiring surgical decompression following repeated cervical steroid injections for chronic pain. Pain **42** (1990) 197–199

97. Winnie, A. P., Hartman, J. T., Meyers, H. L., Ramamurthy, S., Barangan, V.: Pain clinic II: Intradural and extradural corticosteroids for sciatica. Anesth. Analg. **51** (1972) 990–999

98. Zimmermann, G.: The epidural space: The "Carbage Can" or "Gold Mine" in anesthesia. In: ASRA Supplement of the American Society of Regional Anesthesia (1995)

Chapter 39: Caudal anesthesia in adult patients
Chapter 40: Caudal anesthesia in pediatric patients

1. Armitage, E. N.: Caudal block in children. Anaesthesia **34** (1979) 396

2. Armitage, E. N.: Regional Anaesthesia in pediatrics. Clinics in Anaesthesiology **3** (1985) 555

3. Boyd, H. R.: Iatrogenic intraspinal epidermoid. J. Neurosurg. **24** (1966) 105–107

4. Broadman, L. M.: Where should advocacy for pediatric patients end and concerns for patients safety begin? Editorial. Reg. Anesth. **22** (3) (1997) 205–208

5. Busoni, P.: Continuous caudal block. In: Saint-Maurice, C., Schulte Steinberg, O., Armitage, E. (eds.): Regional Anaesthesia in Children. Appleton & Lange, Mediglobe (1990) 88–96

6. Busoni, P., Andreucetti, T.: The spread of caudal analgesia in children: a mathematical model. Anaesth. Intens. Care **14** (1986) 140

7. Busoni, P., Sarti, A.: Sacral intervertebral epidural block. Anesthesiology **67** (1987) 993

8. Desparmet, J., Mateo, J., Ecoffey, C., Mazoit, X.: Efficacy of an epidural test dose in children anesthetized with halothane. Anesthesiology **72** (1990) 249

9. Giaufre, E.: Single shot caudal block. In: Saint-Maurize, C., Schulte Steinberg, O., Armitage, E. (eds.): Regional Anaesthesia in Children. Appleton & Lange, Mediglobe (1990) 81–87

10. Gibson, T., Norris, W.: Skin fragments removed by injection needles. Lancet **2** (1958) 983–985

11. Greenscher, J., Mofenson, H. C., Borofsky, L. G., Sharma, R.: Lumbar puncture in the neonate: A simplified techique. J. Pediatr. **78** (1971)1034

12. Halcrow, S. J., Crawford, P. J., Craft, A. W.: Epidermoid spinal cord tumour after lumbar puncture. Arch. Dis. Child. **60** (1985) 978–979

13. Moore, D. C.: Single-dose caudal block. In: Moore, D. C. (ed.): Regional Block. (4th ed.) Charles Thomas, Springfield (1976)

14. Netter, F. H.: Knöcherne Bedeckung des Gehirns und des Rückenmarks. In: Krämer, G. (Hrsg.): Farbatlanten der Medizin (Band 5). Nervensystem I: Neuroanatomie und Physiologie. Georg Thieme Verlag, Stuttgart-New York (1987)

15. Reisner, L., Ellis, J.: Epidural and caudal puncture. In: Benumof, L. J. (ed.): Clinical procedures in anesthesia and intensive care. Lippincott, Philadelphia (1992) 681

16. Schulte Steinberg, O.: Kaudalanästhesie – transsacrale Anästhesie – sacral-intervertebrale Epiduralanästhesie. In: Niesel, H. C. (Hrsg.): Regionalanästhesie, Lokalanästhesie, Regionale Schmerztherapie. Georg Thieme Verlag, Stuttgart-New-York (1994)

17. Shaywitz, B.: Epidermoid spinal cord tumors and previous lumbar punctures. J. Pediatr. **80** (1972) 638–640

18. Willis, R.: Caudal epidural blockade. In: Cousins, M. J., Bridenbaugh, P. O. (eds.): Neural Blockade. (2ⁿᵈ ed.) Lippincott, Philadelphia (1988) 361–383

Chapter 41: Adjuncts to local anesthesia in neuraxial blocks

1. Abdel-Ghaffar, M. E. Abdulatif, M. A., al Ghamdi, A., Mowafi, H., Anwar, A.: Epidural ketamine reduces post-operative epidural PCA consumption of fentanyl / bupivacaine. Can. J. Anaesth. **45** (2) (1998) 103–109

2. Adams, H. A., Werner, C.: Vom Razemat zum Eutomer: (S)-Ketamin. Renaissance einer Substanz? Anaesthesist **46** (1997) 1026–1042

3. Bastigkeit, M.: S(+)-Ketamin: Mehr Wirkung – weniger Nebenwirkung. Rettungsdienst **2** (1998) 114–119

4. Bastigkeit, M.: Ketamin: Chirales Pharmakon mit vielen Facetten. Pharmazeutische Zeitung **4** (1997) 40–47

5. Borgbjerg, F., M., Svensson, B. A., Frigast, C., Gordh, T.: Histopathology after repeated intrathecal injections of preservative-free ketamine in rabbit: A light and electron microscope examination. Anesth. Analg. **79** (1994) 105–111

6. Chambers, W. A., Littlewood, D. G., Logan, M. R., Scott, D. B.: Effect of added epinephrine on spinal anesthesia with lidocaine. Anesth. Analg. **60** (1981) 417

7. Chambers, W. A., Littlewood, D. G., Scott, D. B.: Spinal anesthesia with bupivacaine: Effect of added vasoconstrictors. Anesth. Analg. **61** (1982) 49

8. Chia, Y. Y., Liu, K., Liu, Y. C., Chang, H. C., Wong, C. S.: Adding ketamine in a multimodal patient-controlled epidural regimen reduces postoperative pain and analgesic consumption. Anesth. Analg. **86** (6) (1998) 1245–1249

9. Choe, H., Choi, Y. S., Kim, Y. H., Ko, S. H., Choi, H. G., Han, Y. J., Song, H. S.: Epidural morphine plus ketamine for upper abdominal surgery: improved analgesia from preincisional versus postincisional administration. Anesth. Analg. **84** (3) (1997) 560–563

10. Dripps, R. D., Vandam, L. D.: Long term follow-up of patients who recieved 10098 spinal anesthetics. I. Failure to discover major neurological sequelae. JAMA **156** (1954) 1486

11. Findlow, D., Aldridge, L. M., Doyle, E.: Comparison of caudal block using bupivacaine and ketamine with ilioinguinal nerve block for orchidopexy in children. Anaesthesia **52** (11) (1997) 1110–1113

12. Fogarty, D. J., Carabine, U. A., Milligan, K. R.: Comparison of the analgesic effects of intrathecal clonidine and intrathecal morphine after spinal anesthesia in patients undergoing total hip replacement. Br. J. Anaesth. **71** (1993) 661–664

13. Freye, E.: Peridurale Analgesie mit Opioiden. In: Freye, E.: Opioide in der Medizin. Wirkung und Einsatzgebiete zentraler Analgetika. Springer Verlag (1995)

14. Gebhardt, B.: Pharmakologie und Klinik der peridu- ralen und intrathekalen Anwendung von Ketamin. Anaesthesist. **43** (2) (1994) 34–40

15. Hawksworth, C., Serpell, M.: Intrathecal anesthesia with ketamine. Reg. Anesth. and Pain Med. **23** (3) (1998) 283–288

16. Hays, R. L., Palmer, C. M.: Respiratory depression af- ter intrathecal sufentanil during labor. Anesthesi- ology **81** (1994) 511–512

17. Jamali, S., Monin, S., Begon, C., Dubousset, A. M., Ecoffey, C.: Clonidine in pediatric caudal anesthe- sia. Anesth. Analg. **78** (1994) 663–666

18. Kabeer, A. A., Hardy, P. A.: Long-term use of sub- arachnoid clonidine for analgesia in refractory sym- pathetic dystrophy. Case report. Reg. Anesth. **21** (3) (1996) 249–252

19. Kawana, Y., Sato, H., Shimada, H., Fujita, N., Hayashi, A., Araki, Y.: Epidural ketamine for postoperative pain relief after gynecologic operations: a double- blind study and comparison with epidural mor- phine. Anesth. Analg. **66** (8) (1987) 735–738

20. Knight, B.: Comment on case report of Kabeer and Hardy. Reg. Anesth. **22** (5) (1997) 485–486

21. Le Polain, B., De Kock, M., Scoltes, J. L., Vanleirde, M.: Clonidine combined with sufentanil and bupi- vacaine with adrenaline for obstetric analgesia. Br. J. Anesth. **71** (1993) 657–660

22. Lin, T. C., Wong, C. S., Chen, F. C., Lin, S. Y., Ho, S. T.: Long-term epidural ketamine, morphine and bu- pivacaine attenuate reflex sympathetic dystrophy neuralgia. Can. J. Anaesth. **45** (2) (1998) 175–177

23. Lund, P. C.: Principles and practice of spinal anes- thesia. IL. Charles Thomas, Springfield (1971)

24. Muller, A., Lemos, D.: Cancer pain: Beneficial effect of ketamine addition to spinal administration of mor- phine-clonidine-lidocaine mixture. Ann. Fr. Anesth. Reanim **15** (3) (1996) 271–276

25. Naguib, M., Adu-Gyamfi, Y., Absood, G. H., Farag, H., Gyasi, H. K.: Epidural ketamine for postoperative anal- gesia. Can. Anaesth. Soc. J. **33** (1) (1986) 16–21

26. Nikolajsen, L., Hansen, C. L., Nielsen, J., Keller, J., Arendt-Nielsen, L., Jensen, T. S.: The effect of keta- mine on phantom pain: A central neuropathic dis- order maintained by peripheral input. Pain **67** (1) (1996) 69–77

27. Rawal, N.: Klinischer Einsatz der rückenmarksna- hen Opioidanalgesie. Teil 1. Der Schmerz **10** (1996) 176–189

28. Rawal, N.: Klinischer Einsatz der rückenmarksnahen Opioidanalgesie. Teil 2. Der Schmerz **10** (1996) 226– 236

29. Rockemann, M. G., Seeling, W.: Epidurale und in- trathekale Anwendung von alpha-2-Adrenozep- tor-Agonisten zur postoperativen Analgesie. Der Schmerz **10** (1996) 57–64

30. Rockemann, M. G., Seeling, W., Georgieff, M: Stellen- wert der alpha-2-Agonisten in Anästhesie und Inten- sivmedizin. Anästh. Intensivmed. **35** (1994) 176–184

31. Rowlingson, J.: Toxicity of local anesthetic additives. Reg. Anesth. **18** (1993) 453–460

32. Semple, D., Findlow, D., Aldridge, L. M., Doyle, E.: The optimal dose of ketamine for caudal epidural blockade in children. Anaesthesia **51** (12) (1996) 1170–1172

33. Spivey, D. L.: Epinephrine does not prolong lido- caine spinal anesthesia in term parturients. Anaesth. Analg. **64** (1985) 468

34. Stevens, R. A., Petty, R. H., Hill, H. F., Kao, T. C., Schaffer, R., Hahn, M. B., Harris, P.: Redistribution of sufentanil to cerebrospinal fluid and systemic cir- culation after epidural administration in dogs. Anesth. Analg. **76** (1993) 323–327

35. Takahashi, H., Miyazaki, M., Nanbu, T., Yanagida, H., Morita, S.: The NMDA-receptor antagonist ke- tamine abolishes neuropathic pain after epidural ad- ministration in a clinical case. Pain **75** (2–3) (1998) 391–394

36. Vercauteren, M., Lauwers, E., Meese, G., de Heert, S., Adriaensen, H.: Comparison of epidural sufen- tanil plus clonidine with sufentanil alone for post- operative pain relief. Anaesthesia **45** (1990) 531

37. Wong, C. S., Liaw, W. J., Tung, C. S., Su, Y. F., Ho, S. T.: Ketamine potentiates analgesic effect of mor- phine in postoperative epidural pain control. Reg. Anesth. **21** (6) (1996) 534–541

38. Wong, C. S., Lu, C. C., Cherng, C. H., Ho, S. T.: Pre- emptive analgesia with ketamine, morphine and epidural lidocaine prior to total knee replacement. Can. J. Anaesth. **44** (1) (1997) 31–37

39. Wong, C. S., Shen, T. T., Liaw, W. J., Cherng, C. H., Ho. S. T.: Epidural coadministration of ketamine, morphine and bupivacaine attenuates postherpetic neuralgia – a case report. Acta Anaesth. Sin. **34** (4) (1996) 151–155

40. Yaksh, T. L.: Epidural Ketamine: A useful, mechanis- tically novel adjuvant for epidural morphine. Reg. Anesth. **21** (6) (1996) 508–513

41. Yang, C. Y., Wong, C. S., Chang, J. Y., Ho, S. T.: In- trathecal ketamine reduces morphine requirements in patients with terminal cancer pain. Can. J. Anaesth. **43** (4) (1996) 379–383

42. Zenz, M., Donner, B.: Regionale Opioidanalgesie. In: Niesel, H. C.: Regionalanaesthesie, Lokalanaesthesie, Regionale Schmerztherapie. Thieme Verlag (1994)

Subject index

Page numbers in **bold type** refer to figures and/or tables.

Survey of the records and checklists